TEACHING IN NURSING AND ROLE OF THE EDUCATOR

Marilyn H. Oermann, PhD, RN, ANEF, FAAN, is the Thelma M. Ingles Professor of Nursing and director of Evaluation and Educational Research at Duke University School of Nursing, Durham, North Carolina. She is the author/coauthor of 18 nursing education books and many articles on teaching and evaluation in nursing, and on writing for publication. She is the editor of *Nurse Educator* and the *Journal of Nursing Care Quality* and is past editor of the *Annual Review of Nursing Education*. Dr. Oermann received the National League for Nursing Award for Excellence in Nursing Education Research, the Sigma Theta Tau International Elizabeth Russell Belford Award for Excellence in Education, and the American Association of Colleges of Nursing Scholarship of Teaching and Learning Excellence Award.

Jennie C. De Gagne, PhD, DNP, RN-BC, CNE, ANEF, is an associate professor at Duke University School of Nursing, Durham, North Carolina. She has provided consultation to a variety of nursing schools, including in South Korea, Ghana, South Africa, Sri Lanka, India, and Taiwan, on program development, continuing education, and faculty development. As an expert in educational technology and online education, Dr. De Gagne has focused her research on effective use of instructional technology as well as cybercivility in nursing education across the curriculum and guidelines. Her scholarly work includes nearly 100 authored or coauthored publications, 40 of them in peer-reviewed journals, and more than 70 national and international presentations.

Beth Cusatis Phillips, PhD, RN, CNE, is an associate professor at the Duke University School of Nursing. She has over 20 years of teaching experience at the undergraduate level and also teaches at the master's level in nursing education. Dr. Phillips is a proponent for innovation in teaching and preparing the new generation of nurses for the future. Dr. Phillips presents nationally on nursing education topics including clinical decision making among prelicensure nursing students, interprofessional education, and faculty development.

TEACHING IN NURSING AND ROLE OF THE EDUCATOR

THE COMPLETE GUIDE TO BEST PRACTICE IN TEACHING, EVALUATION, AND CURRICULUM DEVELOPMENT

SECOND EDITION

MARILYN H. OERMANN, PHD, RN, ANEF, FAAN
JENNIE C. DE GAGNE, PHD, DNP, RN-BC, CNE, ANEF
BETH CUSATIS PHILLIPS, PHD, RN, CNE

EDITORS

SPRINGER PUBLISHING COMPANY
NEW YORK

Springer Publishing Company, LLC
11 West 42nd Street
New York, NY 10036
www.springerpub.com

Acquisitions Editor: Margaret Zuccarini
Composition: diacriTech

ISBN: 978-0-8261-4013-5
e-book ISBN: 978-0-8261-4014-2
Instructor's PowerPoints ISBN: 978-0-8261-4017-3
Instructor's Manual ISBN: 978-0-8261-4015-9

Instructor Materials: Instructors may request supplements by emailing textbook@springerpub.com

17 18 19 20 / 5 4 3 2 1

Library of Congress Cataloging-in-Publication Data
Names: Oermann, Marilyn H., editor. | De Gagne, Jennie C., editor. |
    Phillips, Beth Cusatis, editor.
Title: Teaching in nursing and role of the educator : the complete guide to
    best practice in teaching, evaluation, and curriculum development /
    Marilyn H. Oermann, Jennie C. De Gagne, Beth Cusatis Phillips, editors.
Description: Second edition. | New York, NY : Springer Publishing Company,
    LLC, [2018] | Includes bibliographical references and index.
Identifiers: LCCN 2017030284 | ISBN 9780826140135 | ISBN 9780826140142
    (e-book) | ISBN 9780826140173 (instructor's PowerPoints) |
    ISBN 9780826140159 (instructor's manual)
Subjects: | MESH: Education, Nursing—methods | Faculty, Nursing | Teaching
Classification: LCC RT90 | NLM WY 18 | DDC 610.73071/1—dc23 LC record available at
    https://lccn.loc.gov/2017030284

Printed in the United States of America by McNaughton & Gunn.

To nurse educators and students preparing for a future role as a teacher in nursing

Contents

Contributors

Darlene E. Baker, MSN, RN, CNE
Assistant Director
Education-Innovation-Simulation Learning
  Environment
School of Nursing
University of North Carolina at Chapel Hill
Chapel Hill, North Carolina

Donna L. Boland, PhD, RN, ANEF
Associate Professor Emeritus
Indiana University
School of Nursing
Indianapolis, Indiana

Jamie L. Conklin, MSLIS
Research and Education Librarian
Liaison to the School of Nursing
Duke University Medical Center
  Library & Archives
Durham, North Carolina

Helen B. Connors, PhD, RN,
  FAAN, ANEF
E. Jean M. Hill Endowed Professor
The University of Kansas School of Nursing
  and Center for Health Informatics
Kansas City, Kansas

Martha A. Dawson, DNP, RN, FACHE
Assistant Professor and Specialty
  Coordinator for Nursing and Health
  Systems Administration, Family,
  Community and Health Systems
The University of Alabama at
  Birmingham School of Nursing
Birmingham, Alabama

Jennie C. De Gagne, PhD, DNP,
  RN-BC, CNE, ANEF
Associate Professor
Duke University School of Nursing
Durham, North Carolina

Kristina T. Dreifuerst, PhD, RN,
  CNE, ANEF
Associate Professor
College of Nursing
Marquette University
Milwaukee, Wisconsin

Dawne Marie Dunbar, MSN/Ed, RN,
  CNE, CHSE
Associate Professor of Nursing
Director of Clinical Simulation
Westbrook College of Health Professions
University of New England
Portland, Maine

Carol F. Durham, EdD, RN,
  ANEF, FAAN
Professor
Director, Education-Innovation-
  Simulation Learning Environment
School of Nursing
University of North Carolina at
  Chapel Hill
Chapel Hill, North Carolina

Katherine Foss, MSN, RN
Supervisor, Clinical Entry Programs
University of Colorado Hospital
Aurora, Colorado

Betsy Frank, PhD, RN, ANEF
Professor Emerita
School of Nursing, College of Health and
    Human Services
Indiana State University
Terre Haute, Indiana

Kathleen B. Gaberson, PhD, RN,
    CNOR, CNE, ANEF
Owner and Nursing Education Consultant
OWK Consulting
Pittsburgh, Pennsylvania

C. Ann Gakumo, PhD, RN
Associate Professor
Acute, Chronic and Continuing Care
The University of Alabama at
    Birmingham School of Nursing
Birmingham, Alabama

Karen L. Gorton, PhD, RN, MS
Assistant Professor and Assistant Dean
    of Undergraduate Programs
College of Nursing
University of Colorado
Aurora, Colorado

Katie A. Haerling, PhD, RN
Associate Professor
Nursing and Healthcare Leadership
University of Washington Tacoma
Tacoma, Washington

Debra Hagler, PhD, RN, ACNS-BC,
    CNE, CHSE, ANEF, FAAN
Clinical Professor
College of Nursing and Health Innovation
Arizona State University
Phoenix, Arizona

Pamela R. Jeffries, PhD, RN, ANEF,
    FAAN
Professor and Dean
School of Nursing
George Washington University
Washington, DC

Sarah B. Keating, EdD, RN, FAAN
Professor and Dean Emeritus
Samuel Merritt University,
    School of Nursing
Oakland, California

Shelley Cohen Konrad, PhD, LCSW,
    FANP
Professor, Director, School of Social Work
Director, Interprofessional Education
    Collaborative
University of New England
Portland, Maine

Brenda Morris, EdD, RN, CNE
Clinical Professor
College of Nursing and Health
    Innovation
Arizona State University
Phoenix, Arizona

Marilyn H. Oermann, PhD, RN, ANEF,
    FAAN
Thelma M. Ingles Professor of
    Nursing
Director of Evaluation and Educational
    Research
Duke University School of Nursing
Durham, North Carolina

Karen T. Pardue, PhD, RN, CNE,
    ANEF
Professor of Nursing
Associate Dean for Academic Affairs
Westbrook College of Health
    Professions
University of New England
Portland, Maine

Beth Cusatis Phillips, PhD, RN,
    CNE
Associate Professor
Duke University School of Nursing
Durham, North Carolina

Kathy Tally, MS
National Consultant for Online
    Quality Assurance
Overland Park, Kansas

Theresa M. "Terry" Valiga, EdD, RN,
    CNE, ANEF, FAAN
Professor, Director of Institute for
    Educational Excellence
Chair of Division of Clinical Systems
    and Analytics
Duke University School of Nursing
Durham, North Carolina

Lynda Wilson, PhD, RN
Professor Emerita
The University of Alabama at
   Birmingham School of
   Nursing
Birmingham, Alabama

Lisa K. Woodley, MSN, RN
Assistant Professor
School of Nursing
University of North Carolina at
   Chapel Hill
Chapel Hill, North Carolina

Preface

There is a critical need to prepare nurses for roles as educators in schools of nursing and health care settings. This book, in its second edition, is written to meet that need: It is a comprehensive text that provides, under one cover, essential concepts for effective teaching in nursing and carrying out other dimensions of the educator role. The book examines the role of a faculty member in a school of nursing and nurse educator in other settings; theories of learning; teaching methods, including integrating technology in teaching; teaching in online environments, simulation, learning laboratories, and clinical settings; interprofessional education; developing partnerships with clinical agencies; and preparing graduates to contribute to global health. Nurse educators also need to assess learning and performance, and for this reason the book includes chapters on assessment, testing, and clinical evaluation. Teachers in nursing should understand the curriculum and how it is developed and evaluated, also explained in this book. It is important in nursing education that teachers use evidence to guide their educational practices and develop their scholarship; those areas are addressed in the last section of the book. Chapters are written by leading experts who integrate research findings and other evidence in their chapters.

The book was written for students in master's, doctor of nursing practice (DNP), and PhD nursing programs who are preparing themselves for a teaching role; nurses in clinical settings who are transitioning into nurse educator roles or are teaching students in addition to their practice positions; students and nurses learning about nursing education through continuing education and certificate programs; and novice and experienced teachers who want to expand their knowledge about teaching and gain new ideas for their courses. If students are taking only one or two nursing education courses in their graduate program, this book will be of particular value because of its comprehensiveness. One of the goals was to prepare a scholarly book on teaching in nursing that is also practical, and the chapters are written with that goal in mind.

Nurse educators are employed in academic institutions and a variety of health care agencies. They educate nursing students at all levels, and in health care agencies they are responsible for providing nurses and other health care professionals' continuing education and training. Chapter 1 discusses trends supporting careers in nursing education, educational preparation for employment as a faculty member in a school of nursing, and preparation for educator roles in service settings. Competencies and responsibilities of the nurse educator, transition to the educator role, balancing roles, and faculty development are examined in the chapter.

Understanding how students learn is essential to effective teaching. It is also important for the nurse educator to recognize that no two students will have the same background, previous experiences, and preferences for teaching methods, and these differences have a potential effect on their learning. Chapter 2 examines theories of learning and related teaching strategies.

Understanding learners is an important component of quality teaching. Nurse educators need an understanding of the varied attributes of students, which can affect their learning process and outcomes; students' culture; and their learning style preferences—the way in which students approach a particular learning situation. Chapter 3 examines varied attributes of nursing students, learner differences that can influence what and how we teach, and multiple strategies nurse educators can use that take into consideration these different characteristics.

The most important question to ask about any teaching method is whether it is a good fit for the specific learning objectives, learners, teachers, and available resources. Chapter 4 describes a variety of teaching methods and offers guidance in selecting methods to fit the intended outcomes, learner characteristics, and available resources. Teaching methods are considered in relation to supporting learner development in the cognitive, affective, and psychomotor learning domains. Strategies are described for incorporating active learning and for promoting critical thinking.

The rapid advances and constant pace of change in technology create challenges and opportunities for teaching and learning. Successful integration of technology in the nursing curriculum requires a paradigm shift and new competencies for the teacher as the technology continues to evolve. Chapter 5 focuses on technology integration that supports achievement of learning outcomes with attention to curriculum and classroom alignment. The chapter guides nurse educators in exploring and embracing technology tools that support good teaching practices.

Teaching online is not the same as teaching in a classroom. Chapter 6 focuses on the differences between teaching in the traditional classroom and teaching online. The roles of the facilitator and the student are discussed in relation to pedagogy, course content, teaching strategies, reconceptualizing and designing online learning environments, interacting online, and using technology to teach and learn.

Traditionally, simulations have been used to provide opportunities for students to practice patient care in a "safe" environment before going into the clinical setting. However, in the current environment of increasing patient acuity and limited clinical placements, simulation serves a broader role as an adjunct or replacement for traditional clinical experiences. Chapter 7 provides an overview of types of clinical simulations in nursing and how to integrate them into a nursing curriculum. Debriefing approaches, evaluation processes to use when developing and implementing clinical simulations, and evidence on the use of clinical simulations are discussed in this chapter.

The transformation of health care, coupled with alarming patient care outcome data, is heralding a new mandate to prepare nurses for collaborative team-based models of care. This educational reform presents a challenge, as the configuration of most nursing, medicine, and allied health programs reflects singular siloed programs of study. Such design results in nursing and health profession graduates who have little to no knowledge of what their respective colleagues do, and demonstrate little to no skill or experience in interprofessional communication and ways of effectively working together on teams. Chapter 8, a new chapter in the second edition, examines the content and processes for weaving interprofessional education into nursing curricula. Foundational frameworks are provided, along with examples of didactic, simulation, and clinical learning experiences that promote collaborative practice capabilities.

Skills acquisition is an important component of nursing education, beginning early in the curriculum and continuing throughout the nursing program. Learning laboratories provide a safe environment for initial psychomotor skills acquisition while offering opportunities to socialize students into the professional role of a nurse. Chapter 9 examines phases of skill development, deliberate practice, and development of professional confidence; roles of the teacher, staff, mentors, and others in the learning laboratory; expectations for learners; types of learning laboratories and their integration into the curriculum; competency evaluations; and other important topics. The chapter is comprehensive and also describes laboratory organization and management.

The clinical teacher plays a pivotal role in shaping learning for nursing students in the clinical setting. Because of this, it is essential that clinical teachers exhibit effective teaching behaviors, use best practices in teaching nursing, and inspire students. Chapter 10 explains why effective clinical teaching is so critical and the process of clinical teaching. Specific teaching strategies, such as how to create a learning climate that is inviting and supportive to students, how to foster effective relationships in the clinical setting, how to design an effective and inspirational clinical orientation, and how to choose the best patient assignments for students, are discussed.

Academic–practice partnerships exist at several levels for the purpose of preparing the nursing workforce to meet nursing practice realities and contemporary health care challenges. Chapter 11 provides guidelines for establishing and sustaining meaningful partnerships between education and practice to stimulate collaborative models of clinical nursing education. Nurse educator roles and responsibilities are explored. Specific examples are provided to illustrate concepts and strategies to improve the educational preparation of nurses and ultimately the quality and safety of patient care.

Through the process of assessment, the teacher collects information about student learning and performance. With this information, the teacher can determine further learning needs, plan learning activities to meet those needs, and confirm the outcomes and competencies met by the students. Chapter 12 explains assessment, evaluation, and grading in nursing education. Methods are described for assessing learning, and examples are provided of many of these methods.

Tests are a common assessment method used in nursing education, and varied types of test items are described in Chapter 13. A test must produce relevant and consistent results to form the basis for sound inferences about what learners know and can do. Good planning, careful test construction, proper administration, accurate scoring, and sound interpretation of scores are essential for producing useful test results. This chapter describes the process of planning, constructing, administering, scoring, and analyzing tests. Various types of test items are presented with examples of each item.

As students learn about nursing, they develop their knowledge base, higher level thinking skills, and a wide range of practice competencies essential for patient care. Learning concepts in a classroom or an online environment is not sufficient: Students need to apply those concepts and other knowledge to clinical situations and be proficient in carrying out care. Teachers guide student learning in the clinical setting and evaluate their performance in practice. Chapter 14 describes the clinical evaluation process, the importance of giving prompt and specific feedback to students as they are learning, principles that are important when observing and rating performance, and grading clinical practice.

It is vital that nurse educators take into account the context in which teaching takes place. Often, both new and experienced teachers focus on the specific content of the classes or sessions they teach and lose sight of the objectives and how they relate to the overall program. Chapter 15 describes the processes for curriculum development or revision for schools of nursing and for educational programs in health care settings. The chapter reviews the factors that influence educational programs and curricula and provides guidelines for collecting and analyzing data to make informed decisions about revising or developing curricula.

Nurse educators are expected to implement the curriculum that has been approved by the faculty. When starting the process of curriculum review, revision, and/or redesign, it is important for educators to consider a variety of curriculum models. Chapter 16, which builds on the prior chapter, is designed to help faculty consider various models for curriculum design, appreciate how essential it is for the curriculum to be internally consistent for students to be successful in achieving stated program outcomes, and appreciate the significance of a course syllabus.

Evaluation provides decision makers with information about the institution's or program's aims, purpose, and goals and how well it is functioning in relation to these intentions. Chapter 17 focuses on various theories and theoretical frameworks that underpin program evaluation efforts and discusses evaluation models and their use in approaching evaluation systematically. The chapter also examines research methodologies for generating useful evaluative information, especially within the context of nursing programs, connections between accountability and accreditation, and approaches to developing and implementing program evaluation meaningful to nursing programs.

Evidence-based teaching is the use of research findings and other evidence to guide educational decisions and practices. Available evidence should be used when developing the curriculum and courses, selecting teaching methods and approaches to use with students, planning clinical learning activities, and assessing students' learning and performance. Chapter 18 describes evidence-based teaching in nursing, the need for better research in nursing education, and a process for engaging in evidence-based teaching.

The role of the nurse educator includes more than teaching, assessing learning, and developing courses: It also includes scholarship and contributing to the development of nursing education as a science. Scholars in nursing education question and search for new ideas; they debate and think beyond how it has always been done. For the teacher's work to be considered as scholarship, it needs to be public, peer-reviewed and critiqued, and shared with others so they can build on that work. Chapter 19 examines scholarship in nursing education and developing one's role as a scholar. Because of the importance of dissemination to scholarship, the chapter includes a description of the process of writing for publication and other strategies for dissemination. Assessment of teaching, by students and peers, and the scholarship of teaching also are discussed, including development of a teaching portfolio to document teaching excellence and scholarship. This chapter builds on the first chapter, which examines career development as a nurse educator.

In today's increasingly globalized and complex world, nurse educators are in unique positions to prepare students as global citizens who can contribute to global health diplomacy and ensure culturally competent care at local and international levels. Accordingly, schools of nursing must be involved in curriculum changes and pedagogical approaches that support students and faculty and integrate global perspectives across the curriculum. Focusing on the role of nurse educators in preparing nurses for interprofessional work in the globalized world of the 21st century, this last chapter in the book, Chapter 20, examines major global health challenges and the impact of globalization on nursing practice and suggests recommendations for incorporating global health competencies in nursing education programs. This chapter also describes strategies for nurse educators to use to ensure that graduates are prepared to work in a globalized world and to contribute to planetary health.

In addition to this book, we have provided an Instructor's Manual that includes a sample course syllabus; chapter-based PowerPoint presentations; and materials for an online course (with chapter summaries, student learning activities, discussion questions, and assessment strategies). To obtain your electronic copy of these materials, faculty should contact Springer Publishing Company at textbook@springerpub .com. Margaret Zuccarini, our editor at Springer Publishing, deserves a special acknowledgment for her continued support, enthusiasm, and commitment to nursing education.

Marilyn H. Oermann
Jennie C. De Gagne
Beth Cusatis Phillips

I

Nursing Education:
Roles of Teacher and Learner

1

The Process of Becoming a Nurse Educator

MARILYN H. OERMANN AND BETSY FRANK

OBJECTIVES

- Describe the roles and responsibilities of nurse educators in academic and health care settings
- Compare educational requirements for nurse educators in different employment settings
- Examine the transition from clinician to educator and strategies for facilitating that transition

Several recent reports have highlighted the need for more nurse educators. Nurse educators teach in academic institutions and in a variety of health care agencies. They educate nursing students at all levels, from certified nursing assistants (CNAs) to doctorally prepared current and future nurse educators, clinicians, and researchers. Nursing professional development practitioners teach in health care settings and are responsible for providing nurses and other health care professionals with orientation and continuing education and training.

TRENDS SUPPORTING CAREERS IN NURSING EDUCATION

Although the nursing shortage has abated somewhat because of economic trends that led to older nurses staying longer in the workforce, nursing shortages are cyclical and affected by economic conditions, population growth and the aging of the U.S. population, changes in health care reimbursement, and other factors. Shortages of registered nurses (RNs) in hospitals occur when the economy is good and disappear during recessions (W. G. Johnson, Butler, Harootunian, Wilson, & Linan, 2016). The most recent U.S. Department of Health and Human Services, Health Resources and Services Administration (HRSA), workforce analysis projects that by 2025, the supply of RNs and licensed practical nurses will increase more than the demand nationally and in most states (HRSA, National Center for Health Workforce Analysis, 2014). The report emphasizes, however, that many factors will continue to affect the demand and supply of the nurse workforce, including the impact of a nurse educator shortage on student enrollment in nursing education programs. Projections about nursing shortages are difficult to make. Though the number of nurses younger than 30 has increased due to an upsurge in persons choosing careers in nursing, a 2013 report from the HRSA has stated that one third of nurses are older than 50. The retirement of these nurses will not only result in the loss of experienced RNs in the workforce but also will have an impact on the supply of nurses in future years. Furthermore, health care reform, as enacted through the Patient Protection and Affordable Care Act, will increase the demand for all health care services.

Despite an increase in students enrolling in and graduating from nursing programs in the United States, greater demand for health care will require even more nurses to deliver those needed services. As a result, more faculty in academic and service settings will be needed to educate nursing personnel to fulfill current and future roles within the health care system.

To maintain an adequate supply of nurses, schools of nursing need qualified faculty to teach those students. One current issue, which is projected to worsen in future years, is the aging of the nursing faculty workforce. The National League for Nursing (NLN) reported that 76% of full-time educators were older than 45 (NLN, 2014). Not only are nursing faculty aging, with many projected to retire in upcoming years, but an overall nursing faculty shortage exists. In 2015, the American Association of Colleges of Nursing (AACN) reported that 1,236 faculty positions were vacant in colleges and universities offering baccalaureate and graduate degrees in nursing.

Academic nurse educators are not the only educators needed to meet the needs of the health care delivery system. Nursing professional development generalists and specialists in health care settings are also vital. A rapidly changing health care delivery system requires those in the workforce to keep abreast of changing standards of practice, skill competency, and regulatory requirements. Educators in health care agencies play a key role in helping nursing and other staff members keep up to date in their job requirements. They also have an important role in providing interprofessional education and preparing health care teams to work collaboratively (Harper & Shinners, 2016).

As one can see, prospects of long-term employment for nurse educators across all education and service settings are excellent. By choosing a career as a nurse educator, one has the opportunity to be a role model, coach, and mentor for the current and next generation of nurses (Yoder-Wise & Kowalski, 2012).

ROLE PREPARATION

EDUCATIONAL PREPARATION FOR ACADEMIC EMPLOYMENT

Nursing education occurs across the spectrum of educational settings. In the United States, preparation for the NCLEX-RN® occurs in community colleges at the associate degree level, at the diploma level in hospital schools of nursing, and in colleges and universities that award bachelor's, master's, and doctoral degrees. The RNs from these programs work across a range of health care institutions. Increasingly, however, health care agencies are requiring their staff to be baccalaureate prepared or working on a bachelor of science in nursing (BSN) degree. The Institute of Medicine *Future of Nursing* report has called for 80% of the nursing workforce to be prepared at the baccalaureate degree level or higher by the year 2020 (Committee on the Robert Wood Johnson Foundation Initiative on the Future of Nursing at the Institute of Medicine, 2011).

Most practical nursing programs and some CNA programs also take place in community college settings. Many of these occur in career ladder education programs leading to an associate degree in nursing.

Academic credentials for nurse educators employed in postsecondary institutions are set by state Boards of Nursing and accreditation agencies. For example, the Commission on Collegiate Nursing Education (CCNE), an agency that accredits baccalaureate and higher degree programs, requires faculty to have a graduate degree (CCNE, 2013). The Accreditation Commission for Education in Nursing (ACEN) criteria for teaching in schools of nursing does not specify the degrees required. The 2017 accreditation standards indicate that nursing faculty should have the educational qualifications and experience required by the school of nursing and its governing organization, and the state in which the nursing program is located. Nursing faculty need to be qualified to teach the assigned courses (ACEN, 2017). The ACEN also accredits practical nursing programs and has the same standard for nurse faculty.

The NLN Commission for Nursing Education Accreditation (CNEA), the third accrediting agency in nursing education, indicates that nurse faculty at all program levels should be qualified by education, professional credentials, and experience for their assigned teaching responsibilities. They also should meet state and other agency qualifications. The goal is for schools of nursing to employ full- and part-time faculty with a graduate degree in nursing or a relevant field that relates to their teaching role and responsibilities (NLN CNEA, 2016).

Graduate programs in nursing often have nurse educator tracks based on the NLN's *The Scope of Practice for Academic Nurse Educators 2012 Revision* (NLN, 2012). Nurse educator tracks include theoretical content related to nursing education, as well as a teaching practicum, which provides experience teaching in various settings. These tracks are found in master's and post-master's certificate programs. Doctor of nursing practice (DNP) programs are designed for nurses seeking an advanced degree in nursing practice. The DNP is an alternative to research-focused doctoral programs. Doctor of philosophy (PhD) programs prepare students to conduct research. In some PhD programs, though, role development may include educator tracks as well, with a research focus in the science of nursing education. Most PhD programs, however, focus on clinical and nursing systems research. Graduates from DNP and PhD programs often have career goals that include teaching in prelicensure and graduate nursing programs, and should prepare themselves for their role as a faculty member through courses in their doctoral program or continuing education (Oermann, 2017; Oermann, Lynn, & Agger, 2016).

Given the recommendation for a primarily baccalaureate-prepared nursing workforce, more nurse educators will need to be prepared at the doctoral level to meet the educational needs of future nurses. A master's degree with a major in nursing education is a stepping stone for future doctoral study.

The educational path one chooses depends on the type of nursing program in which one wishes to teach. Colleges and universities have specific degree requirements for employment. For example, many universities require a terminal degree (doctoral) for tenure track positions or positions with some guarantee of permanency, provided certain requirements are met. For universities with a Carnegie Classification of Highest Research Activity (The Carnegie Classification of Institutions of Higher Education, n.d.), a PhD is required for a tenure track position. Tenure track faculty in these institutions conduct research and engage in scholarship, teach students often at the graduate level, and participate in service. However, many of these universities also have clinical or teaching tracks, which are non-tenure tracks and have different requirements for faculty. With non-tenure tracks faculty may have yearly or multiyear contracts for employment versus a permanent position that accompanies tenure. Typically their role focuses on teaching, clinical practice, and service, with some scholarship. Full-time clinical and teaching appointments may also require a PhD, DNP, or a master's degree in nursing. Universities that do not have high research missions may have tenure track appointments for faculty with DNPs. Full- or part-time clinical teaching appointments, or those teaching appointments that involve clinical supervision of students, require a master's degree. Community colleges generally do not have tenure track positions. Nevertheless, master's degrees are required to teach full- and part-time in those settings.

When interviewing for employment in an academic institution, it is important to clarify what the job description is and what the expectations are for role performance (Halstead & Frank, 2018). By clarifying these criteria, one can better match career goals to institutional expectations. For example, if a prospective faculty member has expertise in nursing education research, that person should know whether the institution values this type of research when considering promotion and tenure. Table 1.1 summarizes the types of academic appointments and the educational preparation required.

TABLE 1.1 Summary of Educational Requirements for Nurse Educator Employment

Employment Setting	Education Required
Hospitals and other health care agencies	BSN or MSN
Community colleges: Practical Nursing and CNA programs	BSN or MSN
Community colleges: Associate degree programs	MSN
Colleges and universities: Baccalaureate and Master's programs	MSN (clinical teaching) with doctoral degree preferred
Colleges and universities: Doctoral programs	Doctoral degree

BSN, bachelor of science in nursing; CNA, certified nursing assistant; MSN, master of science in nursing.

EDUCATIONAL PREPARATION FOR EMPLOYMENT IN HEALTH CARE SETTINGS

Educators in nursing professional development teach in acute care, long-term care, and community settings. Their role is to facilitate the professional development and growth of nurses and other health care personnel (Harper & Maloney, 2016). Some of these positions may require less than a master's degree. However, having a master's degree in nursing education, or a clinically focused master's degree with elective courses in nursing education, will enhance one's ability to carry out the responsibilities of teaching staff, both nursing and interprofessional. Educators who practice in nursing professional development can be generalists or specialists. The generalist is a bachelor's prepared RN, whereas the specialist has both a graduate degree and certification in nursing professional development (Harper & Shinners, 2016). The broad term for both of these roles is nursing professional development practitioner.

NURSE EDUCATOR COMPETENCIES

The Scope and Practice for Academic Nurse Educators 2012 Revision, developed by the NLN, describes the scope of practice and standards for teaching in schools of nursing (NLN, 2012). This document has served as the guiding force in setting the expectations for the NLN certification as a nurse educator. Although the competencies have been directed at faculty in schools of nursing, they are applicable to educators in nursing professional development roles.

The NLN competencies are as follows:

- Facilitate learning
- Facilitate learner development and socialization
- Use assessment and evaluation strategies
- Participate in curriculum design and evaluation of program outcomes
- Function as a change agent and leader
- Pursue continuous quality improvement in the nurse educator role
- Engage in scholarship
- Function within the educational environment (NLN, 2012, pp. 14–22)

RESPONSIBILITIES OF NURSE EDUCATORS

ACADEMIC NURSE EDUCATORS

Responsibilities of nurse educators differ according to institutional type and whether one teaches primarily at the prelicensure or graduate level. Prior to deciding on a career in nursing education, job shadowing a nurse faculty member or an educator in a clinical setting can provide a realistic view of the role and responsibilities.

Academic institutions require faculty to teach, have some form of scholarly activity, and perform service to the institution and the profession. How one's overall duties are allotted depends on the institutional type. Those who are employed in community colleges will spend most of their time teaching in the classroom, simulation and skills laboratories, and clinical setting, with some time allotted for service and scholarship. Those who teach in undergraduate and graduate programs in colleges and universities will also teach, but will have greater expectations for scholarly productivity, including supporting research through funded grants if in a tenure track position in a school with a research mission. Faculty with doctoral degrees (DNP and PhD) even in non-tenure track positions in most universities will be expected to engage in scholarly activities and publish. Across all schools of nursing, an expectation of nurse faculty is that they participate in service—for example, as a member of a committee—to the school of nursing, college or university, and nursing profession.

When considering employment in an academic setting, one should be clear about the job expectations. Is the position tenure track, or with a renewable yearly or multi-year contract? If the position is part-time and involves only clinical teaching, how much grading of assignments is involved, and is the grading time paid for? If the position is full-time, but on the clinical or teaching track, what kind of scholarship is expected?

Teaching Responsibilities

Teaching involves more than transmitting knowledge through lectures and guiding students in clinical practice. Faculty must have evidence-based knowledge of student learning styles, teaching methods, and methods for evaluating student learning. Facilitating students' assimilation of theory into practice is key. Oermann, Shellenbarger, and Gaberson (2018) have recommended a closer integration of the clinical, simulation, and classroom components of a student's education. Some nursing education programs employ full-time clinical faculty, whose primary role is teaching in the clinical setting and sometimes also in the simulation and skills laboratories. All full- and part-time nurse educators teaching in the clinical setting need to have knowledge of the curriculum and expected learning outcomes. This knowledge helps them facilitate the students' integration of theory with clinical practice.

Aside from the actual classroom, online, and clinical teaching, faculty also have the responsibility of formulating the curriculum that not only meets contemporary standards of practice, but also prepares students for future nursing roles. Curriculum is not static, but constantly needs revision to meet changing licensure examination expectations, societal changes, and changes in the health care delivery system. For example, *The Future of Nursing* report recommended expanded roles for nurses in the health care system (Committee on the Robert Wood Johnson Foundation Initiative on the Future of Nursing at the Institute of Medicine, 2011). This recommendation has led to curriculum revision at both the undergraduate and graduate levels. Faculty in schools of nursing need to develop curricula that will prepare nurses for a changing health care environment and new models of health care delivery (Hendricks, Taylor, Walker, & Welch, 2016). Providing leadership and promoting curriculum change involves ensuring that the curriculum is based on the most current educational standards and competencies, including the core competencies needed by all health care professionals:

- Patient-centered care
- Teamwork and collaboration
- Evidence-based practice
- Quality improvement
- Safety
- Informatics (Cronenwett, Sherwood, & Gelmon, 2009; Dolansky & Moore, 2013; Quality and Safety Education for Nurses [QSEN] Institute, 2014)

Committee work is essential to the process, including leading taskforces within the nursing program and sometimes in the larger institution to shepherd the revised curriculum through the approval process. Nurse educators have an important role in curriculum development and revision in the school and carrying out other activities to provide a quality education for students. They develop innovative learning activities for students, assessment strategies, and tests in their courses; serve on committees to make decisions about admissions and progression in the nursing program; evaluate their courses and nursing program; advise students and support them in their education; and serve in other roles that are essential to offering a quality educational experience for students.

Scholarship Responsibilities

Halstead and Frank (2018) have pointed out that all teachers are scholars. The various accreditation criteria have expectations for scholarship for faculty at all levels of nursing education. These expectations include teachers at all levels of postsecondary education and in service settings. For example, the ACEN accreditation criteria for associate degree programs states that "faculty (full- and part-time) maintain expertise in their areas of responsibility, and their performance reflects scholarship and evidence-based teaching and clinical practices" (ACEN, 2017, Standard 2, p. 2).

Scholarship is more than only traditional research, obtaining grant funding, presenting at professional conferences, and publishing in academic journals. Scholarship is also a "spirit of inquiry"—reflecting on teaching practices, asking if there are better ways of helping students learn, and searching for evidence to improve teaching. A spirit of inquiry involves the ability to search the literature for evidence, and working with colleagues to understand their practices in the classroom, online, and in clinical settings.

This view of scholarship grows out of Boyer's 1990 seminal work, *Scholarship Reconsidered: Priorities of the Professoriate,* which broadened the definition of scholarship. The original work included the scholarship of discovery, integration application, and teaching. In 1996, Boyer added the scholarship of engagement, which for nurse educators could include clinical practice. Oermann (2014) described these categories of scholarship based on the Boyer Model. Table 1.2 lists the forms of scholarship and their definitions, with examples of each form of scholarship.

TABLE 1.2 Summary of Boyer's Categories of Scholarship

Type of Scholarship	Definition	Evidence
Scholarship of Discovery	Conducting original research to gain knowledge about nursing	Grants, peer-reviewed publications, presentations
Scholarship of Integration	Synthesis of research done by others, making connections across disciplines	Peer-reviewed publications of research, syntheses, integrative and literature reviews, policy papers, books, products resulting from interdisciplinary efforts
Scholarship of Application	Development of clinical knowledge, applying knowledge to practice to solve clinical problems, service to profession and scholarship of engagement	Consultations, outcomes of clinical practice, presentations and publications about practice
Scholarship of Teaching	Inquiry that focuses on learning and teaching, developing innovations, curriculum development, and evaluation	New teaching practices that are evaluated, peer-reviewed publications, presentations about teaching innovations and practices, chapters and textbooks

Source: Adapted from Oermann (2014).

Service Responsibilities

Service responsibilities contribute to the functioning of the organization. No matter the academic setting, all full-time faculty will be expected to participate in nursing program committees and committees of the larger institution. Committees include those concerned with faculty issues; student admission, progression, and retention issues; curriculum development; and program evaluation, among others.

Professional service includes leadership within professional organizations and activities such as reviewing manuscripts for journals. Other forms of professional service may include committee work in service settings and the community. Faculty expertise may also be needed to facilitate research in service settings or to assist with quality improvement activities (Halstead & Frank, 2018).

NURSING PROFESSIONAL DEVELOPMENT PRACTITIONERS

Educators in nursing professional development also have teaching, scholarship, and service responsibilities. Although typically the curriculum process is thought of as occurring in the academic setting, educators in health care settings must also formulate, implement, and evaluate various curricula. For example, these educators design and evaluate nurse residency and orientation programs, as well as programs for ensuring continuing competency of staff and promoting teamwork and collaboration. The educator in this setting has a growing role in providing interprofessional education. Knowledge of standards of practice, health care trends, and competencies to be developed by staff are critical for practice in nursing professional development. For example, patient-centered care, a core competency to be developed by all health care providers, can be promoted through educational programs. These educators also have an important role in promoting evidence-based practice in their setting.

In addition to having job responsibilities in the health care setting, some professional development educators might also function as part-time faculty in nursing programs. In serving as part-time faculty, these educators have an important role in developing future nursing professionals (Adelman-Mullally et al., 2013).

Although much scholarship takes place in academic settings, educators in nursing professional development also participate in and facilitate scholarship activities. These include conducting studies that create new knowledge, developing and evaluating practice and educational innovations, and promoting evidence-based practice and quality improvement. Nursing professional development practitioners play a key role in creating programs that help nurses and others to engage in these scholarly activities. In the revised *Nursing Professional Development: Scope and Standards* (Harper & Maloney, 2016), the specialist role, for nurses with graduate degrees and certification, is to develop knowledge and tools to improve care and have a leadership role in promoting evidence-based practice and scholarship in the health care setting.

Educators in nursing professional development are change agents and leaders in their clinical setting and the larger health care delivery system. Through their education of nurses and other health care providers, and their leadership, they work toward improving the quality and safety of care. Nurses in professional development may provide education for the community and promote increased access to health care through their community and professional service efforts. They also may assume a leadership role in a professional organization. Nursing professional development practitioners are guided by their standards for practice (Harper & Maloney, 2016). Exhibit 1.1 suggests some questions for reflection when considering full- or part-time employment as a nurse educator in an academic or health setting.

EXHIBIT 1.1 Questions to Consider Prior to Seeking Employment as a Nurse Educator

1. Do I want to work in an academic environment or health care setting?
2. What are the academic credentials needed for employment?
3. What kind of flexibility do I want and need in setting my work hours?
4. Do I want to work full- or part-time as a nurse educator?
5. Do I want to combine academic and clinical practice responsibilities?

(continued)

EXHIBIT 1.1 Questions to Consider Prior to Seeking Employment as a Nurse Educator (*continued*)

6. In my career, do I want to spend the majority of my time teaching or combining research and teaching?
7. What service activities are expected in the role as an educator?
8. If I seek employment in an academic setting, what level of students and types of courses do I want to teach?
9. If I work in an academic setting, do I want to maintain some practice as a staff nurse, nurse practitioner, or clinical specialist?

TRANSITION TO THE EDUCATOR ROLE

Schoening (2013) found that clinicians who transition to the educator role go through four phases, which are anticipation/expectation, disorientation, information seeking, and identity formation. According to Schoening's Nurse Educator Transition Model, successful transition results in "feeling and thinking like a teacher" (p. 170). This is a similar transition to new graduates as they learn about their role as a professional nurse and gain expertise, moving from novice to expert.

As novice nurse educators transition into the educator role, not only must they learn skills related to classroom and clinical teaching, but they must also learn how to function within an academic setting, be it a community college, college, or university. If teaching in nursing professional development, they need to learn how to function within that setting. Included in this transition is learning how to balance the requirements of the position. The nurse educator in academic settings typically does not function on a day-to-day basis within a particular work shift such as 7 a.m. to 7 p.m. This is also true for educators in a professional development role. Planning for class presentations and assessment and grading of student assignments typically takes place outside of the formal work setting. If one is transitioning to an academic nurse educator role, balancing teaching, scholarship, and service expectations may cause role stress if the scholarship expectations are higher than what was required in prior settings. Some nurse educators may not be well prepared for engaging in scholarship and should seek a mentor to guide their development in this area.

Although educators who have been full-time clinicians are familiar with a health care agency's culture and role expectations, becoming socialized to higher education presents additional challenges. Expectations vary by school of nursing and its mission. Schools with a research mission emphasize scholarship more so than schools with a mission that focuses only on education. In deciding on the setting in which to teach, the goals and mission of the school should be examined in relation to one's own career goals. Furthermore, understanding institutional culture is an important factor in acclimating to the values and norms of the academic setting. Academic preparation for the educator role, through course work, continuing education, or faculty development, is critical for nurses transitioning to teaching in a school of nursing or health care setting. This preparation is important regardless of whether the nurse has a master's, DNP, or PhD degree. Too many nurse faculty and educators in other settings continue to gain their knowledge and competencies for teaching "on the job" (Oermann, 2017). However, with the extensive knowledge and skills needed for the educator role, that model is no longer effective. The more preparation one can get in nursing education, the easier the transition to the educator role. It also is important to find a good mentor to guide the transition process and serve as a resource for the new educator.

Good communication skills are important for adjustment. For example, a clinical nurse educator in a school of nursing must communicate with nursing staff to facilitate the students' clinical learning and make appropriate clinical assignments for students (Oermann, Shellenbarger, & Gaberson 2018). Committee work in the academic and health care setting requires good communication skills to facilitate effective committee functioning. Communication skills are essential for collaborating with other nurse educators and for effective teaching.

Orientation to the role can also ease the transition from clinician to educator. Orientation is critical for all educator roles, but particularly for the part-time clinical educator role in a school of nursing. This educator can feel isolated from the larger academic program. Therefore, knowing expectations and how the clinical practice fits into the curriculum can ease feelings of isolation. Orientation should include not only information on the overall curriculum and course outcomes to be met in the clinical setting, but also on clinical teaching expectations and how to assess and grade student performance (K. V. Johnson, 2016; Oermann et al., 2018). Full-time faculty need orientation to the academic environment, including the curriculum and information regarding the school's promotion, retention, and tenure criteria (Clark, Alcala-Van Houten, & Perea-Ryan, 2010).

BALANCING ROLE RESPONSIBILITIES

Part of the transition to becoming a nurse educator is balancing all dimensions of the role. Whereas nursing professional development practitioners have some autonomy in how to organize responsibilities, they generally have more regular work hours as compared to the educator in an academic setting. Aside from assigned times for teaching and posted office hours, most academic educators can decide when and where work is done. They can typically prepare classes, grade assignments, and do scholarship activities from home.

Clinical expertise is essential for teaching clinical courses, and faculty members need to be clinically competent for their education to be effective. Faculty who need to maintain some clinical practice to maintain specialty certification have special challenges. Beck and Ruth-Sahd (2013) found that faculty want to remain clinically competent to enhance their teaching. Therefore, finding a dedicated time for clinical practice is one way to maintain clinical competence. This dedicated time could occur during the academic year or in the summer, if faculty are not on 12-month contracts. Based on their research, Beck and Ruth-Sahd have advocated including clinical practice within the Boyer (1990) Model of scholarship. They have also recommended the inclusion of clinical practice, in some way, in tenure and promotion criteria.

On the other hand, some faculty members focus more of their time on research (Roberts & Glod, 2013). If faculty focus more on research, their teaching could become separated from the realities of clinical practice unless they find other ways to keep abreast of current practice. Working with clinical partners in research efforts or on health care agency committees are ways to keep clinically grounded.

FACULTY DEVELOPMENT

Transition to the nurse educator role does not end with orientation. All full- and part-time faculty in the academic setting, and educators in health care settings, need continuing education to maintain competency. Although continuing education related to one's clinical specialty is important, so too is continuing education related to the educator competencies. For example, the NLN and AACN offer conferences and webinars for faculty development. Nursing professional development practitioners can attend the Association for Nursing Professional Development annual convention. Like any specialty, nursing education changes with regard to expectations for role performance and standards of practice. Attending professional meetings helps one to stay abreast of new trends and best practices. A list of websites of selected professional organizations that offer continuing education for educators is found in Table 1.3.

TABLE 1.3 Websites of Interest for Nurse Educators

Name of Organization	Mission of Organization Stated on Website	Web Address
National League for Nursing (NLN)	"The National League for Nursing promotes excellence in nursing education to build a strong and diverse nursing workforce to advance the health of our nation and the global community."	www.nln.org
American Association of Colleges of Nursing (AACN)	"The American Association of Colleges of Nursing (AACN) is the national voice for baccalaureate and graduate nursing education. AACN works to establish quality standards for nursing education; assists schools in implementing those standards; influences the nursing profession to improve health care; and promotes public support for professional nursing education, research, and practice."	www.aacn.nche.edu
Organization for Associate Degree Nursing (OADN)	The Organization for Associate Degree Nursing promotes "Associate Degree Nursing through education, leadership, inclusivity, collaboration, and advocacy to ensure excellence in the profession."	www.oadn.org
Association for Nursing Professional Development (ANPD)	"The Association for Nursing Professional Development (ANPD) advances the specialty practice of nursing professional development for the enhancement of health care outcomes. Professional development as a specialty of nursing practice is defined by standards, based on research, and critical to quality patient and organizational outcomes."	www.anpd.org/?page=about

(continued)

TABLE 1.3 Websites of Interest for Nurse Educators (*continued*)

Name of Organization	Mission of Organization Stated on Website	Web Address
Accreditation Commission for Education in Nursing (ACEN)	The Accreditation Commission for Education in Nursing (ACEN) is responsible for the specialized accreditation of nursing education programs (clinical doctorate, master's, baccalaureate, associate, diploma, and practical programs).	www.acenursing .org/mission -purpose-goals
Commission on Collegiate Nursing Education (CCNE)	"The Commission on Collegiate Nursing Education (CCNE) is an autonomous accrediting agency, contributing to the improvement of the public's health. CCNE ensures the quality and integrity of baccalaureate, graduate, and residency programs in nursing."	www.aacn.nche .edu/ccne -accreditation
National League for Nursing Commission for Nursing Education Accreditation (CNEA)	The NLN "Commission for Nursing Education Accreditation (CNEA) promotes excellence and integrity in nursing education globally through an accreditation process that respects the diversity of program mission, curricula, students, and faculty; emphasizes a culture of continuous quality improvement; and influences the preparation of a caring and competent nursing workforce."	www.nln.org/ accreditation -services/the-nln -commission-for -nursing-education -accreditation -(cnea)

SUMMARY

Choosing a career as a nurse educator provides many rewards and presents a few obstacles. Nevertheless, nurse educators in academic and health care settings can have a profound influence on how the current and next generation of nurses function within the health care system. Through their research, nurse educators advance the science of nursing education and build evidence for teaching. In partnership with practitioners, their clinical research improves patient care and strengthens the connection between education, practice, and research. Moreover, no matter the setting, nurse educators function as change agents and leaders.

Balancing one's responsibilities is a challenge, especially in a new role. Included in this balancing act is the ability to give attention to one's personal life. Flexible work hours can enhance the ability to use good time management skills to accomplish all that is expected. Furthermore, the adjustment to new responsibilities is enhanced with good mentors. One particular challenge for those teaching in schools of nursing, however, is salary levels. Generally, nurses in practice have higher salaries than faculty in schools of nursing. Some faculty members who teach 9 or 10 months during the academic year practice over the summer to keep current in their clinical skills and earn extra income.

Finally, making decisions about further education can be daunting. If one's career choice is to teach full-time in a baccalaureate and higher degree program, a doctorate is likely required for promotion, tenure, and retention. The type of doctorate chosen, research (PhD) or practice (DNP), depends on one's career goals, the type of scholarly trajectory desired, and the type of doctorate accepted for the tenure track. Nurse educators prepared at the DNP level are uniquely equipped to make the connection between education and practice through their clinical expertise. These educators have strong clinical skills, which can be used to teach at the prelicensure level and in graduate programs that prepare advanced practice nurses. Those prepared at the PhD level have knowledge and skills in generating new knowledge through more traditional forms of research. These nurse faculty may teach at the prelicensure level and in graduate programs.

The nurse educator role is complex. Each succeeding chapter in this book presents an in-depth discussion of the specific role competencies that are necessary for functioning as a nurse educator across many settings. Understanding all the dimensions of the role will foster the all-important transition from clinician to nurse educator.

REFERENCES

Accreditation Commission for Education in Nursing. (2017). *Accreditation manual: Section III. 2017 standards and criteria.* Atlanta, GA: Author.

Adelman-Mullally, T., Mulder, C. K., McCarter-Spalding, D. E., Hagler, D. A., Gaberson, K. B., Hanner, M. B., . . . Young, P. K. (2013). The clinical nurse educator as leader. *Nurse Education in Practice, 13,* 29–34. doi:10.1016/j.nepr.2012.07.006

American Association of Colleges of Nursing. (2015). Nursing faculty shortage. Retrieved from http://www.aacn.nche.edu/media-relations/fact-sheets/nursing-faculty-shortage

Beck, J., & Ruth-Sahd, L. (2013). The lived experience of seeking tenure while practicing clinically. *Dimensions of Critical Care Nursing, 32,* 37–45. doi:10.1097/DCC.0b013e31826bc6e9

Boyer, E. L. (1990). *Scholarship reconsidered: Priorities of the professoriate.* Princeton, NJ: The Carnegie Foundation for the Advancement of Teaching.

Boyer, E. L. (1996). The scholarship of engagement. *Journal of Public Service and Outreach, 1*(1), 11–20.

The Carnegie Classification of Institutions of Higher Education. (n.d.). About Carnegie Classification. Retrieved from http://carnegieclassifications.iu.edu

Clark, N. J., Alcala-Van Houten, L., & Perea-Ryan, M. (2010). Transitioning from clinical practice to academia: University expectations on the tenure track. *Nurse Educator, 35,* 105–109. doi:10.1097/NNE.0b013e3181d95069

Commission on Collegiate Nursing Education. (2013). Standards for accreditation of baccalaureate and graduate degree nursing programs. Retrieved from http://www.aacn.nche.edu/ccne-accreditation/standards-procedures-resources/baccalaureate-graduate/standards

Committee on the Robert Wood Johnson Foundation Initiative on the Future of Nursing at the Institute of Medicine. (2011). *The future of nursing: Leading change, advancing health.* Washington, DC: National Academies Press.

Cronenwett, L., Sherwood, G., & Gelmon, S. B. (2009). Improving quality and safety education: The QSEN Learning Collaborative. *Nursing Outlook, 57,* 304–312.

Dolansky, M. A., & Moore, S. M. (2013). Quality and Safety Education for Nurses (QSEN): The key is systems thinking. *Online Journal of Issues in Nursing, 18*(3), Manuscript 1. doi:10.3912/OJIN.Vol18No03Man01

Halstead, J. A., & Frank, B. (2018). *Pathways to a nursing education career: Transitioning from practice to academia* (2nd ed.). New York, NY: Springer Publishing.

Harper, M. G., & Maloney, P. (Eds.). (2016). *Nursing professional development: Scope and standards of practice* (3rd ed.). Chicago, IL: Association for Nursing Professional Development.

Harper, M. G., & Shinners, J. (2016). Overview of nursing professional development: Major revisions in 2016. *Journal for Nurses in Professional Development, 32,* 228–230. doi:10.1097/NND.0000000000000270

Hendricks, S. M., Taylor, C., Walker, M., & Welch, J. A. (2016). Triangulating competencies, concepts, and professional development in curriculum revisions. *Nurse Educator, 41,* 33–36. doi:10.1097/NNE.0000000000000198

Johnson, K. V. (2016). Improving adjunct nursing instructors' knowledge of student assessment in clinical courses. *Nurse Educator, 41,* 108–110. doi:10.1097/NNE.0000000000000205

Johnson, W. G., Butler, R., Harootunian, G., Wilson, B., & Linan, M. (2016). Registered nurses: The curious case of a persistent shortage. *Journal of Nursing Scholarship, 48,* 387–396. doi:10.1111/jnu.12218

National League for Nursing. (2012). *The scope of practice for academic nurse educators 2012 revision.* Philadelphia, PA: Wolters Kluwer.

National League for Nursing. (2014). *NLN nurse educator shortage fact sheet.* Retrieved from http://www.nln.org/docs/default-source/advocacy-public-policy/nurse-faculty-shortage-fact-sheet-pdf.pdf?sfvrsn=0

National League for Nursing Commission for Nursing Education Accreditation. (2016). *Accreditation standards for nursing education programs.* Washington, DC: Author.

Oermann, M. H. (2014). Defining and assessing the scholarship of teaching in nursing. *Journal of Professional Nursing, 30,* 370–375. doi:10.1016/j.profnurs.2014.03.001

Oermann, M. H. (2017). Preparing nurse faculty: It's for everyone. *Nurse Educator, 42*(1), 1.

Oermann, M. H., Lynn, M., & Agger, C. A. (2016). Hiring intentions of directors of nursing programs related to DNP- and PhD-prepared faculty and roles of faculty. *Journal of Professional Nursing, 32,* 173–179.

Oermann, M. H., Shellenbarger, T., & Gaberson, K. B. (2018). *Clinical teaching strategies in nursing* (5th ed.). New York, NY: Springer Publishing.

Quality and Safety Education for Nurses Institute. (2014). Competencies. Retrieved from http://qsen.org/competencies

Roberts, S. J., & Glod, C. (2013). Faculty roles: Dilemmas for the future of nursing education. *Nursing Forum, 48,* 99–105. doi:10.1111/nuf.12018

Schoening, A. M. (2013). From bedside to classroom: The Nurse Educator Transition Model. *Nursing Education Perspectives, 34,* 167–172. doi:10.5480/1536-5026-34.3.167

U.S. Department of Health and Human Services, Health Resources and Services Administration, National Center for Health Workforce Analysis. (2014). *The future of the nursing workforce: National- and state-level projections, 2012–2025.* Rockville, MD: Author.

Yoder-Wise, P. S., & Kowalski, K. E. (2012). *Fast facts for the classroom nursing instructor: Classroom teaching in a nutshell.* New York, NY: Springer Publishing.

2

Learning Theories

BETH CUSATIS PHILLIPS

OBJECTIVES

- Describe selected theories of learning
- Explore teaching strategies based on various learning theories

Nurse educators play a key role in the teaching and learning process. They need to be effective teachers not only in the classroom, but also in the nursing skills laboratory, simulation, in the clinical area, and during student advising. Understanding how students learn in each of these settings is paramount to good instruction. Nurse educators need to create instruction that is based on the best evidence of teaching and learning. The value of theory lies in providing insights into the underlying mechanisms of teaching and learning (Masterman, 2013). Theory can guide the creation of learning activities as well as assist in the reflection of the teaching process. Examining the theories of learning is essential to providing quality education. This chapter examines selected learning theories and teaching strategies based on those theories.

The first known writing about teaching and learning dates to 2100 BCE, in the Babylonian Code of Hammurabi, which briefly addressed teaching as an apprenticeship model, where learning was by practical experience (King, n.d.). The Greeks were well known for using the question-and-answer method of teaching, primarily recognized as the Socratic method, which dates back to 300 BCE (Phillips, 2010). Over the past 150 years, scientists and philosophers developed theoretical and conceptual models that represented the learning process. They struggled to understand how learning occurred.

Current neuroscience research has changed forever the theory and practice of education. Now, like no time in the past, we have the capability to see learning happen in the brain. Through the use of positron emission tomography scans and now functional magnetic resonance imaging, one can actually see the components of the brain in action as information is processed. From this research has emerged the concept of

This chapter was prepared based on work by Amy C. Pettigrew, PhD, RN, CNE, ANEF, in the first edition of this book.

brain plasticity, the idea that experience can actually change both the brain's anatomy and physiology (Boyle, 2010). Research related to neurotransmitters in the brain also contributes to insight into how best to structure learning processes.

WHAT IS LEARNING?

Learning is a core element of human existence, and teachers are needed for much of human learning. The puzzle of explaining how we learn, and therefore how to teach, has been in the forefront since the middle of the 19th century. While there are many definitions of *learning*, the following discussion of learning theories is based on Schunk's definition: "Learning is an enduring change in behavior, or in the capacity to behave in a given fashion, which results from practice or other forms of experience" (Schunk, 2012, p. 3).

THEORIES OF LEARNING

Any model of teaching and learning needs to include the teacher, student, personal attributes of each, learning environment, learning content, and teaching strategies (Utley, 2011). Because it has only been in the past 10 years that we have actually seen learning happen in the brain, scientists were left to hypothesize how learning worked, as a means of creating a rationale for an event (learning) that they could not otherwise explain.

The major theories of learning can be categorized as: behaviorism, cognitivism, social cognitivism, humanism, constructivism, and brain-based learning. Early theories were based on direct observation and then elaborated on by further schools of thought. Table 2.1 provides a general overview of the schools of thought.

TABLE 2.1 Major Learning Theories

Schools of Thought	Major Tenets	Major Theorists and Contributors
Behaviorism	Learning is a change in behavior, shaped by an external environment	Pavlov Skinner Thorndike
Cognitivism	Learning is an internal process	Bruner Piaget Gagne
Social Cognitivism	Role of social processes in addition to internal processes	Vygotsky Bandura Lave and Wenger
Humanism	People intentionally act based on perceived needs	Rogers Maslow
Constructivism	Learning is an internal process built on previous learning	Dewey Piaget Kolb Gardner
Brain-Based Learning	Cognitive neuroscience has identified actual neural processes of learning. Teaching methods should focus on how the brain learns	Sousa Jensen

BEHAVIORISM

With no method to see inside the brain and watch learning happen, teachers and scientists were left to hypothesize how people learned. Beginning during the second half of the 19th century and continuing into the early 20th century, scientists looked for ways of changing basic behavior. Behavioral theories defined learning as change in the method or frequency of a behavior due to some interaction in the outer environment. The interaction with the environment is key to learning within these theories. Conditioning plays a role in behaviorism.

Three well-known scientists, Pavlov, Skinner, and Thorndike, examined learning using a behaviorist perspective. Their work focused on learning as behavior change developed by external conditioning and reinforcement (Schunk, 2012).

Ivan Pavlov (1849–1936) is known for his work with *classical conditioning*, a multistep process that entailed introducing an unconditioned stimulus, which brings about an unconditioned response. For Pavlov, this entailed presenting a dog with meat, which in turn resulted in salivation. While training the dog, a metronome would be ticking in the background. Over time the dog would become conditioned to the metronome and would start to salivate when the metronome ticked. "A stimulus that was neutral in and of itself had been superimposed upon the action of the inborn alimentary reflex," Pavlov wrote of the results. "We observed that, after several repetitions of the combined stimulation, the sounds of the metronome had acquired the property of stimulating salivary secretion" (Pavlov, 1927).

Edward Thorndike (1874–1949) is known for his work that focused on learning, individual differences, intelligence, and transfer of knowledge (Hilgard, 1996). Thorndike developed psychological *connectionism*. He hypothesized that learning is the formulation of connections between sensory stimuli and neural impulses that are identified through behavior. He also believed that learning occurred often by trial and error. Thorndike noted that teachers need to help students form good habits and that teaching should contextualize content for students to understand how to apply what they have learned. He also proposed that information should be presented when the student is ready to learn or just before the information can be used in a serviceable way (Thorndike & Gates, 1929).

B.F. Skinner (1904–1990) formulated the theory of *operant conditioning* in the 1930s. Based on the work of Thorndike, Skinner believed that the best way to understand behavior was to examine the causes of an action and its consequences. Skinner created the term operant conditioning, which is changing behavior using reinforcement that follows the desired response. Skinner identified three types of responses that can follow behavior: neutral operants or responses from the environment that neither increase nor decrease the probability of a behavior being repeated; reinforcers, which are responses from the environment that increase the probability of a behavior being repeated; and punishers or responses from the environment that decrease the likelihood of a behavior being repeated.

Positive reinforcement strengthens a behavior by providing a consequence that an individual finds rewarding. The removal of an unpleasant reinforcer can also strengthen behavior. This is known as negative reinforcement because it is the removal of an adverse stimulus. Negative reinforcement strengthens behavior because it stops or removes an unpleasant experience (Skinner, 1953). Punishment inhibits behavior and is the opposite of reinforcement as it is designed to eliminate a response. Like reinforcement, punishment occurs by directly applying an unpleasant stimulus after a response or by removing a potentially rewarding stimulus (McLeod, 2007).

While popular through much of the 20th century, behaviorism is no longer a predominant educational perspective. However, the concepts of positive and negative reinforcement retain their usefulness today. Behavioral objectives, learning contracts, and programmed learning are based on behaviorism. Examples of teaching methods with this educational perspective are listed in Exhibit 2.1.

EXHIBIT 2.1 Examples of Teaching Methods Based on Behaviorism

Guided practice

Lecture without discussion

Programmed learning and instruction

Repetition

Skill exercises

COGNITIVISM

Cognitivism theories are a group of theories that include the work of Bruner, Gagne, Vygotsky, and others. During the 1960s, cognitive aspects of learning were recognized, primarily because the behaviorist perspective could not explain why people organize and make sense of the information they learn. Cognitive Theory defines learning as a semi-permanent change in mental processes or associations. Cognitivists do not require an outward demonstration of learning, instead focusing more on the internal processes and connections that take place during learning.

Cognitivists consider learning as mental structures that provide a base for organizing and building knowledge. Learning is not a change in behavior but a change in mental structures. Changes may be observed in behavior, but the behavior is due to a change in cognition. The locus of control for learning is in the learner, not the environment (Utley, 2011).

Jerome Bruner (1915–2016) proposed the Cognitive Growth Theory to examine intellectual growth of children. He proposed that as children grow, they depend on a widening array of modes of understanding. Infants rely on enactive responses (action) to process and represent information, children 1 to 4 years of age rely on images to process information, and finally children over the age of 4 begin to use language to shape and augment information processing (Bruner, 1964).

A primary focus of cognitive psychology is on memory, a subject that has been studied for thousands of years. Information Processing Theory explains acquisition of knowledge in a step-wise manner. Information processing theorists such as Robert Gagne (1919–2002) are less concerned with external factors and focus on mental processes that come between stimulus and response (Schunk, 2012). These theorists hypothesize that people selectively pay attention to environmental details, transform data into information, and rehearse the information, relating the new information to that already known (Mayer, 2011).

Within the Information Processing Model, Gagne (1985) described four processes: (a) encoding when environmental information is sensed or attended to (generation of neural impulses), (b) processing of information (filtering out of irrelevant information), (c) storage after encoding (may be short term or long term), and (d) retrieval, when the information is needed for a task (action).

Examples of teaching methods based on cognitivism include use of problem solving, reciprocal teaching (activities involving a dialogue between the teacher and students about segments of text to understand its meaning), and scaffolding (providing support such as resources and guides during the learning process to promote a deeper level of learning) (Crutchshank, Metcalf, & Jenkins, 2011; Gagne, Wager, Golas, & Keller, 2005).

SOCIAL COGNITIVISM

Lev Semyonovich Vygotsky (1896–1934) expanded Piaget's basic developmental theory of cognitive abilities of the individual to include the concept of social–cultural cognition, the idea that all learning occurs in a cultural context and involves social interactions. He emphasized the role that culture and language play in developing students' thinking and the ways in which teachers and peers assist learners in developing new ideas and skills. Vygotsky proposed the concept of the zone of proximal development, which suggested that students learn subjects best just beyond their range of existing experience with assistance from the teacher or another classmate. Assistance from others bridges the distance from what students know or can do independently to what they can know or do with assistance (Schunk, 2012).

SOCIAL LEARNING THEORY

Based on the work of Albert Bandura (1925–), this theory focuses on the concept that much of human learning occurs in the environment (Schunk, 2012). Social Learning Theory is built on the importance of observational learning, imitation, and modeling. Bandura's Theory hypothesizes that there is a continuous interaction among behaviors, cognitions, and the environment. The learner and environment are in a reciprocal relationship where one influences the other, and human behavior is learned visually through modeling from observing others (Bandura, 1977, 1986). For a student to learn, three internal processes must occur: attention or observation, retention or processing in memory, and motivation or having a reason to replicate another's behavior.

SITUATED LEARNING THEORY

Jean Lave and Etienne Wenger (1991) suggested that learning takes place in the same situation or environment in which it is applied. Their Situated Learning Theory proposes that learning is more than just a reception of knowledge. Rather, the knowledge is presented in as authentic a context as is possible and social interaction and collaboration among community members is imperative to the learning. Apprenticeship experiences enable the learner to be in the real environment in order to learn. Because nursing education involves social interaction and collaboration, and emphasizes the real practice of nurses, an authentic context is critical. Therefore, selecting teaching strategies that best prepare learners to acquire and retain knowledge is important. Exhibit 2.2 provides examples of teaching methods based on social cognitivism theories.

EXHIBIT 2.2 Examples of Teaching Methods Based on Social Cognitivism

Demonstration/return demonstration

Observational learning

Role modeling

Scaffolding

Apprenticeships in authentic contexts

HUMANISM

Humanistic Theory, largely constructivist, emphasizes both cognitive and affective learning. Within this paradigm learning is viewed as a personal act to fulfill one's potential (Schunk, 2012). The five basic principles of humanistic education include the promotion of self-direction and independence; development of the ability to take responsibility for what is learned; development of creativity; curiosity; and an interest in the arts (Huitt, 2009).

HIERARCHY OF NEEDS

The Hierarchy of Needs Theory, first discussed by Maslow in 1943, posits that all human actions are directed toward goal attainment. Most human actions are based on hierarchical needs, with lower order needs taking precedence over higher-order needs (Maslow, 1968). The lowest order need is physiological needs such as food, air, and water. Safety needs become predominant when there are environmental threats. Love and belonging needs become important once physiological and safety needs are met. Esteem needs are based on acceptance, achievement, and respect from others. The highest level is the need for self-actualization, which leads to self-fulfillment and personal growth (Maslow, 1943).

The first four needs are deficiency needs, which motivate people to resolve them (Maslow, 1968). Self-actualization is considered a growth or being need and, according to Maslow (1943), can only be reached by those individuals who have satisfied all lower level needs and are then able to "become everything that one is capable of becoming" (Maslow, 1943, p. 382). In 1970, Maslow expanded the hierarchy to include cognitive, aesthetic (1970a), and transcendence needs (1970b). Encouraging learners to meet their deficiency needs will allow them to strive for all they are able to achieve (McLeod, 2016).

Carl Rogers (1902–1987) concurred with Maslow and extended Maslow's work by concluding that for people to grow, they need an environment that provides genuineness, acceptance, and empathy. Rogers believed that every person could achieve their goals, wishes, and desires in life; self-actualization took place when, or if, they did (McLeod, 2012). Examples of teaching methods based on humanism include participatory and discovery methods, allowing students choices and opportunities for their learning, and providing resources and encouragement for learning (Schunk, 2012).

CONSTRUCTIVISM

A reaction to didactic approaches such as behaviorism and programmed instruction, constructivism states that learning is an active, contextualized process of constructing knowledge through experiencing and reflecting on the experience rather than acquiring it. Knowledge is constructed based on personal experiences and hypotheses. Learners continuously test these hypotheses through social interaction. Each person has a different interpretation and construction of knowledge process. The learner is not a "blank slate" but brings past experiences and cultural factors to a situation (Bruning, Schraw, Norby, & Ronning, 2010).

John Dewey (1859–1952) was one of the 20th century's most influential educators. His ideas of experiential education placed an emphasis on meaningful activity in learning and participation in the classroom (Schunk, 2012). Unlike earlier models of teaching, which relied on a teacher-centered classroom and rote learning, Dewey's idea of progressive education asserted that students must be invested in what they are learning.

He proposed that curriculum should be relevant to students' lives. He viewed experiential learning of practical life skills as crucial to education (Schunk, 2012).

Jean Piaget (1896–1980) was the first to state that learning is a developmental process and that children create knowledge rather than learn from the teacher. He recognized that children construct knowledge based on practice, which is related to biological and developmental maturation. Piaget observed young children and mapped out four stages of growth: sensorimotor (birth to about 2 years), preoperational (ages 2–7), concrete operations (ages 7–14), and formal operations (beginning around ages 11–15 and extending into adulthood). His work recognized the importance of some rote learning while also hypothesizing that other activities that support students' exploration are essential (Hilgard & Bower, 1975; Huitt & Hummel, 2003).

In the early 1970s, David Kolb and Roger Fry (1975) developed the *Experiential Learning Model* composed of four elements: concrete experience, observation of and reflection on that experience, formation of abstract concepts based on the reflection, and testing of the new concepts. These four elements are the basis of a cycle of learning that can begin with any one of the four elements, but typically begins with a concrete experience. He named his model to emphasize its links to ideas from John Dewey, Jean Piaget, and other writers of the cognitivist paradigm. His model was developed predominantly for use with adult education but has had widespread pedagogical influence in higher education. Kolb (1984) created a graphic representation of his model using two perpendicular continua, one related to process and the other related to perception.

Howard Gardner (1943–) argued that learning occurred in a variety of ways based on eight different intelligences. The *Multiple Intelligences Theory* suggests that human beings have a number of relatively discrete intellectual capacities (Gardner, 2011). This theory postulates that all humans possess the capacity to develop several intelligences and each has a unique and distinct profile. From the educator's perspective, this theory implies that all people are individuals and that each should be taught in a way that best fits his or her intellectual profile. In addition, this theory lends itself well to the idea that teaching should be done using multiple ways in order to reach more students. Gardner's eight intelligences are spatial, bodily-kinesthetic, musical, linguistic, logical-mathematical, interpersonal, intrapersonal, and naturalistic. See Exhibit 2.3 for a detailed description of each intelligence. Some examples of teaching methods based on constructivism are in Exhibit 2.4.

EXHIBIT 2.3 Gardner's Multiple Intelligences

Spatial

The ability to conceptualize and manipulate large-scale spatial arrays (e.g., airplane pilot) or more local forms of space (e.g., chess player).

Bodily-Kinesthetic

The ability to use one's whole body or parts of the body (like the hands or the mouth) to solve problems or create products (e.g., dancer).

Musical

Sensitivity to rhythm, pitch, meter, tone, melody, and timbre. May entail the ability to sing, play musical instruments, and/or compose music (e.g., musical conductor).

Linguistic

Sensitivity to the meaning of words, the order among words, and the sound, rhythms, inflections, and meter of words (e.g., poet). Sometimes called language intelligence.

(continued)

EXHIBIT 2.3 Gardner's Multiple Intelligences (*continued*)

Logical-Mathematical

The capacity to conceptualize the logical relations among actions or symbols (e.g., mathematicians, scientists).

Interpersonal

The ability to interact effectively with others. Sensitivity to others' moods, feelings, temperaments, and motivations (e.g., negotiator). Sometimes called social intelligence.

Intrapersonal

Sensitivity to one's own feelings, goals, and anxieties, and the capacity to plan and act in light of one's own traits. Intrapersonal intelligence is not particular to specific careers; rather, it is a goal for every individual in a complex modern society, where one has to make consequential decisions for oneself. Sometimes called self-intelligence.

Naturalistic

The ability to make consequential distinctions in the world of nature as, for example, between one plant and another, or one cloud formation and another (e.g., taxonomist). Sometimes called nature intelligence.

Source: From Gardner (2011).

EXHIBIT 2.4 Examples of Teaching Methods Based on Constructivism

Case-based learning

Discovery learning

Inquiry-based learning

Problem-based learning

Project-based learning

Class discussions and debates

Cooperative learning

Field trips

Guided experimentation

Peer tutoring

Research projects

Simulation

BRAIN-BASED LEARNING

Based on the rapid influx of information from brain research over the past 20 years, a new paradigm that bridges research and education has emerged. *Brain-based learning* is "the active engagement of purposeful strategies based on principles derived from an understanding of the brain" (Jensen, 2008, p. 4). According to cognitive neuroscientists, learning literally changes the brain. An increased rate of signaling by cortical neurons generates an increased number of branches in the neo-cortex, which in turn increases the density of cellular material and enhances connections with other neurons (creating more synapses). The changes only happen in the areas of the brain that are stimulated. The synapses increase because of the repeated firing of the particular neurons engaged in learning in the presence of emotion chemicals such as adrenaline and serotonin around the neurons.

The longevity of learning is in proportion to the number of neocortical areas that are engaged (Sousa, 2011). Jensen (2013) established seven guiding principles for brain-based learning that are significant for nurse educators to understand (Exhibit 2.5). Exhibit 2.6 lists examples of teaching strategies based on concepts of brain-based learning.

EXHIBIT 2.5 Guiding Principles for Brain-Based Learning

1. Brains are dynamic, not static.
2. Human brains are unique.
3. Brains use active construction of learning.
4. Human brains are social brains.
5. The physical and the cognitive are interconnected.
6. Uniqueness is the rule, not the exception.
7. Brains are designed for "gist" processing.

EXHIBIT 2.6 Examples of Teaching Strategies Based on Brain-Based Learning

Preexpose learners to content and context a week before the lesson

Teach less content and more in depth on important concepts

Provide frequent, nonjudgmental feedback

Provide some form of feedback to each student during the class

Engage students socially and physically

Empower learners by providing choices

Set high standards

Encourage peer support

Ensure the classroom is safe for risk-taking

Manage high levels of student stress

Allow students time to practice prior to testing

Maintain a variety of teaching methods that complement diverse learning styles

Celebrate successes

Source: From Jensen (2008).

SUMMARY

For many years, parents, educators, psychologists, and more recently cognitive neuroscientists have explored the concepts of teaching and learning. The science of teaching and learning, going back to Pavlov in the 19th century, has now evolved from theories based on observation to knowing which parts of the brain are activated by different stimuli. We now know that the brain is constantly learning by creating new connections. The question still remains, however: What is the ideal way to assist students in the learning process?

Nursing faculty members also should be aware of the need to teach students how to learn, and how to be successful in their courses. What are the best ways to motivate students to learn? What are the best ways to engage students in the classroom and online environment to encourage the deep understanding of material? How can nursing faculty use learning theory to help students learn and develop?

An engaged classroom, with students actively participating in the process of learning, is our challenge. Nurse educators must accept this challenge by finding new and different ways of teaching to reach all students and creating prepared and equipped nurses for the future.

REFERENCES

Bandura, A. (1977). *Social learning theory.* New York, NY: General Learning Press.

Bandura, A. (1986). *Social foundations of thought and action: A social cognitive theory.* Englewood Cliffs, NJ: Prentice Hall.

Boyle, T. (2010). The brain: Changing the adult mind through the power of plasticity. Retrieved from http://www.brainhq.com/media/news/brain-changing-adult-mind-through-power-plasticity

Bruner, J. (1964). The course of cognitive growth. *American Psychologist, 19,* 1–15.

Bruning, R. H., Schraw, G. J., Norby, M. M., & Ronning, R. R. (2010). *Cognitive psychology and instruction* (5th ed.). Upper Saddle River, NJ: Pearson.

Crutchshank, D., Metcalf, K., & Jenkins, D. (2011). *The act of teaching.* San Francisco, CA: McGraw-Hill.

Gagne, R. M. (1985). *The conditions of learning and theory of instruction* (4th ed.). New York, NY: Holt, Rinehart and Winston.

Gagne, R. M., Wager, W. W., Golas, F. C., & Keller, J. M. (2005). *Principles of instructional design* (5th ed.). Belmont, CA: Thomas/Wadsworth.

Gardner, H. (2011). *Frames of mind: The theory of multiple intelligences.* New York, NY: Basic Books.

Hilgard, E. R. (1996). Perspectives on educational psychology. *Educational Psychology Review, 8,* 419–431.

Hilgard, E. R., & Bower, G. H. (1975). *Theories of learning.* Englewood Cliffs, NJ: Prentice Hall.

Huitt, W. (2009). Humanism and open education. Retrieved from http://www.edpsycinteractive.org/topics/affect/humed.html

Huitt, W., & Hummel, J. (2003). Piaget's theory of cognitive development. Retrieved from http://www.edpsycinteractive.org/topics/cognition/piaget.html

Jensen, E. (2008). *Brain-based learning* (2nd ed.). Thousand Oaks, CA: Corwin Press.

Jensen, E. (2013). Guiding principles for brain-based education: Building common ground between neuroscientists and educators. Retrieved from http://www.brainbasedlearning.net/blog

King, L. (n.d.). Ancient history sourcebook: Code of Hammurabi. Retrieved from http://www.fordham.edu/halsall/ancient/hamcode.asp

Kolb, D. (1985). *Learning style inventory.* Boston, MA: McBer.

Kolb, D. A., & Fry, R. E. (1975). Toward an applied theory of experiential learning. In C. Cooper (Ed.), *Theories of group processes* (pp. 33–57). New York, NY: Wiley.

Lave, J., & Wenger, E. (1991). *Situated learning: Legitimate peripheral participation.* Cambridge, UK: Cambridge University Press.

Maslow, A. H. (1943). A theory of human motivation. *Psychological Review, 50,* 370–396.

Maslow, A. H. (1968). *Toward a psychology of being* (2nd ed.). New York, NY: Van Nostrand Reinhold.

Maslow, A. H. (1970a). *Motivation and personality.* New York, NY: Harper & Row.

Maslow, A. H. (1970b). *Religions, values, and peak experiences.* New York, NY: Penguin.

Masterman, L. (2013). The challenge of teachers' design practice. In H. Beetham & R. Sharpe (Eds.), *Rethinking pedagogy for a digital age* (pp. 64–67). New York, NY: Routledge.

Mayer, R. E. (2011). *Applying the science of learning.* Boston, MA: Pearson.

McLeod, S. A. (2007). B.F. Skinner operant conditioning. Retrieved from http://www.simplypsychology.org/operant-conditioning.html

McLeod, S. A. (2012). Carl Rogers. Retrieved from http://www.simplypsychology.org /carl-rogers.html

McLeod, S. A. (2016). Maslow's hierarchy of needs. Retrieved from https://www.simplypsychology.org/maslow.html

Pavlov, I. (1927). *Conditioned reflexes.* London, UK: Oxford University Press.

Phillips, C. (2010). *Socrates café*. New York, NY: W. W. Norton.

Schunk, D. H. (2012). *Learning theories: An educational perspective*. Boston, MA: Pearson.

Skinner, B. F. (1953). *Science and human behavior*. New York, NY: Free Press.

Sousa, D. (2011). *How the brain learns* (4th ed.). Thousand Oaks, CA: Corwin Press.

Thorndike, E. L., & Gates A. I. (1929). *Elementary principles of education*. New York, NY: MacMillan.

Utley, R. (2011). *Theory and research for academic nurse educators*. Boston, MA: Jones & Bartlett.

3

Understanding the Learner

BETH CUSATIS PHILLIPS

OBJECTIVES

- Describe the varied attributes that learners bring to the nursing program
- Analyze learner differences that can influence teaching nursing students
- Explore strategies that nurse educators can use to enhance learning

Understanding learners is an important component of quality teaching. Ideally, nurse educators use a learner-centered approach when preparing lessons to teach; during class and when teaching in simulation, clinical practice, and other settings; and for assessment. Nurse educators need an understanding of the varied attributes of students, which can affect their learning process and outcomes; students' culture and ethnicity; and their learning style preferences, the way in which students approach a particular learning situation. Students' age, gender, motivation, and self-regulation for learning are other characteristics that can influence our teaching approaches. This chapter examines varied attributes of nursing students, learner differences that can influence what and how we teach, and multiple strategies nurse educators can use that take into consideration these different characteristics.

LEARNER ATTRIBUTES

Learners come to the nursing program from varied backgrounds and with different perspectives, life experiences, desires, and needs. They have different aspirations, preferences, and resources (Beetham & Sharpe, 2013). The way in which students learn varies as well; some are methodical, analytical learners, while others are more intuitive. Some students learn better by "doing" and some by "seeing." Students vary in culture, ethnicity, learning preferences, age, gender, motivation, economic background, previous life experiences, and many other factors, which can have an influence on learning.

Currently the majority of students in nursing education programs are White, non-Hispanic (about 66%), female (85%), and younger than the age of 30 (National League for Nursing [NLN], 2014). As the United States becomes more diverse, so must our nursing education programs.

CULTURE AND ATTRIBUTES

Our increasingly global society brings with it diversity as never before experienced in higher education. Understanding the culture and ethnicity of learners aids nurse educators in teaching them more effectively and appropriately. According to the United States Department of Education National Center for Education Statistics (2016a), the percentage of public school students who were learned English as a second language was higher in 2013–2014 (9.3%, or an estimated 4.5 million students) than 10 years earlier (8.8%, or an estimated 4.2 million students). The rising complexity of teaching a diverse class of nursing students requires that faculty members be attuned to the learning needs of each student, recognizing that effective teaching should incorporate multiple methods to meet the range of needs.

In North America, we are immersed in a Western perspective of learning and knowing. Western perspectives value the individual learner over the collective, promote autonomy and independence of thought and action, and emphasize scientific research (Merriam & Bierema, 2014). However, nurse educators need to recognize this ethnocentrism and develop courses with multicultural perspectives. Valuable lessons in education come out of both Western and Eastern perspectives (Smith & Hu, 2013).

Faculty members can no longer assume that they understand and know the students in their courses. One of the major cultural differences is communication (Svinicki & McKeachie, 2013). For example, looking away rather than establishing eye contact with a faculty member is indicative of careful attention rather than inattention or anger in Asian and Native American cultures (Akechi et al., 2013). Nonparticipation, such as not answering questions to clarify a concept and not questioning the teacher, may be related to a cultural norm of showing respect to elders in certain cultures (Suinn, 2013). In a situation such as this, the teacher can use tools such as audience response system (clickers) or a 1-minute paper, which may assist the students and give the faculty member more input as to student comprehension.

Another important cultural difference is related to collectivism (the better good of the whole) or individualism (a focus on the individual). Western norms relate to individualism, but many cultures, such as Asian and certain African, Latin American, and Native American cultures, value the success of the whole more than individual success (Merriam & Kim, 2008). Small group activities in the classroom and projects may assist in deeper learning for these groups. Study groups also are helpful for this population of students.

Students from other countries and cultures may have a lower level of verbal fluency (Suinn, 2013). Students whose native language is not English may have an easier time with reading and writing than with verbal communication. In this situation, having class sessions video and audio digitally archived and available to students out of class may be of help to students. Other strategies include having content available in written format and using activities such as simulation, which provide kinesthetic as well as auditory and visual cues. Examples of teaching strategies for use in multicultural classrooms are provided in Exhibit 3.1.

EXHIBIT 3.1 Teaching Strategies for Inclusion in Multicultural Classrooms

Become aware of your own cultural biases

Treat each student as different from other students in the course

Maintain a culturally neutral classroom

Recognize the complexity of diversity

Foster intergroup relations

Be concrete

Monitor your use of idioms

Be accessible

Digitally archive videos or audio files of classes for students to review

Use culturally integrated examples, pictures, case studies, and so on

Encourage sharing of culturally diverse life experiences

LEARNING STYLE PREFERENCES

The concept of learning styles or preferences has been studied for more than 50 years. In the literature, the verbiage used varies from learning style to learning preference, but Anderson (2016) explained: "A learning style is a preference rather than something that is fixed and is influenced by previous learning experiences" (p. 55). A *learning style preference* is the preference for a particular style for learning; it is the manner in which an individual approaches a learning situation, which has implications for teaching. Do students learn and retain more when teaching methods match their learning style preference? Does purposeful matching of teaching to learning style preference improve learning outcomes? Learning style preference models were developed to guide students' understanding of how they prefer to learn, but preference is not the only way they can learn (Davis, 2009). In fact, expanding one's way of learning builds a stronger, more flexible learner by increasing the "cognitive repertoire and processes" (Davis, 2009, p. 273). Identification of learning style preferences has been a useful tool for students to examine their own preferences, develop better study methods, and identify particular ways to improve their learning outcomes.

There are many models of learning style preferences. Popular theorists such as Kolb (1984) and Fleming and Mills (1992) have described learning styles and learner preferences, using different theoretical and physiological perspectives. Using the concepts of his Experiential Learning Model, Kolb hypothesized that each of the four quadrants of the perceiving and processing continua could be interpreted as four preferred learning preferences.

Divergers (concrete and reflective) view concrete experiences from multiple perspectives and adapt by thinking rather than doing. *Convergers* (abstract and active) prefer the practical application of problem solving and technical tasks over personal issues. *Assimilators* (abstract and reflective) focus more on ideas than people and integrate multiple ideas into a conceptual whole. *Accommodators* (concrete and active) are comfortable with people and tend to use trial and error in problem solving (Kolb, 1984) (Figure 3.1).

In 1992, Fleming and Mills introduced the VARK Learning Preference Model, which introduces four learning style preferences: visual, auditory, read/write, and kinesthetic (VARK). They suggested that these learning style preferences relate to only one component of learning: how to take in and give out information.

FIGURE 3.1 Kolb's learning cycle and learning styles.

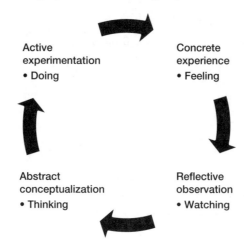

Source: Adapted from Kolb (1984).

Each mode is measured using the VARK tool (Fleming, 2012). The four learning style preference modes are:

- A *visual* preference is a preference for information in graphic formats such as maps, charts, and flow charts rather than in text format.
- An *aural/auditory* preference describes a preference for information that is language based (heard or spoken).
- A *read/write* preference indicates an inclination for information in text format.
- A *kinesthetic* learner prefers information that is concrete and experience-based.

Pashler, McDaniel, Rohrer, and Bjork (2008) undertook a comprehensive meta-analysis of the research supporting the concept of learning style preferences and application of learning styles to improve instruction. Their review found evidence that individuals, if asked, will express preferences for how material is presented to them. However, they also found that there was no evidence to support the hypothesis that matching teaching methods to learning style preferences will lead to improved learning outcomes. Leite, Svinicki, and Shi (2010) studied the VARK Model. They found validity in its measurement of learning preferences but recognized it as only one of many ways to assess learning.

No single assessment of learning style preference guarantees that a student's learning needs will be satisfied. The teacher should create learning environments that address the content and concepts to be learned using a multitude of methods rather than trying to match instruction to each student's learning style preference. Being aware of one's own style preference can help guide the student in ways to study. In addition, when teachers use multiple approaches, students are challenged to learn in different ways that enhance their learning. The teacher's own personal learning style preference is often not taken into consideration (Sternberg, Grigorenko, & Zhang, 2008) but could be shared in order to role model ways to strengthen learning by using different modes. For example, teachers who are auditory learners could share that they challenge themselves to practice kinesthetically to strengthen their knowledge base and skill. Additionally, material presented with a variety of methods keeps students engaged with the content and learning. Exhibit 3.2 provides examples of teaching strategies for diverse learning style preferences.

EXHIBIT 3.2 Examples of Teaching Strategies for Diverse Learning Style Preferences

Vary teaching methods, assignments, and learning activities

Include individual and group activities

Use discussion in the classroom, online environment

Use color, charts, and graphics in visual presentations

Use role play and simulations

Provide opportunities to learn by doing

Provide opportunities for the diverse learning style preferences in the course and laboratory

Encourage learners to challenge themselves to use other styles in learning

Do not teach solely using your personal learning style preference

AGE

Over the past 60 years, the age makeup of the student population in higher education has changed significantly. Starting with the returning veterans of World War II, colleges have seen rapid increases in the number of adult learners. Adult learners are considered to be nontraditional college students. *Nontraditional* refers to any student who delays starting college for a year or more, attends college on a part-time basis, works full time, has dependents, is a single parent, is financially independent, or does not have a high school diploma (Pelletier, 2010). Nontraditional students are the majority on college campuses today (Center for Postsecondary and Economic Success, 2015; Taliaferro, 2017; Ross-Gordon, 2011). Research on learners has shown that adults come from a wide variety of backgrounds and bring many different perspectives to the classroom (Wlodkowski, 2010). Although adults as learners are often classified into one group, adult learners today are comprised of Traditionalists, Baby Boomers, GenXers, and Millennials based on birth date, with Gen Z preparing to enter college in the next 3 years (Table 3.1). Much is published about learning, values, motivation, and preferences for delivery methods for each of these generations. However, there is little actual research other than general surveys to support these differences.

TABLE 3.1 Generational Differences in Values, Learning, and Teaching Methods

Generation	Ages	Values	Learning Motivation	Delivery Methods	Feedback
Baby Boomer	1945–1964	Optimistic, involved, hard workers	Public and peer recognition, relevance to career goals	Lecture, small group discussion	Well-documented feedback all at once
Generation X	1965–1979	Informal, skeptical, self-reliant	Relevance to personal goals, recognition by faculty	On-the-job training, e-learning, active learning	Regular ongoing feedback

(continued)

TABLE 3.1 Generational Differences in Values, Learning, and Teaching Methods (*continued*)

Generation	Ages	Values	Learning Motivation	Delivery Methods	Feedback
Millennial	1980–2000	Realists, confident, frequent use of social networking	Fast track to success, structured assignments with clear deadlines	E-learning, blogs, wikis, podcasts, mobile apps, hands-on learning	Frequent feedback
Generation Z	2001–present	Ethnically diverse, globally aware, conservative, volunteerism, environmental concerns	Digital natives, content abundance, technology dependent, collaborative	Dislike traditional classroom format, multitaskers, want learning to be fun	Instant feedback

In nursing education, 42% of students in associate degree programs are over the age of 30 compared to 18% of baccalaureate students. Sixty-four percent of RN to bachelor of science in nursing (BSN) students, 60% of master's nursing students, and 84% of doctoral nursing students are older than the age of 30 (NLN, 2014).

It is important to examine adult learners based on their unique learning needs. In 1973, Malcolm Knowles introduced the term "andragogy," outlining differences between children and adult learners (Knowles, 1973). Andragogy focuses on learning needs of adult learners. Knowles identified six assumptions about adult learning:

1. *Need to Know:* Adults prefer to know why they are learning particular content at the outset of learning. Teachers should assist adults to contextualize the learning to recognize its importance.
2. *Learner's Self-Concept:* Adult self-concept is dependent on progress toward self-direction. Adults need to be approached as capable and self-directed learners.
3. *Role of the Learner's Experiences:* Adults enter into education with prior experiences, which provide them with additional valuable resources. The richest resource for learning resides within; therefore, developing active learning strategies that build on adults' experiences is beneficial (Svinicki & McKeachie, 2013).
4. *Readiness to Learn:* Adults become ready to learn when they can use their learning to deal with real-life situations or perform a task. They want to learn what they can apply to current situations.
5. *Orientation to Learning:* Adults are life-centered (task-centered, problem-centered) in their orientation to learning. They want to learn what will help them perform tasks or deal with problems they confront in everyday situations and those presented in the context of application to real life.
6. *Motivation:* Adults are responsive to some external motivators (e.g., a better job and higher salaries), but the most potent motivators are internal (e.g., desire for increased job satisfaction and self-esteem (Knowles, Holton, & Swanson, 2011).

Nursing faculty members are faced with intergenerational classrooms and concurrently the needs of traditional and adult learners. Well-organized classes, with introductions that contextualize the content, relate it to clinical practice, and contain active learning exercises address the needs of both traditional and adult students. The use of technology also should be considered, as the Millennial and Gen Z students have grown up using the Internet and receiving immediate answers to questions.

In clinical situations, it is important to assist the nursing staff and preceptors to understand the difference in generational learners. In 2013, the average age of RNs was 50 years old (National Council of State Boards of Nursing, 2013). That means that Baby Boomers are working with Gen X and Millennial nurses. For example, students may be embracing technology with nursing reference books accessible on cell phones, a behavior that some older nursing staff may interpret as texting and indifference on the part of the student. Exhibit 3.3 lists teaching strategies for use in multigenerational classrooms.

EXHIBIT 3.3 Examples of Teaching Strategies for Multigenerational Classrooms

Clarify the essentials when preparing the syllabus, assignments, and evaluation tools
Contextualize the content
Offer choices for assignments
Create multigenerational team assignments
Provide frequent feedback
Use simulation activities and case studies
Use web-enhanced (hybrid) classes when feasible
Encourage sharing of varying viewpoints
Balance technology usage

Source: From Wilson and Gerber (2008).

GENDER

Nationally, 9.6% of the RN workforce is male (United States Census Bureau, 2013). Only 5% of full-time faculty teaching in baccalaureate and higher degree programs are men (Robert Wood Johnson Foundation, 2012). In nursing programs, 15% of students enrolled in associate degree and BSN programs are male, 14% are male in RN to BSN programs, and 13% are male in master's and doctoral programs (NLN, 2014).

As more men enter nursing education programs, faculty members need to take into account gender differences in learning, expectations, and perspectives. Throughout recent history, nursing has been a career that is undertaken primarily by females. Our classrooms have been filled with female students with female faculty members. The word "nurse" often has a female connotation. However, over the past 15 years the number of men in nursing education programs has increased, and creating a gender-neutral classroom is a necessity (Robert Wood Johnson Foundation, 2012).

Through the 1990s, there was a flurry of research investigating how male and female students differed in the college classroom. Rocca (2010) conducted an analysis of literature on student participation in the general college classroom and found continued subtle gender biases. Male college students tended to participate and be more engaged in the classroom, especially when the faculty member was male, and female students were more likely to participate with a female faculty member. Faculty members tended to ask male students more abstract questions and female students more factual questions. Male students speak more frequently and longer in class discussions, and female students receive less feedback on answers than do males (Columbia University Graduate School of Arts & Sciences Teaching Center, 2012).

To promote a gender-neutral classroom, nursing faculty members should assess their own gender biases and create a classroom that addresses males and females equally. Language needs to remain gender neutral, not assuming that every nurse is a female, including on examinations. Exhibit 3.4 provides some strategies for nurse educators to use to create a gender-neutral teaching situation.

EXHIBIT 3.4 Teaching Strategies to Create a Gender-Neutral Learning Environment

Treat all students equally, making no assumptions with regard to gender

Get to know the names of all students and pronounce them correctly

Set ground rules for discussions in class and online

Use gender-neutral language in case studies, examples, and exam questions

Ask questions of all students

Give students time to answer questions

Do not allow a few students to dominate discussion

Assess how you respond to students

Avoid interrupting student responses

Do not allow students to interrupt or intimidate each other

Use group activities to foster student confidence

Provide all students with feedback and encouragement

Promote a respectful climate in the classroom and online environment with acceptance of differences

Use diverse examples rather than ones that assume a certain background or experience

Be sure examples include both male and female references

Be consistent in addressing all students either by first or last names

Ensure that male and female students are held to the same academic standards

Be aware of the type of humor used in teaching to ensure that it is not offensive

SOCIAL DETERMINANTS OF HEALTH

Students' inherent genetic makeup defines a component of their ability to learn and acquire knowledge. The environment in which they were raised, including the way they were taught, the games they played as children, and their support systems, affect their ability to learn (Dewar, 2014; Wolfgang, Stannard, & Jones, 2001). In higher education, minorities and the poor fare worse than their peers, reinforcing inequality, and college is unaffordable for too many (Bowen & McPherson, 2016). Learning is influenced by the resources learners have available to aid them, not only from a technological perspective, but also from the perspective of physical and social determinants of health (Healthy People 2020, 2017). A nursing student who is hungry and tired from not getting adequate nutrition and housing may not process information as quickly or as well as others. Similar to Maslow's Hierarchy of Needs, discussed in Chapter 2, basic need attainment allows for increased cognitive processing and achievement of growth and development. Understanding the importance of basic need fulfilment by nurse educators may assist students in attaining their goals through successful education. The social determinants of health can affect students' access to and quality of education. Exhibit 3.5 lists the determinants of health according to Healthy People 2020 (2017).

EXHIBIT 3.5 Social Determinants of Health

Five areas that reflect critical components of social determinants of health

- Economic Stability
  - Poverty
  - Employment
  - Food Security
  - Housing Stability
- Education
  - High School Graduation
  - Enrollment in Higher Education
  - Language and Literacy
  - Early Childhood Education and Development
- Social and Community Context
  - Social Cohesion
  - Civic Participation
  - Discrimination
  - Incarceration
- Health and Health Care
  - Access to Health Care
  - Access to Primary Care
  - Health Literacy
- Neighborhood and Built Environment
  - Access to Healthy Foods
  - Quality of Housing
  - Crime and Violence
  - Environmental Conditions

Source: From Healthy People 2020 (2017).

MOTIVATION AND ACADEMIC SELF-REGULATION

The interaction of evidence-based teaching strategies and students' strategic use of learning methods, motivation, and self-regulation leads to good learning outcomes (Weinstein, Acee, & Jung, 2010). Many students begin higher education without the specific skills needed to study a particular discipline. As students learn content, they also need to learn the skills to be successful in studying the discipline (Weinstein et al., 2013). Strategic learners are active learners and are persistent in reaching learning goals. They know when they do not understand content and seek out resources to help them understand it. They recognize that learning is under their own control (Schunk & Zimmerman, 2012).

Strategic learners are effective learners who set reasonable and attainable goals for learning, which motivate them to continue studying (Schunk, Pintrich, & Meece, 2008).

Students who consciously set learning goals tend to be self-reflective, use metacognitive processes, are self-aware, and have higher levels of self-efficacy than other students (Kitsantas, Winsler, & Huie, 2008). They attribute success to effort, time management, and learning skills rather than luck (Weinstein et al., 2010). Strategic learners are motivated learners who want to learn (Zimmerman, 2011). A final key component needed for strategic learning is self-regulation, the use of executive control functions (Weinstein et al., 2010; Zimmerman & Schunk, 2011).

MOTIVATION

Motivation is a key dimension of self-regulated learning and a prerequisite for meaningful learning (Ginsberg, 2005; Mayer, 2011). Motivation as a biological phenomenon is a process that mediates how much energy and attention the brain allocates to a given stimulus. Motivation as a social science phenomenon is an internal state that begins and sustains goal-directed behavior. Motivation is based on multiple factors, which include goal orientation, interest, self-efficacy, and causal attribution (Mayer, 2011; Zimmerman & Schunk, 2012).

Goal orientation can be learning or performance based. Research has shown that students with stronger learning goals use deep learning skills more frequently. They also recover from a poor grade and improve performance to a higher degree than students with a performance goal orientation (Zimmerman & Schunk, 2012).

Interest is another contributor to motivation and is a precursor to learning. Students will work harder to learn when the content is of interest or related to their career plans (individual) or of high personal value at the time (situational) (Mayer, 2011; Zimmerman & Schunk, 2012).

Self-efficacy, the individual's self-assessed ability to complete tasks needed to achieve goals, is believed to be a strong element of motivation (Kitsantas, Winsler, & Huie, 2008; Wlodkowski, 2010). Self-efficacy is generally situation based and future oriented, but based on previous experiences.

Causal attributions are a student's beliefs about the causation of academic outcomes. These are students' perceptions rather than actual causes. Attributions are influenced by preexisting factors such as self-efficacy and by external environmental factors such as rewards (Zimmerman & Schunk, 2012). Students who make effort-based attributions are likely to put forth effort during learning to be successful (Mayer, 2011). A number of strategies to increase motivation are presented in Exhibit 3.6.

EXHIBIT 3.6 Teaching Strategies to Increase Student Motivation

Maintain a high level of enthusiasm for the content

Maintain a cohesive course structure

Keep content relevant to the intended outcome

Maintain a positive learning environment

Foster good lines of communication

Assist students to transfer previously achieved skills

Connect learning to the real world

Use lots of examples

Use active learning strategies

(continued)

Hold students to high expectations

Use appropriate assessment tools

Focus class and assessments on conceptual understanding

Provide many opportunities for graded assessments

Use rubrics for grading

Limit the use of high-stakes testing

Source: From Nilson (2010).

SELF-REGULATION

Self-regulation is "the process by which learners personally activate and sustain cognitions, affects, and behaviors that are systematically oriented to the attainment of learning goals" (Schunk & Zimmerman, 2012, p. vii). Self-regulation is employed as students recognize that there might be improved ways to accomplish a goal and change their learning strategies (Winne & Hadwin, 2012). With self-regulated learning, students are motivated to learn and can transform their cognitive abilities into improved academic performance.

Litchtinger and Kaplan (2011) suggested that self-regulation was essential for success in higher education and that motivation was a key component of the first component of self-regulation, forethought. When students set mastery goals, they are more likely to engage in self-regulation than if they set performance goals. Self-awareness and motivation begin the process of self-regulation.

Current literature supports a model of self-regulated learning that has three main phases (Weimer, 2010; Zusho & Edwards, 2011; Zimmerman, 2008). The first phase, forethought, includes the processes of goal setting and task-planning. The second phase is the action phase, which entails the processes of monitoring, controlling, and evaluating learning. The final phase of self-regulation is management, during which the student engages in reaction and reflection (Zusho & Edwards, 2011). Self-efficacy and an interest in learning motivate learners. Self-reflection after learning, to ensure that learners are satisfied with their performance, enhances motivation to continue to learn.

TEACHER-STUDENT RELATIONSHIPS

Student engagement, in both curricular and co-curricular activities, is a strong predictor of student success in higher education, and student contact with faculty is associated with the development of key relationships and better outcomes (National Survey of Student Engagement [NSSE], 2012). An excellent predictor of student satisfaction with college is the extent to which students believe the campus environment is supportive of their curricular and co-curricular needs (NSSE, 2012). Nurse educators need to understand that one of the major hallmarks of the supportive learning environment is student–faculty interaction. Interaction includes discussing ideas from class, clinical practice, and other environments of learning with students both in and out of those settings; giving prompt feedback on student work; discussing grades; talking about career plans with students; working with students on activities other than coursework; and engaging students in their own research projects outside of course requirements (NSSE, 2012).

Academic advising and the relationship built between a learner and advisor plays a key role in student retention, satisfaction, and overall influence on future career goals

(Vianden, 2016). In addition, satisfied students promote their school of nursing to others and bind the students to the school as alumni. Creasey, Jarvis, and Knapcik (2009) reported that students who had a strong sense of connection and nonthreatening associations with faculty members had less anxiety than their peers who felt less connected.

There is current attention on instructional immediacy (Walkem, 2014), the behavior that brings the instructor and students closer together in terms of perceived distance (Mehrabian, 1971). Nonverbal immediacy includes behaviors such as smiling, gesturing, eye contact, and having relaxed body language. Verbal immediacy refers to calling the students by name, using humor, and encouraging student input and discussion. Both verbal immediacy and nonverbal immediacy have a positive effect on student motivation (Kerssen-Griep & Witt, 2014; Velez & Cano, 2008).

Cox and Orehovec (2007) identified five types of faculty–student interactions in a residential college designed to increase faculty–student interaction. Disengagement, where interaction did not occur, was a common finding. Incidental or unintentional interactions were perfunctory polite greetings or recognition. Functional interactions occurred for a specific purpose such as asking a question, which led frequently to more interaction. Personal interaction was often the outcome of functional interactions and was highly valued by students, often leading to the beginning of a relationship between teacher and student. Mentoring, a rare outcome of interaction, occurred when a faculty member provided direct assistance with professional development, emotional and psychosocial support, and role modeling (Cox & Orehovec, 2007, p. 356).

Smyth (2011) found that respect was the most important attribute students wanted and the factor that encouraged them to learn. Based on a study by Delaney, Johnson, Johnson, and Treslan (2010), students in both online and face-to-face courses valued respect over all other faculty characteristics. For online students, faculty who were responsive and knowledgeable were ranked next, whereas students in courses that were face to face valued faculty who were knowledgeable and approachable. To understand the learner, faculty should know what students want and need from them. Exhibit 3.7 provides strategies to promote student engagement.

EXHIBIT 3.7 Teaching Strategies to Promote Student Engagement

Improve students' self-beliefs by giving them some control over learning processes
Give students opportunities to work alone, cultivating intrinsic motivation
Be approachable, sensitive to student needs, and well prepared
Create learning experiences that include active and collaborative learning components
Create challenging learning activities that push students to grow in abilities
Ensure that your course (classroom, online, laboratory, simulation, clinical practice, other settings) is welcoming to diverse students

Source: From Weimer (2012).

STUDENTS WITH DISABILITIES

More and more, students with disabilities are entering college. Eleven percent of undergraduate college students who enrolled in the 2012–2013 school year reported having a disability (United States Department of Education National Center for Education Statistics, 2016b). These students may be unsure of their ability to get the accommodations they require and deserve (Grasgreen, 2014). Disabilities vary from physical limitations to emotional and psychological problems. The U.S. Department of Education listed reported disabilities as: a specific learning disability, visual impairment, hard of hearing, deafness, a speech impairment, an orthopedic impairment, and a health impairment. Faculty should be educated on their responsibilities in teaching this population. Once a student receives accommodations for a disability, it is up to the faculty member to ensure that his or her course and teaching are consistent with the requirements. Students should not have to constantly remind faculty members of their needs. For example, a hearing-impaired student whose accommodations require closed captioning of all video recordings should not have to ask for transcripts or closed captioning.

However, students share the responsibility for ensuring that their needs are met. According to the U.S. Department of Education Office for Civil Rights (2011), the attitudes and self-advocacy skills of students with disabilities play an important role in the success or failure of their education.

SUMMARY

Nurse educators are in an ideal position to have a significant impact on students' learning. The diversity of our classrooms no longer allows a "one-size-fits-all" approach to teaching. To effectively engage students in the learning process, nurse educators need to understand multiple factors. First, the teacher should assess the diversity of the students. Cultural heritage and ethnicity, age, gender, learning style, motivation, disabilities, and ability to self-regulate are only a few of the significant differences among students. The teacher also should assess the content of the course and outcomes to be met. What is the goal of the learning? How will most students in the course best learn the concepts and other types of material? What do the students already know about the subject? How can the teacher best connect the new content to the material the students have already learned? Understanding the learner encourages growth and learning by all and creates an open and welcoming environment to learn.

REFERENCES

Akechi, H., Senju, A., Uibo, H., Kikuchi, Y., Hasegawa, T., & Hietanen, J. (2013). Attention to eye contact in the west and east: Autonomic responses and evaluative ratings. *PLOS ONE, 8*(3), e59312. doi:10.1371/journal.pone.0059312

Anderson, I. (2016). Identifying different learning styles to enhance the learning experience. *Nursing Standard, 31*(7), 53–63. doi:10.7748/ns.2016.e10407

Beetham, H., & Sharpe, R. (2013). *Rethinking pedagogy for a digital age: Designing for 21st century learning.* Hoboken, NJ: Taylor & Francis.

Bowen, W. G., & McPherson, M. S. (2016). *Lesson plan: An agenda for change in American higher education.* Princeton, NJ: Princeton University Press.

Center for Postsecondary and Economic Success. (2015). Yesterday's non-traditional student is today's traditional student. Retrieved from http://www.clasp.org/resources-and-publications/publication-1/CPES-Nontraditional-students-pdf.pdf

Columbia University Graduate School of Arts & Sciences Teaching Center. (2012). Gender issues in the college classroom. Retrieved from http://gsas.columbia.edu/content/handouts

Cox, B., & Orehovec, E. (2007). Faculty-student interaction outside the classroom: A typology from a residential college. *The Review of Higher Education, 30,* 343–362.

Creasey, G., Jarvis, P., & Knapcik, E. (2009). A measure to assess student-instructor relationships. *International Journal for the Scholarship of Teaching and Learning, 3*(2), Article 14. doi:10.20429/ijsotl.2009.030214

Davis, B. (2009). *Tools for teaching.* San Francisco, CA: Jossey Bass.

Delaney, J. G., Johnson, A. N., Johnson, T. D., & Treslan, D. L. (2010). *Students' perceptions of effective teaching in higher education.* St. Johns, Newfoundland, Canada: Distance Education and Learning Technologies.

Dewar, G. (2014). The cognitive benefits of play: Effects on the learning brain. *Parenting Science.* doi:10.1080/03634520903505936

Fleming, N. (2017). VARK: A guide to learning styles. Retrieved from http://www.vark-learn.com

Fleming, N., & Mills, C. (1992). Not another inventory, rather a catalyst for reflection. *To Improve the Academy, 11,* 137.

Ginsberg, M. B. (2005). Cultural diversity, motivation, and differentiation. *Theory Into Practice, 44,* 218–225.

Grasgreen, A. (2014). Dropping the ball on disabilities: Inside Higher Ed. Retrieved from https://www.insidehighered.com/news/2014/04/02/students-disabilities-frustrated-ignorance-and-lack-services

Healthy People 2020. (2017). Social determinants of health. Retrieved from https://www.healthypeople.gov/2020/topics-objectives/topic/social-determinants-of-health

Kerssen-Griep, J., & Witt, P. L. (2014). *Instructional feedback III: How do instructor facework tactics and immediacy cues interact to predict student perceptions of being mentored?* Communication Studies Faculty Publications and Presentations, University of Portland Pilot Scholars. Retrieved from http://pilotscholars.up.edu/cgi/viewcontent.cgi?article=1006&context=cst_facpubs

Kitsantas, A., Winsler, A., & Huie, F. (2008). Self-regulation and ability predictors of academic success: A predictive validity study. *Journal of Advanced Academics, 20,* 42–68.

Knowles, M. S. (1973). *The adult learner: A neglected species.* Houston, TX: Gulf Publishing.

Knowles, M. S., Holton, E. F., & Swanson, R. A. (2011). *The adult learner: The definitive classic in adult education and human resource development* (7th ed.). London, UK: Elsevier.

Kolb, D. A. (1984). *Experiential learning: Experience as the source of learning and development.* Englewood Cliffs, NJ: Prentice Hall.

Kolb, D. A., Rubin, I. M., McIntyre, J. M. (1974). *Organizational psychology: A book of readings* (2nd ed.). Englewood Cliffs, NJ: Prentice Hall.

Leite, W. L., Svinicki, M., & Shi, Y. (2010). Attempted validation of the scores of the VARK: Learning styles inventory with multitrait-multimethod confirmatory factor analysis models. *Educational and Psychological Measurement, 70,* 323–339.

Litchtinger, E., & Kaplan, A. (2011). Purposes of engagement in academic self-regulation. *New Directions for Teaching & Learning, 2011*(126), 9–17. doi:10.1002/tl.440

Mayer, R. E. (2011). *Applying the science of learning.* Boston, MA: Pearson.

Mehrabian, A. (1971). *Silent messages.* Belmont, CA: Wadsworth.

Merriam, S. B., & Bierema, L. L. (2014). *Adult learning: Linking theory and practice.* San Francisco, CA: Wiley.

Merriam, S. B., & Kim, Y. S. (2008). Non-Western perspectives on learning and knowing. *New Directions for Adult and Continuing Education, 2008*(119), 71–81. doi:10.1002/ace.307

National Council of State Boards of Nursing. (2013). NCSBN & the forum of state nursing workforce centers 2013 national workforce survey of RNs. Retrieved from https://www.ncsbn.org/2013_Poster_graphics.pdf

National League for Nursing. (2014). *Nursing student demographics.* Retrieved from http://www.nln.org/newsroom/nursing-education-statistics/nursing-student-demographics

National Survey of Student Engagement. (2012). *Promoting student learning and institutional improvement: Lessons from the NSSE at 13.* Bloomington: Indiana University Center for Postsecondary Research.

Nilson, L. (2010). *Teaching at its best* (3rd ed.). San Francisco, CA: Jossey-Bass.

Pashler, H., McDaniel, M., Rohrer, D., & Bjork, R. (2008). Learning styles: Concepts and evidence. *Psychological Science in the Public Interest, 9,* 106–119.

Pelletier, S. (2010). Success for adult students. *Public Purpose.* Retrieved from http://www.aascu.org/uploadedFiles/AASCU/Content/Root/MediaAndPublications/PublicPurposeMagazines/Issue/10fall_adultstudents.pdf

Robert Wood Johnson Foundation. (2012). Men slowly change the face of nursing education. Retrieved from http://www.rwjf.org/en/about-rwjf/newsroom/newsroom-content/2012/04/men-slowly-change-the-face-of-nursing-education.html

Rocca, K. (2010). Student participation in the college classroom: An extended multidisciplinary literature review. *Communication Education, 59,* 185–213.

Ross-Gordon, J. (2011). Research on adult learners: Supporting the needs of a student population that is no longer nontraditional. *Peer Review, 13*(1), 26–29. Retrieved from https://www.aacu.org/publications-research/periodicals/research-adult-learners-supporting-needs-student-population-no

Schunk, D. H., Pintrich, P. R., & Meece, J. L. (2008). *Motivation in education: Theory, research, and applications* (3rd ed.). Upper Saddle River, NJ: Prentice Hall.

Schunk, D. H., & Zimmerman, B. (2012). *Motivation and self-regulated learning: Theory, Research, and implications.* New York, NY: Routledge.

Smith, J., & Hu, R. (2013). Rethinking teacher education: Synchronizing eastern and western views of teaching and learning to promote 21st century skills and global perspective. *Education Research and Perspectives, 40,* 86–108.

Smyth, E. (2011). What students want: Characteristics of effective teachers from the students' perspective. *Faculty Focus.* Retrieved from http://www.facultyfocus.com/articles/philosophy-of-teaching/what-students-want-characteristics-of-effective-teachers-from-the-students-perspective

Sternberg, R., Grigorenko, E., & Zhang, L. (2008). Styles of learning and thinking matter in instruction and assessment. *Perspectives on Psychological Science, 3,* 486–506.

Suinn, R. (2013). Teaching culturally diverse students. In M. Svinicki & W. McKeachie (Eds.), *McKeachie's teaching tips: Strategies, research, and theory for college and university teachers* (14th ed., pp. 150–171). Belmont, CA: Wadsworth.

Svinicki, M., & McKeachie, W. (2013). *McKeachie's teaching tips: Strategies, research, and theory for college and university teachers* (14th ed.). Belmont, CA: Wadsworth.

Taliaferro, W. (2017). Today's students, yesterday's financial aid policies. Retrieved from http://www.clasp.org/issues/postsecondary/in-focus/todays-students-yesterdays-financial-aid-policies

U.S. Census Bureau. (2013). *Men in nursing occupations: American community survey highlight report.* Retrieved from http://www.census.gov/people/io/files/Men_in_Nursing_Occupations.pdf

U.S. Department of Education National Center for Education Statistics. (2016a). Postsecondary education. In *Digest of education statistics: 2014* (Chapter 3). Retrieved from https://nces.ed.gov/programs/digest/d14/ch_3.asp

U.S. Department of Education National Center for Education Statistics. (2016b). *The condition of education 2016: English language learners in public schools.* Retrieved from https://nces.ed.gov/programs/coe/indicator_cgf.asp

U.S. Department of Education Office for Civil Rights. (2011). *Transition of students with disabilities to postsecondary education: A guide for high school educators,* Washington, DC: Author. Retrieved from https://www2.ed.gov/about/offices/list/ocr/transitionguide.html#keys

Velez, J., & Cano, J. (2008). The relationship between teacher immediacy and student motivation. *Journal of Agriculture Education, 49*(3), 76–86.

Vianden, J. (2016). Ties that bind: Academic advisors as agents of student relationship management. *NACADA Journal, 36*(1), 19–29.

Walkem, K. (2014). Instructional immediacy in elearning. *Collegian, 21,* 179–184.

Weimer, M. (2010). What it means to be a self-regulated learner. *Faculty Focus.* Retrieved from http://www.facultyfocus.com/articles/teaching-and-learning/what-it-means-to-be-a-self-regulated-learner

Weimer, M. (2012). Ten ways to promote student engagement. *Faculty Focus.* Retrieved from http://www.facultyfocus.com/articles/effective-teaching-strategies/10-ways-to-promote-student-engagement

Weinstein, C. E., Acee, T. W., & Jung, J. H. (2010). Learning strategies. In B. McGaw, P. L. Peterson, & E. Baker (Eds.), *International encyclopedia of education* (3rd ed., pp. 323–329). New York, NY: Elsevier.

Weinstein, C. E., Acee, T. W., Stano, N., Meyer, D., Husman, J., McKeachie, W., & King, C. (2013). Teaching students how to become more strategic and self-regulated learners. In M. Svinicki, & W. McKeachie (Eds.), *McKeachie's teaching tips: Strategies, research, and theory for college and university teachers* (14th ed., pp. 291–304). Belmont, CA: Wadsworth.

Wilson, M., & Gerber, L. (2008). How generational theory can improve teaching: Strategies for working with the "millennials." *Currents in Teaching and Learning, 1*(1), 29–44. Retrieved from http://www.worcester.edu/WorkArea/DownloadAsset.aspx?id=5366

Winne, P. H., & Hadwin, A. F. (2012). The weave of motivation and self-regulated learning. In D. Schunk & B. Zimmerman (Eds.), *Motivation and self-regulated learning: Theory, research, and implications* (pp. 297–314). New York, NY: Routledge.

Wlodkowski, R. (2010). Enhancing adult motivation to learn: A comprehensive guide for teaching all adults. *Journal of Adult Education, 39*(2), 40–43.

Wolfgang, C. H., Stannard, L. L., & Jones, I. (2001). Block play performance among preschoolers as a predictor of later school achievement in mathematics. *Journal of Research in Childhood Education, 15*(2), 173–180.

Zimmerman, B. J. (2008). Investigating self-regulation and motivation: Historical background, methodological developments, and future prospects. *American Educational Research Journal, 45*(1), 166–183.

Zimmerman, B. J. (2011). Motivational sources and outcomes of self-regulated learning and performance. In B. J. Zimmerman & D. H. Schunk (Eds.), *Handbook of self-regulation of learning and performance* (pp. 408–425). New York, NY: Taylor & Francis.

Zimmerman, B. J., & Schunk, D. H. (2011). *Handbook of self-regulation of learning and performance.* New York, NY: Taylor & Francis.

Zimmerman, B. J., & Schunk, D. H. (2012). Motivation: An essential dimension of self-regulated learning. In D. H. Schunk & B. J. Zimmerman (Eds.), *Motivation and self-regulated learning: Theory, research, and implications* (pp. 1–30). New York, NY: Routledge.

Zusho, A., & Edwards, K. (2011). Self-regulation and achievement goals in the college classroom. *New Directions for Teaching & Learning, 2011*(126), 21–31. doi:10.1002/tl.441

Teaching and Teaching Methods

4

Learning Environment and Teaching Methods

DEBRA HAGLER AND BRENDA MORRIS

OBJECTIVES

- Describe characteristics of a supportive learning environment
- Select teaching/learning activities to support cognitive, affective, and psychomotor learning
- Describe a variety of teaching methods suitable for nursing education

Teaching takes place in formal and informal settings, as part of personal and professional roles. A teacher may be working alongside a student caring for a patient in a health setting, organizing group work in a classroom, facilitating a reflection session after a high-fidelity simulation, leading a discussion via webinar, or responding to learners asynchronously. This chapter describes the teacher's role in developing a supportive learning environment and using a variety of teaching methods, with guidance for selecting methods to fit the intended outcomes, learner characteristics, and available resources. Teaching methods are considered in relation to supporting learner development in the cognitive, affective, and psychomotor learning domains. Strategies are described for incorporating active learning and for promoting critical thinking. Expanded information on the use of educational technology is presented in Chapter 5 and on teaching through simulation in Chapter 7. Teaching methods for specific settings are described in later chapters as well: teaching in online environments in Chapter 6, teaching in the learning laboratory in Chapter 9, and clinical teaching in Chapter 10.

DEVELOPING A LEARNING ENVIRONMENT

People can, and often do, learn without being taught—that is, people can learn without a teacher. However, teachers cannot teach unless there are learners. Distance technologies and other innovations have afforded a shift from direct face-to-face instruction in real time to providing more flexible options for both learners and teachers. Teachers may not be physically present in the same location as their students, and learners may be reviewing information well after the teacher developed and provided the instruction. Regardless of the physical distance and time separation from their students, teachers need to demonstrate a supportive presence and help their learners construct knowledge.

Recent changes in educational policy, progressing from emphasis on the teacher's actions to focusing more on students' learning outcomes, mirror health care systems' progress from emphasizing care provision to a focus on patient outcomes. In education and health care, there is still much work to be done in prioritizing learner and patient outcomes.

Teachers can make a significant difference in outcomes for learners by establishing a supportive learning environment. Students face significant stresses from numerous sources in their personal and academic roles. Prelicensure nursing students have identified suggestions to improve student–faculty relationships that could be implemented by faculty members: striving for effective and respectful communication, engaging in shared faculty–student activities, seeking balance and clarity for assignments and testing, and providing encouragement (Clark, Nguyen, & Barbosa-Leiker, 2014).

The connections that students make with other students in the class can also support learning outcomes. While the teacher can role-model and encourage respectful communication, the support and validation of peers are additional powerful sources of motivation for learners to participate in in-class activities and accept the risks of contributing diverse viewpoints (Barr, 2016). Establishing shared expectations for respectful civil interaction from the beginning helps a group of learners focus on learning together. Ambrose, Bridges, DiPietro, Lovett, and Norman (2010) have recommended research-based strategies such as those in Exhibit 4.1 for creating a productive classroom climate.

EXHIBIT 4.1 Strategies That Promote Student Development and a Productive Climate

- Make uncertainty safe
- Resist a single right answer
- Incorporate evidence into performance and grading criteria
- Examine your assumptions about students
- Be mindful of low-ability cues
- Do not ask individuals to speak for an entire group
- Reduce anonymity
- Model inclusive language, behavior, and attitudes
- Use multiple and diverse examples
- Establish and reinforce ground rules for interaction
- Make sure course content does not marginalize students
- Use the syllabus and first day of class to establish the course climate
- Set up processes to get feedback on the climate
- Anticipate and prepare for potentially sensitive issues
- Address tensions early
- Turn discord and tension into a learning opportunity
- Facilitate active learning

Source: From Ambrose et al. (2010). Used with permission.

SELECTING TEACHING METHODS

It is unreasonable to expect that a teacher should be skilled in using every teaching method. The teacher's own comfort level with teaching methods is important to consider so that the focus of attention stays on learners and the learning process. However, expanding a teacher's comfort range to reflect on assumptions about learning can "open the door" to contemplating new teaching methods (Weimer, 2010). There is more than one way to teach any topic.

The most important question to ask about a teaching method is whether it is a good fit for the specific learning objectives, learners, teachers, and available resources. If the goal is to support students in mastering key course concepts and developing learning-related attitudes, values, beliefs, and skills (Slavich & Zimbardo, 2012), then the same teaching method will not work equally well for all situations. Nurse educators who would be appalled at the idea of treating each patient with identical interventions regardless of patients' individual needs might not appear as concerned about using identical teaching methods for all learners and instructional purposes. Yet, choosing teaching methods congruent with specific learner needs and desired educational outcomes is critical to effective instruction. The single most important factor in choosing a teaching method is whether that method will help students meet the intended learning outcomes or objectives.

DOMAINS OF LEARNING

Learning can be described as development in one or more of three different domains: cognitive, affective, and psychomotor. Cognitive development, which involves thinking, cannot be directly observed but is seen through the behaviors or products of thinking. Affective development, which involves values and beliefs, cannot be directly observed either, so it is seen through attitudes, behaviors, and choices that express values. Psychomotor development, which involves skilled movement, is directly observable in physical action. Program outcomes, course objectives (also referred to as outcomes), and module or daily objectives are written to reflect expected development across the three domains of learning. Nurses in practice rely on all three domains to provide care, so nurse educators need to design instruction, teach, and assess for student development in all three domains (Oermann & Gaberson, 2017).

Patients can view the physical care that nurses provide (psychomotor knowledge) and recognize that nurses have high ethical standards (Gallup, 2016) reflecting nursing values and beliefs (affective knowledge). Patients, however, may not be aware of the intense thinking and planning that nurses engage in to promote health and prevent harm (cognitive knowledge). Despite the hidden nature of the thinking process in our observable work, the cognitive domain is often the easiest domain to address in writing objectives and in choosing teaching methods. In some teaching/learning situations, the affective and psychomotor aspects of learning are ignored or expected to develop without much attention, but educators who plan only for cognitive development should not be surprised when learners' beliefs and physical skills do not change with accumulation of information alone. Development in affective values and physical skills is needed in concert with cognition in order to change behavior.

Some teaching strategies support learning in all three domains, whereas other strategies are more specific to learning in only one or two of the domains. Strategies chosen for a single class meeting do not need to represent each of the domains, but all domains should be included regularly for integrative experiences. It is important to note the hierarchical nature of each domain and to align the levels of learning objectives, teaching strategies, and evaluation methods. Descriptions of the levels within each learning domain and examples of activities that might be used for teaching in that domain are in Tables 4.1 to 4.3.

TABLE 4.1 Activities to Support Learning in the Cognitive Domain

Level	Definition	Examples of Teaching Strategies/Learning Activities
Remembering	Recall previous information.	Practice definitions with flash cards, matching games.
Understanding	Comprehend the meaning.	Complete a crossword puzzle, represent images with words, or words with images.
Applying	Use a concept in a new situation, carry out a procedure.	Interpret an equianalgesic chart to compare doses of two different narcotics.
Analyzing	Distinguish between facts and inferences.	Discuss what is known versus what can be inferred about a patient's health situation.
Evaluating	Make judgments about the value of ideas or materials.	Compare a patient's activity plan with the collaborative goals set by the patient and health team.
Creating	Build a structure or pattern from diverse elements.	Develop self-care learning materials for a patient or group of patients.

Source: Adapted from Anderson et al. (2001).

TABLE 4.2 Activities to Support Learning in the Affective Domain

Level	Definition	Examples of Teaching Strategies/Learning Activities
Receiving	Open to experience, willing to hear.	Listen to a lecture or story, watch a film.
Responding	React and participate actively.	Participate in discussions, ask questions, suggest interpretations.
Valuing	Attach values and express personal opinions.	Write a plan for personal health improvement.
Organization or creation of value system	Reconcile internal conflicts; develop value system.	Write a philosophy of nursing including examples of behaviors that reflect the philosophy.
Internalization of or characterized by values	Adopt belief system and philosophy.	Carry out a plan for personal health improvement.

Source: Adapted from Krathwohl, Bloom, and Masia (1964).

TABLE 4.3 Activities to Support Learning in the Psychomotor Domain

Level	Definition	Examples of Teaching Strategies/Learning Activities
Imitation	Copy action of another; observe and replicate.	Watch a demonstration of how to safely position a patient and repeat the action.
Manipulation	Reproduce activity from instruction or memory.	Practice positioning a patient with verbal coaching or written instructions for reference.
Precision	Execute skill reliably, independent of help.	Demonstrate coordination in using a walker.
Articulation	Adapt and integrate expertise to satisfy a nonstandard objective.	Transfer patients from beds to chairs in a variety of situations.
Naturalization	Automated, unconscious mastery of activity and related skills at strategic level.	Practice taking blood pressures until able to accurately hear the pulse, watch the dial, and manipulate the equipment simultaneously.

Source: Adapted from Dave (1970).

Coaching students practicing tracheal suctioning on task trainer manikins in the learning laboratory might support psychomotor skill development, but the activity lacks the context of care for a valued individual. Listening to an audio-recorded interview with a patient who has a debilitating disease with ineffective airway clearance might work well for supporting the affective objectives of valuing the patient perspective and cognitive objectives related to disease management, but not for psychomotor skill development. However, a carefully planned experience of providing care for an authentic patient in the clinical environment, a standardized patient in the clinical laboratory, or a simulated patient in the simulation laboratory can support development across all three domains.

LEARNER CHARACTERISTICS

The characteristics of the intended learners, including their social and cognitive cultures, are important to consider in choosing teaching methods. Students who are not comfortable interacting with peers or learning in cooperation with peers need support to develop knowledge, skills, and attitudes for professional-level communication and collaboration. Disagreeing in a way that remains respectful and still furthers the discussion is a complex communication skill to develop, yet planning for that development may be ignored, based on an assumption that students begin higher education with such skills. Beginning clinical students often express levels of anxiety that require enormous skill, time, and effort to manage (Hutchinson & Goodin, 2013). Teachers can anticipate and plan for additional attention on helping students learn to manage their anxiety, rather than being surprised when the learner's anxieties overtake the scheduled learning session.

When teaching strategies do not fit well with the characteristics of the learners, there is a greater need for resources to reach learning goals. When learners have not developed the prerequisite knowledge and skills to support them toward a later learning goal, the need for other resources, such as instructional time, increases. For example, if students admitted to an online program are familiar and comfortable with online technology, then orientation and learning related to the technology do not require as much instructional time or focused attention. However, when students admitted to an online program have little previous experience with online learning, teachers will need to plan for extra time and effort to support the learners in developing skills as new technologies are introduced.

RESOURCES

Teaching method choices are sustainable when they are realistic for the reasonably available resources. Resources to consider in choosing teaching methods include time, space, support staff, technology, and materials.

Time is a most precious resource—for both teachers and learners. The teacher's time plan for using a particular teaching method should include the time in preparation, direct instruction, and providing formative feedback/coaching students. The students' time to be considered includes accessing the materials needed, preparatory assignments, instructional time, and any follow-up assignments. An experience that requires extensive instructional time should be planned only to meet the most important course and program goals.

Physical spaces and course enrollment can facilitate interaction or constrain teaching methods and activities. Large-class sections and lecture rooms make group interaction challenging, but not impossible. Even in lecture halls with unmovable desks, students can interact in pairs or clusters.

Availability and access to *support staff* can make the difference in the outcomes of some learning activities. Librarians can be amazing resource persons for students and faculty struggling to search for clinical evidence. Writing center staff can be helpful for students learning to write in the discipline of nursing and for faculty developing writing assignments. Technology experts can help assure that classroom plans for new software use or online resources go smoothly. In settings without support staff, the teacher should plan learning activities with the understanding that troubleshooting library database searches, coaching students to use software, or managing other technical challenges will add to the teacher's responsibilities.

Technology is a resource and a means to an end. When students are learning to manipulate a stethoscope, it is reasonable to focus both on developing auscultation skills and on the stethoscope as a tool, because nurses can expect to use stethoscopes throughout their careers for obtaining assessment data that will support clinical decisions. At times, however, technology that is not the direct focus of a learning objective becomes the focus of a misguided instructional effort. For example, leadership students learning the important skill of realistically budgeting for a clinical project might be directed to use a specific format or software for an assignment. If the format or software that learners are directed to use will require live instruction or tutorials and extensive practice, the teacher must consider whether learning to use the tool is a reasonable investment of student time. A larger investment in time and effort might be appropriate when learners will use the software program or other technology in the future workplace; however, that high level of investment is generally not worthwhile for a single assignment.

Elaborate *materials* and plans might not be a better fit than simple and inexpensive materials and methods for supporting a particular objective. For example, when students are practicing their first urinary catheter insertions, catheterizing a high-fidelity human patient simulator may not improve learning over working with a simple and far less costly Static Pelvic Model. However, when the students are integrating assessments and interventions in more complex situations, being able to hear the simulated patient speak and express discomfort may add a level of realism that engages the student and improves the overall learning experience (Rystedt & Sjöblom, 2012).

PLANNING FOR ACTIVE LEARNING

Higher education has often been associated with a type of learning where students passively listen to their teachers' wise thoughts. Promoting more active learning requires student engagement far beyond mere attendance. A focus on learner engagement and active learning is aligned with a general trend away from teacher-centered strategies and toward strategies focused on what helps students learn (Ambrose et al., 2010).

Safe nursing practice relies heavily on application of the sciences. According to the President's Council of Advisors on Science and Technology (2012), approaches that engage students in active learning (as compared to lecture) lead to improved information retention, critical thinking development, and student persistence in science, technology, engineering, and mathematics (STEM) fields. Nursing students who are learning to base their practice on evidence from the sciences can benefit from active learning strategies as well.

Lecture, a frequently used teaching method in higher education, may call to mind an image of a teacher on the auditorium stage talking at an audience of students while the students doze off to sleep. Nurse educators individually may assert that they do not rely on lecture. However, Shindell (2011) surveyed nurse educators who had recently taught one or more prelicensure didactic courses in accredited prelicensure U.S. nursing programs. In that study, 75% of the 375 responding educators reported lecturing for at least half of their average class sessions. Lecture can be insidious in settings outside the classroom as well: When the postclinical conference, the clinical laboratory session, or the simulation debriefing time involves the teacher doing most of the talking, those sessions have been subtly converted to extra lectures. The students have slipped from their intended roles as active participants back to being more passive recipients.

When teaching consists only of delivering a lecture, educators seem to expect that students can transform the lecturer's words directly into the students' authentic nursing actions. However, telling a student to remember and employ a list of airway clearance measures for their future patients is very different from asking the student to determine what types of airway clearance measures might be suitable for a specific elderly patient with an abdominal incision who is unable to sit up or walk. Applying principles and concepts to new situations requires active practice and coaching.

ACTION AND REFLECTION

Two processes are important for active learning: action and reflection. Taking part in meaningful activity followed by reflecting on the learning processes and outcomes transforms the learner from a passive recipient of someone else's thoughts to an active constructor of knowledge and meaning. This does not mean that all passive strategies should be abandoned. Interposing active and passive strategies together can create a rich opportunity for students to actively participate in learning and practice doing what they are expected to learn. For instance, a class session on substance abuse might be changed from continuous lecture to a series of activities: students completing a classroom survey of attitudes, pairing for brief discussion, participating in a large group discussion, viewing a related film clip, analyzing a short case study in a small group, synthesizing recommendations from the case analysis, and summarizing key learning points.

The passive activities of reading textbook chapters or watching a film can be shifted to more active learning by pairing those activities with specific reflection activities and expectations. Simple instructions can help the student become an active participant. "While you read this passage (or watch this film clip) about a recent news event, identify at least three specific opportunities for health promotion at the individual, family, and community level. Bring your list for discussion to the next class session." Rather than the teacher identifying extensive lists of examples for new concepts, asking the learners to identify and share additional examples of the concept in the environment tests their understanding of the concept and helps them find individual meanings for a concept.

Professional nursing organizations have recently emphasized the importance of planning reflection activities such as debriefing after many types of learning activities (National League for Nursing [NLN], 2015). Debriefing has gained recent attention because of its use in educational simulation, but debriefing also is effective in the classroom and during postclinical conferences.

DEVELOPING HIGHER LEVEL THINKING

Educators highly value critical thinking and aim to foster the development of critical thinking abilities among their graduates. Elder and Paul (2010) define critical thinking as "the process of analyzing and assessing thinking with a view to improving it" (p. 38). Terms that have similar meanings to critical thinking and are occasionally used interchangeably include higher order or higher level thinking, metacognition, critical reflection, and reflective thinking.

There are two aspects of critical thinking: ability and disposition. *Critical thinking ability* involves using higher level thinking skills such as conceptualizing, applying, analyzing, interpreting, inferring, explaining, evaluating, and synthesizing. *Critical thinking disposition* defines the characteristics of the ideal critical thinker: being habitually inquisitive, open-minded, mindful of alternatives, well-informed, fair-minded, and honest in facing personal biases (Ennis, 2010). Critical thinking incorporates the elements of thought and applies the universal intellectual standards.

The ability to think critically is discipline neutral; however, the context in which critical thinking is applied may be discipline specific. For example, how a nursing graduate applies critical thinking to nursing practice is very different from how an engineering graduate applies critical thinking to engineering practice. Both of these graduates may use similar higher order thinking skills; however, the context in which these thinking skills are applied will be different.

TEACHING METHODS TO PROMOTE CRITICAL THINKING

There are many teaching methods that promote the development of critical thinking, including case studies, concept mapping, collaborative learning, problem-based learning (PBL), service learning, and gaming. Teachers can structure learning activities to develop critical thinking by focusing attention on reflection, providing reasons, and developing alternatives.

Teachers may support learners to reflect on a situation or experience by posing questions or structuring a written assignment to include reflection. Posing questions such as "How do you know?" and "What are the reasons?" help learners identify the reasons for their views and remind them to seek reasons for others' views (Ennis, 2010). To encourage learners to develop alternative hypotheses and evaluate alternate points of view, the teacher can prompt the learner to explain from a different perspective. Universal intellectual standards are standards that can be used to assess the quality of one's own thinking and reasoning about a problem, an issue, or a situation (Elder & Paul, 2010). Thinking critically and arriving at sound clinical judgments require use of these standards. Including targeted questions such as those in Table 4.4 help learners apply the Universal Intellectual Standards to their thinking (Elder & Paul, 2010).

TABLE 4.4 Questions Based on Universal Intellectual Standards Essential to Sound Clinical Reasoning

Standard	Questions
Clarity	Could you elaborate further on that point? Could you express that point in another way? Could you give me an illustration? Could you give me an example?
Accuracy	Is that really true? How could we check that out? How could we find out if that is true? What evidence is there to support the validity of your clinical thinking?
Precision	Could you give me more details? Could you be more specific?
Relevance	How is that connected to the question? How does that bear on the issue?
Depth	How does your answer address the complexities in the question? How are you taking into account the problems in the question? Are you dealing with the most significant factors?
Breadth	Do we need to consider another point of view? Is there another way to look at this question? What would this look like from the point of view of a conflicting theory, hypothesis, or conceptual scheme?
Logic	Does this really make sense? Is this consistent with what we know about the issue or problem?
Significance	Is this the most important problem to consider? Is this the central idea to focus on? Which of these facts are most important?
Fairness	Do I have a vested interest in this issue? Am I representing the viewpoints of others in a way that is fair and balanced?

Source: From Hawkins, Elder, and Paul (2010). Reprinted with permission.

TEACHING METHODS

In the following section, a variety of teaching methods are described in categories such as independent learning methods, small-group methods, and large-class methods. However, each of the methods can be used in more than one way. For instance, reading is described as an independent learning activity, but there may be times that reading aloud in the classroom suits the instructional purpose. Discussion can take place in pairs, small groups of three to four, or with the entire class.

INDEPENDENT LEARNING METHODS

Reading

Assigning passages for students to read in a textbook or scholarly journal is a simple instructional plan, but many students find that reading is a difficult way to learn. Learning through reading requires understanding, then interpreting and synthesizing the text into useful application.

Students often report that they begin the assigned reading for the week, reading part of the assignment each day, but never finishing a week's reading before the next week's assigned chapters are due. By default, the chapters at the end of each week's list are the least likely to have been read. Two simple instructional strategies can improve the reading-to-learn experience: limiting the assignment to the most pertinent readings, and identifying the recommended sections by priority order rather than sequential order. Rather than assigning 10 chapters totaling 800 pages each week, assigning only the most important passages from each chapter or the most important chapters improves the possibility that students might be able to finish a week's reading assignment. Prioritizing the passages among the assigned readings that are required versus those recommended for enrichment or review helps students make informed choices and use their time efficiently.

Teachers also help students improve reading comprehension by suggesting specific comprehension strategies along with reading assignments. Levels of support for comprehension increase as the teacher introduces reading strategies, provides the rationale for a particular strategy, and even models the strategy (Zhang, 2011). Three broad categories of reading strategies include problem-solving strategies, support strategies, and global strategies. Problem-solving strategies deal with cognitive and metacognitive approaches such as reading slowly and carefully or paying close attention. Support strategies include approaches such as taking notes while reading or paraphrasing/summarizing text. Global strategies invoke the meaning and purpose of the reading, and the use of context. Poole (2014) surveyed 272 junior and senior university students, native English speakers, about their use of reading strategies. Students with a grade point average (GPA) higher than 3.6 reported using some comprehension strategies significantly more often than their classmates with a GPA less than 2.7. Those strategies used more commonly by the group with a higher GPA included reading for purpose, getting back on track, adjusting reading speed, deciding what to read or ignore, using graphics, rereading, and using context clues.

Strategies that teachers can recommend or model for improving reading comprehension beyond the freshman year are listed in Table 4.5. Many of the strategies can be incorporated in both classroom and online activities.

Writing

Clear writing is important for many nursing roles "Nurses document patient care, communicate via writing with each other and colleagues in other disciplines, create

TABLE 4.5 Teaching Strategies for Improving Reading Comprehension

Strategy	Rationale	Activities to Recommend and Model
Activate prior knowledge	Connecting learners' existing information and experiences to a new topic improves understanding and memory.	Preview headings or key concepts, make predictions.
Use graphic organizers	Using visual representations helps students identify, organize, and remember important ideas.	Create timelines, framed outlines, concept maps, story maps, and Venn diagrams.
Teach comprehension monitoring strategies	Students keeping track of their understanding as they read and implementing "fix-up" strategies when identifying breakdown.	Keeping track: Note confusing or difficult words and concepts, create images, stop after each paragraph to summarize, and generate questions. When understanding breaks down: reread, re-state, use context to figure out unknown words or ideas.
Teach summarization skills	Consolidating large amounts of information (several paragraphs or passages) into key ideas.	Identify topic sentences, identify words or concepts that represent a list of related terms, practice summarizing, and use graphic organizers to summarize.
Teach students to ask and answer questions	Asking questions before, during, and after reading supports engagement and understanding.	Ask explicit and inferential questions, identify whether the answers to teacher's questions are likely to be found in text or require an inference.
Multicomponent comprehension strategy Instruction	Combining several comprehension strategies into an organizational system for reading.	Teach students to independently use strategies. Support students in generalizing strategy use across contexts and courses. Actively engage students in using comprehension strategies through cooperative learning, group discussions, and other interactions.

Source: From Boardman et al. (2008).

educational materials for patients and staff, develop organizational policies and procedures, and compose material for publication" (Troxler, Vann, & Oermann, 2011, p. 280). Writing effectively is a means for health care career progression: crystallizing complex and sometimes opposing ideas into a coherent written message is a critical leadership skill. Exhibit 4.2 identifies core competencies that can be developed through writing.

However, communicating effectively in writing is not easy. The basic writing skills that students attain in secondary schools do not extend to the types of writing needed for professionals. Examples of common writing assignments used in higher education to prepare nurses for professional writing are provided in Exhibit 4.3.

EXHIBIT 4.2 Core Competencies of Advanced Writing

• Organization	• Process
• Argument, evidence, and logic	• Accuracy
• Audience and voice	• Scholarly identity
• Content	• Sources
• Mechanics, grammar	• Expression
• Conceptualization and development of ideas	• Critique

Source: From Ondrusek (2012). Reprinted with permission.

EXHIBIT 4.3 Types of Writing Assignments

• Appraisal	• Narrative
• Book report	• Pamphlet
• Blog	• Patient instructions
• Care plan	• Poetry
• Case analysis	• Policy/Procedure
• Critique	• Process reflection
• Evidence synthesis	• Project proposal
• Film report	• Research paper
• Journal	• Summary
• Letter	• Technical description
• Memo	• Wiki

Students are admitted to nursing programs with a wide range of writing skills. Nursing faculty members can expect to teach students how to write using vocabulary and formatting requirements specific to health professions as well as to support students in remediating basic writing skills. Many schools have student support services available for writing development and remediation, but those services do not take the place of nursing faculty emphasizing written communication consistently throughout the curriculum.

There are a number of strategies for helping students develop effective writing skills, including the use of assignment rubrics, successive drafts, and feedback from peers and instructors. Table 4.6 indicates teaching strategies that support students' writing skills development.

Reflection

Benner, Sutphen, Leonard, and Day (2009) describe the process of helping students learn to identify what is important in a given situation as *teaching for salience*. One of the key strategies they describe as an exemplar of good teaching is that of helping learners reflect on practice. Reflecting on clinical practice allows students to examine clinical experiences and determine which actions were effective and were not effective.

TABLE 4.6 Strategies for Improving Writing and Structuring Writing Assignments

Strategy	Teacher's Action	Rationale
Detailed rubrics	Provide specific criteria for content and quality.	Communicate expectations.
Exemplar papers	Share excellent papers written by previous students (with their permission) as examples.	Clarify intended level and scope of assignment.
Drafts with feedback	Provide feedback on successive versions of the work.	Expect revision of the initial draft.
Sequential section writing	Provide feedback and guidance on one section or aspect of a larger project before the next section is written.	Redirect efforts early.
Peer coaching	Facilitate student peers in providing feedback to one another and revising their own work before they submit for teacher feedback.	Learn from how others conceptualize. Learn to give and receive effective feedback about writing.

Source: From Peinhardt and Hagler (2013); Sallee, Hallett, and Tierney (2011); Troxler et al. (2011).

EXHIBIT 4.4 Questions to Frame Reflection

- What is new to you about this material?
- What did you already know?
- Does any point contradict what you already knew or believed?
- What patterns of reasoning (or data) does the speaker/author offer as evidence?
- How convincing do you find the speakers'/authors' reasoning or data?
- Is there any line of reasoning that you do not follow?
- Is this reasoning familiar to you from other courses?
- What don't you understand?
- What questions remain in your mind?

Source: From Nilson (2010). Reprinted with permission.

The process of reflection facilitates increased self-awareness and enhances learning (Wanda, Fowler, & Wilson, 2016).

Coaching for reflection requires active engagement of the teacher, whereas reflecting requires active engagement of the learner. Strategies such as incorporating regular opportunities for reflective discussion, using structured reflection, providing individual student feedback on the reflection, and providing clear guidelines on the reflective activity will assist students to engage in reflective learning practices (Wanda et al., 2016). Exhibit 4.4 provides a list of questions that could frame reflection in a dialogue or in a writing activity such as journaling or blogging.

Contract Learning

There are several variations to contract learning, depending on the format of the course, the level of learners, and the purpose. These include a team learning contract, a course learning contract, an integrated learning contract, or an individual learning contract with a student.

Team Learning Contract. Teachers may use a team learning contract to specify performance behaviors for members completing a group assignment. A team learning contract is helpful because the learners define what behaviors and outcomes are acceptable to the team, and the team is accountable for enforcing the contract standards among members (Nilson, 2010). This type of approach is useful with adult learners who want to set performance parameters and team behavior expectations.

Course Learning Contract. Educators may use a contract learning approach to managing a course. Using this approach, the teacher provides the learner with a menu of options available to demonstrate course learning outcomes, and establishes the minimum standards for satisfactory performance. The learner contracts with the teacher for the number and types of learning assignments that will be completed to achieve the desired level of performance. This approach allows the motivated, self-directed learner the ability to contract with the teacher to complete a series of learning assignments that demonstrate a high level of course performance (Nilson, 2010). One drawback to this approach is that it may be challenging for learners who are less motivated, not self-directed, or unable to articulate learning needs.

Integrated Learning Contract. An integrated learning contract may be used to provide a structured approach for practicum experiences where a Precepted Clinical Education Model is used. The purpose of the integrated learning contract is to provide a consistent framework for the application of didactic content with practice experiences. The integrated learning contract allows for the faculty, preceptor, and learner to establish mutually agreed upon learning outcomes that facilitate the transfer of didactic knowledge to the practice setting. Additionally, the integrated learning contract facilitates evaluation of learning and attainment of competencies by defining the learning objectives and the evaluation parameters for the student's field experience (Boitel & Fromm, 2014).

Individual Learning Contract. A learning contract specifies what the learner must accomplish to meet the course outcomes. The learning contract will specify individual student learning objectives, learning assignments, evaluation methods, and deadlines. The teacher may initiate the learning contract, or the learner may initiate it, depending on the structure of the course and the purpose of the learning contract. Teachers may initiate the learning contract as a tool to clarify requirements with a student who is not meeting course expectations. In contrast, a student-initiated learning contract allows the self-directed student to individualize a learning experience. Learning contracts are frequently used to guide directed or independent study courses, graduate courses, and fieldwork.

The principles of andragogy support the use of learning contracts to help facilitate adult learning. A well-written learning contract includes the following items: measurable learning objectives; learning activities and resources required to meet the objectives; deliverables or evidence to demonstrate that the outcomes have been met; and the specific criteria for evaluation.

Concept Mapping

Concept mapping is commonly used as an instructional method to facilitate the development of critical thinking by allowing the learner to integrate new concepts into an existing cognitive structure, fostering meaningful learning. A concept map provides a visual representation of a concept and the interrelationships between the central concept and subconcepts. A commonly used structure for concept mapping involves placing the major concept in the center of the map and locating the subconcepts around the major concept, then connecting the subconcepts and major concept to show interrelationships. Concept mapping encourages learners to build upon previous knowledge, integrate new concepts, and explore the interconnections between concepts (Biniecki & Conceicão, 2016). It is important to note that each learner's concept map will be different because learners construct knowledge based upon their previous knowledge.

Concept maps may be unstructured or highly structured. The educator should match the amount of structure for the concept map to the purpose of the concept map. In some circumstances, it may be desirable to use a highly structured approach to concept mapping, whereas it may be preferable to use an unstructured approach when the goal of the teaching method is for the learners to construct their own knowledge. The concept map helps the educator assess a student's understanding of the concept and the connections among subconcepts. Concept mapping is an appropriate teaching strategy when the faculty member is teaching cognitive information and wants to facilitate active learner participation.

In nursing education, concept mapping may be used to help students organize assessment data, integrate interventions and the nursing process, and understand the interrelationships among data. One advantage of concept mapping is that it allows students to build on prior knowledge and assimilate new information in a way that is meaningful to the student. Other advantages include facilitation of active engagement with content, the development of deductive and inductive reasoning, and the ability to cluster information. Concept mapping is effective for visual learners.

Variations of concept mapping include mind mapping and argument mapping. Mind maps use a high level of abstraction and use lines and associative words to link pictures, words, and diagrams to form a map of the associations between ideas (Zipp & Maher, 2013). Argument maps have a low level of abstraction and use boxes, lines, and linking words to show the inferences between claims and supporting evidence. These different forms of knowledge mapping help foster meaningful learning, allow learners to scaffold or build upon previous learning, and facilitate critical thinking.

Self-Paced Modules/Reusable Learning Objects

A reusable learning object (RLO) is a small, self-contained educational unit that may include objectives, content, interactive learning activities, animations, narrated text, visual images, self-assessments, and feedback tools. RLOs may be used to introduce new content, reinforce or clarify existing content, or provide demonstrations (Nilson, 2010). They may be used independently or combined with other RLOs to teach larger content areas. Some teachers use RLOs when they "flip" the classroom by having the learners review the RLO prior to coming to class, then use class time for more active learning activities.

When developing and designing an RLO, it is important for the teacher to keep the RLO focused on a small area of content, clearly define the scope of the RLO, and incorporate strategies that facilitate ease of navigation and interactivity. Some teachers use a storyboard approach to help facilitate the development of RLOs. Most RLOs are between 2 and 15 minutes in length.

RLOs developed by publishing companies are available for purchase or may be included when students purchase textbook packages. The role of the teacher in using RLOs developed by others is to assure that the RLO is congruent with the course objectives, is of sufficient quality to meet student learning needs, and is used in compliance with copyright restrictions.

The benefits of RLOs include the ability of the student to engage in self-paced learning, actively engage with content, review content, and perform self-assessment to identify learning needs. Learners highly value the flexible anytime and anywhere access that RLOs afford and appreciate the opportunity to review challenging content while advancing at their own pace (Williams, O'Connor, Windle, & Wharrad, 2015). For these reasons. RLOs can be more effective than traditional lecture.

SMALL-GROUP METHODS

Discussion

A good discussion is engaging, explores diverse ideas, and helps participants clarify their own thinking in the face of colleagues' alternative ideas. However, poorly planned classroom discussions can take up a large amount of time with little learning impact. Even after a well-focused discussion, students may not understand what points in the discussion are important to remember or apply in future work. Periodic restatements and summaries by group members can help everyone stay on track and remember key points.

A clear learning objective and agreed-upon ground rules help frame a discussion. Will students raise their hands, speak out at will, or indicate in some other way that they would like to have the floor? Is participation required or optional? How will the group manage those who dominate the discussion, avoid participation, move off topic, or show disrespectful behavior to other group members? Another variable to consider when planning online or in-class discussions is the size of the group. Akcaoglu and Lee (2016) found that a small-group size of three to five learners was optimal to facilitate asynchronous online discussions. In small groups, learners perceived higher levels of sociability, social space, and cohesion which allowed the learners to get to know the group and think more deeply through the connections among group learners (Akcaoglu & Lee, 2016). The process of setting group discussion norms collaboratively creates a good starting point for a respectful and scholarly discussion. Examples of teacher responses that enhance discussion are in Table 4.7.

TABLE 4.7 Teacher Responses That Facilitate Discussion

If Student Contribution Is . . .	Possible Teacher's Response to Facilitate Discussion
Accurate	Provide some reinforcement such as a nod or brief affirming statement.
Correct but only one of many	Ask another student to extend or add to the response; avoid early closure.
Incomplete	Follow up with a question that directs the student to include more information.
Unclear	Try to rephrase it, then ask if this is what the student means.
Seemingly wrong	Follow up with one or more gentle Socratic questions designed to lead the student to discover the error. Invite the student to explain, clarify, or elaborate.

Source: Adapted from Nilson (2010). Reprinted with permission.

Experiential Learning

Activities that engage the senses help learners understand and recall concepts. Trying to breathe through a straw for several minutes evokes both physical sensations to remember and a beginning sense of understanding how arduous and frightening it can be to feel short of breath. Taking part in a group exercise such as building a bridge with dry spaghetti or assembling a puzzle can open frank discussion about the dynamics of working in groups to complete tasks. Sorting a collection of items in three different ways helps promote understanding of competing classification systems or nomenclatures. Although doing kinesthetic activities in class takes time, the additional understanding that learners develop through the activity and facilitated reflection promotes lasting learning.

Case Study

A case study is a descriptive analysis of a person or event (Kaylor & Strickland, 2015). Case studies are often created or adapted based upon life experiences. Case studies may be included in a lecture, discussion, or small-group learning activity in classroom or online environments. Case studies actively engage learners by providing opportunities to apply concepts or content to real or simulated scenarios, facilitating knowledge transfer and increasing learner confidence (Cleveland, Carmona, Paper, Solis, & Taylor, 2015). Effective case studies are relevant, are realistic, promote student engagement, and provide a cognitive challenge for the learners (Cleveland et al., 2015).

Case studies may present a one-time snapshot of the situation or a continuous, unfolding story over time. Some case studies use a sequential-interactive approach where the learners move through the case study by making decisions or narrowing down solutions and requesting additional information from the teacher to ultimately solve the case (Nilson, 2010). Whatever approach is used for the case study, it is important for the teacher to debrief the learners by discussing the problems and solutions identified through the case study with the learners. In larger classes, educators can use an audience response system to engage learners and increase interaction around case decisions.

In nursing education, case studies can provide practice opportunities in assessing situations and making decisions. Case studies vary in length from short bullet-style cases (two to three sentences), through minicases or vignettes (two to three paragraphs), to lengthy multipage cases (Nilson, 2010). Teachers may purchase or create the case studies; frequently, nurse educators develop their own case studies based on prior clinical practice experiences. When creating a case study, the teacher develops objectives and questions that correspond with the case study to engage the learner and foster the development of higher level thinking abilities (analysis, synthesis, evaluation).

Cooperative Learning

Cooperative learning encourages students to work interdependently to answer questions or solve problems, while still maintaining individual accountability for learning. Cooperative learning increases retention, engages learners, facilitates critical thinking, and promotes deeper learning. Teachers create a cooperative learning environment by assigning tasks that cannot be completed alone and require small groups of learners to work together (Millis, 2010). Educators build individual accountability into cooperative learning activities by having learners complete self, peer, and group evaluation of contributions to the group's project and functioning. Learners who participate in cooperative learning activities learn group processing skills such as managing group dynamics, ensuring participation by all group members, treating each group member's contributions with respect, and arriving at group consensus.

The teacher's role in cooperative learning is to provide a structure that facilitates problem solving, assists learners in managing group process, and helps learners to synthesize and apply their learning. It is important for the teacher to clearly articulate the purpose of the cooperative learning activity, help the learners understand the value of the learning activity, provide clear instructions, and facilitate closure on completion of the learning activity. Ideally, small groups of two to four students work best for cooperative learning activities. It is important for the teacher to intentionally incorporate heterogeneity into cooperative learning by forming groups with diversity in characteristics such as individual ability, perspective, gender, academic major, or age. Group heterogeneity provides the opportunity to work with and learn from others who are different. Cooperative learning groups also need to work together long enough to form effective working relationships. Teaching methods that promote cooperative learning can be used in traditional classroom or online learning environments, including think-write-pair-share, group investigations, three-step interviews, wikis, blogs, threaded discussions, and the use of clickers for interactive academic gaming.

Team learning contracts may be used in conjunction with cooperative learning strategies to delineate the learning process for faculty and students. The collective learning agreement defines the "preferred actions, processes, behaviors, and methods for both the student and faculty to facilitate learning" (Coy, 2014, p. 229). Collective learning agreements encourage students to be more responsible for their own learning and to actively engage in the learning process because they participated in the creation of the learning environment structure.

Team-Based Learning

Team-based learning (TBL) is a form of cooperative learning, that is, an instructor-led, learner-centered approach to teaching that facilitates active learning (Kim, Song, Lindquist, & Kang, 2016). It is comprised of three phases: preparation, readiness assurance, and application of concepts. During the first phase, preparation, students are assigned to review course materials prior to class. In the second phase, assessment of individual and group readiness to participate in the TBL activities is completed. This is frequently accomplished through the use of multiple-choice questions directed toward assessing student readiness. During the third phase, the learners apply course concepts to case-based scenarios and respond to questions as a team. The teams then share their answers and discuss how they reached their conclusions with the whole class. TBL has been found to improve academic performance, increase problem solving, and enhance perceptions of teamwork (Huitt, Killins, & Brooks, 2015). Additionally, TBL has been associated with an increase in problem-solving ability, knowledge, and clinical performance in undergraduate nursing students (Kim et al., 2016).

Problem-Based Learning

PBL is a student-centered learning method that allows learners to be actively engaged in their learning, acquire new information in the context for their use, and create a link between theory and practice. Benefits of PBL include development of critical thinking, leadership, teamwork, and self-directed learning skills (Kong, Qin, Zhou, Mou, & Gao, 2014). Some programs use PBL as a learning method to deliver the entire curriculum, whereas other programs use PBL techniques to deliver selected learning experiences.

PBL has been used as a teaching–learning method in traditional theory-based, online, and clinical practice courses. The many different approaches to PBL share common attributes, including that (a) problems are used as the central focus to initiate or motivate learning, (b) students collaborate in small groups and work over a period of time to solve problems, (c) the teacher serves as a facilitator of learning instead of a disseminator of content, (d) the teacher coaches teams for managing group processes, and (e) students initiate and direct learning.

There are four basic stages in implementing a PBL method. The first stage is problem analysis, where introductory information is given to the students, and the group identifies what is known and unknown about the situation. The second stage is brainstorming, where the group identifies resources to meet learning needs. During this stage, the group may also pose questions to the facilitator or their peers to clarify the situation. The third stage is self-directed learning, where each group member researches and gathers information to share. The final stage is solution testing, which is an iterative process where group members share resources and information to test solutions by applying new knowledge to solve the situation.

PBL requires the teacher to actively facilitate group learning rather than deliver content. Because PBL relies on students building upon prior content knowledge, PBL may not be the most effective teaching method for entirely new content. It can take students time to adapt to active teaching methods, such as PBL, if they have been previously socialized to more passive teaching methods. To help students transition, the teacher can introduce PBL gradually and explain how the roles of educator and student are different in PBL.

Simulation, Standardized Patients, Role-Play, Imagined Script Writing, and Drama

"Simulation is a technique, not a technology, to replace or amplify real experiences with guided experiences, often immersive in nature, that evoke or replicate substantial aspects of the real world in a fully interactive fashion" (Gaba, 2007, p. 126). The range of fidelity, or faithfulness, to reality in simulation is wide. At the low-fidelity end, learners practice injecting a medication into a practice pad or even a piece of fruit to feel the sense of puncturing through a barrier, while at the high end of simulation fidelity, learners provide care to standardized patients enacting health conditions or manikins programmed with realistic physiologic responses.

Simulation can support learning in the cognitive, affective, and psychomotor domains. Simulation is a powerful teaching method. Several studies have found that the use of simulation may increase clinical nursing judgment, deductive reasoning, and student self-confidence (Bobianski, Aselton, & Cho, 2016; Chmil, Turk, Adamson, & Larew, 2015; Hayes, Power, Davidson, Daly, & Jackson, 2015). Teaching with clinical simulation is described in detail in Chapter 7.

Standardized patients are used in nursing education to provide students with simulated patient encounter experiences to practice skills such as performing physical assessment, communication, and patient interviewing (Rutherford-Hemming & Jennrich, 2013). The use of clinical experiences with standardized patients provides the faculty with an opportunity to assess student learning and evaluate student preparation for live clinical patient encounters. Formative and summative evaluation of student clinical performance may also be conducted with the assistance of standardized patients. Many advanced practice nursing programs use objective structured clinical examinations (OSCEs) staffed with standardized patients to evaluate learner competencies.

Role-play is a teaching method that allows the learner to portray the role of another individual, anticipating how that individual will respond in a given situation. In nursing education, role-play may be used to teach therapeutic communication, conflict resolution skills, and other competencies. It is important for the teacher to create a safe environment to help learners feel comfortable engaging in role-play. Role-play helps the learner train for specific roles by learning to anticipate what an individual might say or do in a situation and preparing how to respond to that individual (Zazkis & Nejad, 2014). It is challenging to use role-play as a teaching method in large enrollment classes, because only a few learners will have the opportunity to actively participate in the role-play activity, whereas the majority of learners may observe as members of the audience.

Imagined script writing is a variation of role-play that can be used with large enrollment classes. In imagined script writing, the learner writes a script for dialog between two characters in a situation (Zazkis & Nejad, 2014). Imagined script writing is similar to role-play in that it helps the learner anticipate how another individual will respond in a given situation; however, this approach has the advantage of allowing the learner to have time to think about and formulate the best response to the situation (Zazkis & Nejad, 2014).

Participating in a scripted *drama* or theatrical presentation is a specific type of role-play that has been used to help nursing students learn about communication, end-of-life care, and ethical or legal issues. Students may participate in the drama as actors or they may watch the drama as observers. Role-playing and drama are most effective for learning experiences when followed by thoughtful debriefing and reflection. The use of drama as a teaching method is a cost-effective alternative for providing experiential learning around situations that are difficult to arrange in the clinical environment (Arveklev, Wigert, Berg, Burton, & Lepp, 2015).

Teaching Others and Making Presentations

There is nothing like developing a presentation to encourage immersion in a topic. Through preparing and giving presentations, students have the opportunity to learn the same way that many teachers have learned unfamiliar content. Organizing a presentation forces thinking about what information is needed, what the audience already knows, and how to explain a complex topic. Presentations focus on information in a chosen or assigned content area but have the additional advantage of providing real practice in the authentic workplace skill of teaching or explaining a concept to others.

Although the student presenter has an active role in learning through the preparation and delivery of a presentation, the other students observing the presentation stay in the positions of passive learners unless their roles are restructured. Assigning the audience members to some of the roles traditionally held by the teacher, such as moderator, timekeeper, provider of positive feedback, and provider of suggestions for further improvement changes the experience of the audience members to active participants in the learning. Engaging each of the students in some role helps adjust the experience to be more collegial and improves the learning potential for both the student presenter and the student audience.

Recording their presentations provides students the opportunity to see how they look and sound as presenters, and it allows for repeated or asynchronous viewing. Class members can provide feedback live or through online interactive video software programs.

Service Learning

Service learning, a form of experiential education, provides students with the opportunity to apply theory to practice while meeting an identified community need (Murray, 2013; Taggart & Crisp, 2011). The evidence suggests that student participation in service learning increases engagement in learning, promotes a positive attitude toward civic involvement, enhances cultural competence, and improves academic outcomes such as persistence, retention, and course completion (Kohlbry, 2016; Murray, 2013; Taggart & Crisp, 2011). Service learning is distinguished from volunteer work by the primary goal of learning through providing service.

To effectively implement service learning, the teacher facilitates discovery learning and critical reflection to ensure that new knowledge, concepts, and skills are meaningfully linked to the learner's personal experiences. Characteristics of effective service-learning experiences include joint planning between the academic institution and community partner, reciprocity between partners, clearly defined roles and responsibilities, effective communication among all parties, and a comprehensive student orientation to the service-learning project.

LARGE-CLASS METHODS

Lecture

A well-organized and enthusiastic lecture can be an inspiring event, while a lecture in which the presenter reads the slides aloud can lead to learners daydreaming. Some advantages of lecturing include that it is an efficient method for delivering content to large groups of students and that students receive the same information. Additionally, lecturing provides the teacher with a sense of control over the learning environment. Lectures may also be used to supplement other learning materials.

Teachers organizing and preparing lectures may learn about the intended content through their own active engagement in the process; however, the students attending a lecture often remain passive. Teachers who are afraid they might not know the answers to student questions might be relieved to read from slides or notes without much interaction. Learners who are uncomfortable with communication might be relieved to listen to a lecture and avoid interacting with peers or teachers. However, unless students are engaged, they are unlikely to remain attentive and retain information from the lecture.

The key to keeping students engaged is to divide a longer lecture into several mini-lectures and stop talking every few minutes while students participate in active thinking tasks. Tasks that help students understand what they are hearing might be generating examples of the concept under discussion, taking part in a kinesthetic activity related to the concept, or applying the concept to solve a problem. For lecture to be effective, it is important to integrate active learning techniques and to summarize critical information. Exhibit 4.5 describes teacher actions that improve the effectiveness of lectures.

EXHIBIT 4.5 Suggestions for an Effective Lecture

- Determine intended learning outcomes
- Budget extra time for questions and interaction
- Subdivide content in 15-minute chunks
- Intersperse lecture with learning activities
- Use attention grabbers to begin
- Incorporate visuals, examples, and restatements
- Engage students in recapping key points

Source: Adapted from Nilson (2010). Reprinted with permission.

Questioning

Questions are a powerful tool for understanding what learners are thinking and helping learners organize and expand their thinking. However, a teacher's question can strike fear into the heart of a learner who is overly worried about what answer the teacher expects.

Brookfield (2012) describes supporting development of critical thinking through asking learners first about the general ideas or concepts being presented, then later asking more direct questions about the learner's own ideas. He suggests a process of asking learners questions related to identifying their assumptions, checking their assumptions, seeing multiple viewpoints, and taking informed actions.

One strategy to improve teaching skill in questioning is to identify pertinent questions related to Paul's Elements of Thought and ask the individual or group to respond to them. Table 4.8 provides examples of questions teachers might ask to facilitate deeper and more expansive thought on a clinical situation or other topics.

TABLE 4.8 Using a Checklist for Clinical Reasoning to Generate Questions

Element of Reasoning	Example Questions
All clinical reasoning has a PURPOSE.	Can you state your purpose clearly? What is the objective of your clinical reasoning? Does your reasoning focus throughout on your clinical goal? Is your clinical goal realistic?
All clinical reasoning is an attempt to figure something out, to settle some QUESTION, to solve some PROBLEM.	What clinical question are you trying to answer? Are there other ways to think about the question? Can you divide the question into subquestions? Is this a question that has more than one right answer, or can there be more than one reasonable answer? Does this question require clinical judgment rather than facts alone?
All clinical reasoning is based on ASSUMPTIONS.	What assumptions are you making? Are they justified? How are your assumptions shaping your point of view? Which of your assumptions might reasonably be questioned?
All clinical reasoning is done from some POINT OF VIEW.	What is your point of view? What insights is it based on? What are its weaknesses? What other points of view should be considered in reasoning through this problem? What are the strengths and weaknesses of these viewpoints? Are you fairmindedly considering the insights behind these viewpoints?
All clinical reasoning is based on DATA, INFORMATION, and EVIDENCE.	To what extent is your reasoning supported by relevant data? Do the data suggest explanations that differ from those you have given? How clear, accurate, and relevant are the data to the clinical question at issue? Have you gathered data sufficient to reach a valid conclusion?
All clinical reasoning is expressed through, and shaped by, CONCEPTS and THEORIES.	What key concepts and theories are guiding your clinical reasoning? What alternative explanations might be possible, given these concepts and theories? Are you clear and precise in using clinical concepts and theories in your reasoning? Are you distorting ideas to fit your agenda?

(continued)

Element of Reasoning	Example Questions
All clinical reasoning contains INFERENCES or INTERPRETATIONS by which we draw CONCLUSIONS and give meaning to data.	To what extent do the data support your clinical conclusions? Are your inferences consistent with each other? Are there other reasonable inferences that should be considered?
All clinical reasoning leads somewhere, that is, has IMPLICATIONS and CONSEQUENCES.	What implications and consequences follow from your reasoning? If we accept your line of reasoning, what implications or consequences are likely? What other implications or consequences are possible or probable?

Source: From Hawkins et al. (2010). Reprinted with permission.

Not all queries are posed in the form of a question. A request that begins with "please share . . ." or "tell me more . . ." implies a question, yet may sound less threatening than a direct question. A specific type of questioning is Socratic questioning, in which the teacher leads the student or group to uncover their knowledge and make connections among concepts through a series of exploratory questions.

Demonstration/Return Demonstration

Demonstration, a teaching method frequently used in clinical practice and laboratory settings, may be incorporated into classroom sessions through display of experiments or problem-solving techniques (Nilson, 2010). Demonstration facilitates learning for students who learn through assimilation or convergence, or who consider themselves visual learners. A return demonstration by the learner supports a kinesthetic preference in learning. Demonstration is discussed more fully in Chapter 9.

Educational Games

Educational games are effective in reinforcing knowledge, motivating effort, building a sense of community, and creating a relaxed atmosphere that facilitates comprehension of content (Abdulmajed, Park, & Tekian, 2015; Blakely, Skirton, Cooper, Allum, & Nelmes, 2009). Many students perceive games as positive and motivational; however, some learners experience anxiety, embarrassment, and intimidation with the peer competition aspect of gaming (Blakely et al., 2009). Educational games provide immediate formative feedback to the learners and allow the teacher to assess the amount of learning that has occurred (Abdulmajed et al., 2015).

Educational games can be high or low technology and are classified by genre such as adventure, music, puzzle, racing, role-play, simulation, sports, and strategy. Learners playing high-tech simulation or strategy games may use virtual reality or interactive video gaming to experience real-life situations or events that facilitate learning and decision making. Low-tech games such as question-and-answer board games, team quizzes, card games, and tossing the ball to answer the question on-the-spot are effective in reinforcing learning.

The teacher should assess and match the fit between the goal for the education session (i.e., delivering new content or reinforcing information) and the readiness of the learners to participate in the game. To effectively use gaming, teachers should be confident in their ability to lead the gaming session and be able to adjust it, dependent on the learners' responses. Logistical factors such as the amount of time, class size, and the teaching environment might be constraints to implementing gaming.

Film

Cinemeducation is the use of movies or film clips to teach concepts, facilitate discussion, and foster critical thinking (Wilson, Blake, Taylor, & Hannings, 2013). Movies create a controlled learning environment to facilitate learning and an opportunity to experience some situations firsthand (Wilson et al., 2013). One drawback of using movies is that learners may make unsupported inferences about what they observe, and they may not have the opportunity to ask questions as they would in a live practice situation. The teacher can ask specific questions to guide learners in identifying inferences from the movie and considering additional information they would obtain if they could interact with the characters.

The teacher should preview the film and ensure that it supports the desired concept, then provide learners with objectives to guide the experience and reflective questions to stimulate critical thinking. The students might submit responses to the teacher for evaluation or discuss responses with peers. Another approach is to have them write about specific concepts seen in the movie. Wilson et al. (2013) used this type of approach to teach family assessment; after viewing a full-length film that depicted a problem affecting a family or public health, learners completed a formal family assessment based on data presented in the film.

Debate

Debate helps learners develop communication skills, structure logical arguments, and engage in rebuttals. Teachers can use debate with small or large groups of learners. A common format for debate involves assigning groups of learners opposing positions on a controversial topic. The teacher provides the structure, facilitates learners' argument development, poses logical questions, manages group dynamics and interpersonal communications, and facilitates learners' reflection. Nurse educators frequently use debate to facilitate thinking about ethical issues. Debate encourages learners to develop logical arguments and impromptu fact-based responses about controversial issues.

Narrative Pedagogy/Storytelling

The use of stories for teaching and learning is naturally engaging and highly flexible. Storytelling formats can range from a simple face-to-face verbal or audio recording recounting an experience to a polished multimedia production. "Narrative requires readers to produce rich and complex mental representations. It offers one of the major means through which the experiences of other people, different cultures, and distant times may be conveyed, and it expands our virtual experience of the world. Typically, narratives manipulate not only our knowledge of things, but also our impressions of how people feel, judge, and react in a multitude of situations" (Sanford & Emmott, 2012, p. xi).

The same experience can be told as a story from different perspectives and with different themes in mind. For example, stories told on a nursing unit to newly hired staff may have the purpose of a cautionary tale, an orientation to the unit culture, establishment of a hierarchy, or providing other information. Exhibit 4.6 describes features common to narratives and stories used to teach.

EXHIBIT 4.6 Typical Features of Narratives/Stories

- Specific rather than generic events
- Specific time and place settings
- People are involved in the events
- Include moment-by-moment thoughts, feelings, and sensory perceptions
- Include a setting, theme, plot, and resolution
- Audience members feel as if they have entered a different world

Source: From Sanford and Emmott (2012).

Although storytelling is common to many purposes, educators have systematically investigated the use of narrative in nursing. Narrative pedagogy is a unique approach that calls upon teachers to "create opportunities to talk with students about their thinking, how they understand (interpret) the situations they encounter, and what this means to their emerging nursing practice" (Ironside, 2015, p. 85).

The wide availability of digital media has provided many options for narratives, including videos and podcasts. A simple recording of a story in the patient's own voice could provide the prompt for an engaging class discussion or other assignment. Teachers need to obtain written permission from the storyteller before recording and sharing narratives.

SUMMARY

Teachers can make a significant difference in outcomes for learners by establishing a supportive learning environment. Encouraging a positive class climate and respectful interactions among peers promotes the development of an effective environment for learning.

The educator selecting a teaching method should consider the fit of that method with the learning objectives, learner and teacher characteristics, and available resources. Of these factors, the single most critical aspect in choosing a teaching method is judging the fit of that method with the intended learning outcomes or objectives.

Learning can be described as development in one or more of three different domains: cognitive, affective, and psychomotor. Some teaching strategies support learning in all three domains, whereas other strategies are more specific to learning in only one or two of the domains.

The characteristics of the intended learners, including their social and cognitive cultures, are important to consider in choosing teaching methods. A teacher does not have to be skilled in using every method. It is important for the teacher to be comfortable with the methods chosen so that the focus of attention stays on learners and the learning process. Choices of teaching method are sustainable when they are realistic for the reasonably available resources. Resources to consider in choosing teaching methods include time, space, support staff, technology, and materials.

A focus on learner engagement and active learning is aligned with a general trend away from teacher-centered strategies and toward strategies focused on what students learn. Two processes are important for active learning: action and reflection. Taking part in some meaningful activity followed by reflecting on the learning processes and outcomes transforms the learner from a passive recipient of someone else's thoughts to a constructor of knowledge and meaning. There are many teaching methods for active learning that promote the development of critical thinking. These include case studies, concept mapping, collaborative or team learning, PBL, service learning, and gaming.

Teaching methods were categorized in this chapter as independent learning, small-group, and large-class methods. However, each of the methods can be used in more than one way. Independent learning methods include reading; writing; reflection; contract learning (including a team learning contract, contract learning approach to a course, and an individual learning contract); concept mapping; and RLOs. Small-group methods presented in the chapter were discussion; experiential methods; case study; cooperative learning; PBL; simulation (including standardized patients, role-play, imagined script writing, and drama); presentations; and service learning. Large-class methods include lecture, questioning, demonstration, educational games, film (and other media), debate, and narrative pedagogy/storytelling. Each of these teaching methods was discussed in the chapter.

REFERENCES

Abdulmajed, H., Park, Y., & Tekian, A. (2015). Assessment of educational games for health professions: A systematic review of trends and outcomes. *Medical Teacher, 37*, S27–S32. doi:10.3109/0142159X.2015.1006609

Akcaoglu, M., & Lee, E. (2016). Increasing social presence in online learning through small group discussions. *The International Review of Research in Open and Distributed Learning, 17*(3). doi:dx.doi.org/10.19173/irrodl.v17i3.2293

Ambrose, S., Bridges, M., DiPietro, M., Lovett, M., & Norman, M. (2010). *How learning works: Seven research-based principles for smart teaching.* San Francisco, CA: Jossey-Bass.

Anderson, L. W., Krathwohl, D. R., Airasian, P., Cruikshank, K. A., Mayer, R. E., Pintrich, P., & Wittrock, M. (2001). *A taxonomy for learning, teaching, and assessing: A revision of Bloom's taxonomy of educational objectives.* New York, NY: Longman.

Arveklev, S., Wigert, H., Berg, L., Burton, B., & Lepp, M. (2015). The use and application of drama in nursing education—An integrative review of the literature. *Nurse Education Today, 35,* e12–e17. doi:10.1016/j.nedt.2015.02.025

Barr, J. J. (2016). *Developing a positive classroom climate. IDEA Paper #61.* The IDEA Center. Retrieved from http://www.ideaedu.org/Research/IDEA-Paper-Series

Benner, P., Sutphen, M., Leonard, V., & Day, L. (2009). *Educating nurses: A call for radical transformation.* San Francisco, CA: Jossey-Bass.

Biniecki, S., & Conceicão, S. (2016). Using concept maps to engage adult learners in critical analysis. *Adult Learning, 27*(2), 51–59. doi:10.1177/1045159515604148

Blakely, G., Skirton, H., Cooper, S., Allum, P., & Nelmes, P. (2009). Educational gaming in the health sciences: Systematic review. *Journal of Advanced Nursing, 65,* 259–269. doi:10.1111/j.1365–2648.2008.04843.x

Boardman, A., Roberts, G., Vaughn, S., Wexler, J., Murray, C., & Kosanovich, M. (2008). *Effective instruction for adolescent struggling readers: A practice brief.* Portsmouth, NH: RMC Research Corporation, Center on Instruction.

Bobianski, K., Aselton, P., & Cho, K. (2016). Home care simulation to teach culturally based competencies in end-of-life care. *Journal of Nursing Education, 55,* 49–53. doi:10.3928/01484834-20151214-12

Boitel, C., & Fromm, L. (2014). Defining signature pedagogy in social work education: Learning theory and the learning contract. *Journal of Social Work Education, 50,* 608–622. doi:10.1080/10437797.2014.947161

Brookfield, S. (2012). *Teaching for critical thinking: Tools and techniques to help students question their assumptions.* San Francisco, CA: Jossey-Bass.

Chmil, J., Turk, M., Adamson, K., & Larew, C. (2015). Effects of an experiential learning simulation design on clinical nursing judgment development. *Nurse Educator, 40,* 228–232. doi:10.1097/NNE.0000000000000159

Cleveland, L., Carmona, E., Paper, B., Solis, L., & Taylor, B. (2015). Baby boy jones interactive case-based learning activity: A web-delivered teaching strategy. *Nurse Educator, 40,* 179–182. doi:10.1097/NNE.0000000000000129

Clark, C., Nguyen, D., & Barbosa-Leiker, C. (2014). Student perceptions of stress, coping, relationships, and academic civility: A longitudinal study. *Nurse Educator, 39*, 170–174. doi:10.1097/NNE.0000000000000049

Coy, P. (2014). Collective learning agreements as democratic practice and joint empowerment. *Conflict Resolution Quarterly, 31*, 229–256. doi:10.1002/crq.21087

Dave, R. H. (1970). Developing and writing educational objectives (psychomotor levels). In R. J. Armstrong (Ed.), *Developing and writing behavioral objectives*. Tucson, AZ: Educational Innovators Press.

Elder, L., & Paul, R. (2010). Universal intellectual standards. Retrieved from http://www.criticalthinking.org/pages/universal-intellectual-standards/527

Ennis, R. (2010). A super-streamlined conception of critical thinking. Retrieved from http://www.criticalthinking.net/definition.html

Gaba, D. M. (2007). The future vision of simulation in healthcare. *Simulation in Healthcare, 2*(2), 126–135. doi:10.1097/01.sih.0000258411.38212.32

Gallup. (2016). Honesty/ethics in professions. Retrieved from http://www.gallup.com/poll/1654/honesty-ethics-professions.aspx

Hawkins, D., Elder, L., & Paul, R. (2010). *Thinker's guide to clinical reasoning*. Dillon Beach, CA: Foundation for Critical Thinking.

Hayes, C., Power, T., Davidson, P., Daly, J., & Jackson, D. (2015). Nurse interrupted: Development of a realistic medication administration simulation for undergraduate nurses. *Nurse Education Today, 35*, 981–986. doi:10.1016/j.nedt.2015.07.002

Huitt, T. W., Killins, A., & Brooks, W. S. (2015). Team-based learning in the gross anatomy laboratory improves academic performance and students' attitudes toward teamwork. *Anatomical Sciences Educator, 8*(2), 95–103. doi:10.1002/ase.1460

Hutchinson, T. L., & Goodin, H. J. (2013). Nursing student anxiety as a context for teaching/learning. *Journal of Holistic Nursing, 31*(1), 19–24. doi:10.1177/0898010112462067

Ironside, P. (2015). Narrative pedagogy: Transforming nursing education through 15 years of research in nursing education. *Nursing Education Perspectives, 38*, 83–88. doi:10.5480/13-1102

Kaylor, S., & Strickland, H. (2015). Unfolding case studies as a formative teaching methodology for novice nursing students. *Journal of Nursing Education, 54*, 106–110. doi:10.3928/01484834-20150120-06

Kim, H., Song, Y., Lindquist, R., & Kang, H. (2016). Effects of team-based learning on problem-solving, knowledge and clinical performance of Korean nursing students. *Nurse Education Today 38*, 115–118. doi:10.1016/j.nedt.2015.12.003

Kohlbry, P. (2016). The impact of international service-learning on nursing students' cultural competency. *Journal of Nursing Scholarship, 48*, 303–311. doi:10.1111/jnu.12209

Kong, L. N., Qin, B., Zhou, Y., Mou, S., & Gao, H. M. (2014). The effectiveness of problem-based learning on development of nursing students' critical thinking: A systematic review and meta-analysis. *International Journal of Nursing Studies, 51*, 458–469. doi:10.1016/j.ijnurstu.2013.06.009

Krathwohl, D. R., Bloom, B. S., & Masia, B. B. (1964). *Taxonomy of educational objectives: The classification of educational goals. Handbook II: Affective domain*. New York, NY: David McKay.

Millis, B. (2010). *New pedagogies and practices for teaching in higher education: Cooperative learning in higher education: Across the disciplines, across the academy*. Sterling, VA: Stylus.

Murray, B. (2013). Service–learning in baccalaureate nursing education: A literature review. *Journal of Nursing Education, 52*, 621–628. doi:10.3928/01484834-20131014-08

National League for Nursing. (2015). *NLN vision series: Debriefing across the curriculum*. Retrieved from http://www.nln.org/docs/default-source/about/nln-vision-series-(position-statements)/nln-vision-debriefing-across-the-curriculum.pdf?sfvrsn=0

Nilson, L. B. (2010). *Teaching at its best: A research-based resource for college instructors*. San Francisco, CA: Jossey-Bass.

Oermann, M. H., & Gaberson, K. B. (2017). *Evaluation and testing in nursing education* (5th ed.). New York, NY: Springer Publishing.

Ondrusek, A. (2012). What the research reveals about graduate students' writing skills: A literature review. *Journal of Education for Library and Information Science, 53*, 176–188.

Peinhardt, R. D., & Hagler, D. (2013). Peer coaching to support writing development. *Journal of Nursing Education, 52*, 24–28. doi:10.3928/01484834-20121121-02

Poole, A. (2014). Successful and struggling students' use of reading strategies: The case of upperclassmen. *Learning Assistance Review, 19*(2), 59–80.

President's Council of Advisors on Science and Technology. (2012). Engage to excel: Producing one million additional college graduates with degrees in science, technology, engineering, and mathematics. Retrieved from https://obamawhitehouse.archives.gov/sites/default/files/microsites/ostp/pcast-engage-to-excel-final_2-25-12.pdf

Rutherford-Hemming, T., & Jennrich, J. (2013). Using standardized patients to strengthen nurse practitioner competency in the clinical setting. *Nursing Education Perspectives, 34,* 118–121. doi:10.5480/1536-5026-34.2.118

Rystedt, H., & Sjöblom, B. (2012). Realism, authenticity, and learning in healthcare simulations: Rules of relevance and irrelevance as interactive achievements. *Instructional Science, 40,* 785–798. doi:10.1007/s11251-012-9213-x

Sallee, M., Hallett, R., & Tierney, W. (2011). Teaching writing in graduate school. *College Teaching, 59*(2), 66–72.

Sanford, A. J., & Emmott, C. (2012). *Mind, brain and narrative.* Cambridge, UK: Cambridge University Press.

Shindell, D. L. (2011). *Factors which influence the use of active learning strategies by nursing faculty* (Dissertation). Available from ProQuest dissertations and theses database (UMI No. 3494746).

Slavich, G. M., & Zimbardo, P. G. (2012). Transformational teaching: Theoretical underpinnings, basic principles, and core methods. *Educational Psychology Review, 24,* 569–608. doi:10.1007/s10648-012-9199-6

Taggart, A., & Crisp, G. (2011). Service learning at community colleges: Synthesis, critique, and recommendations for future research. *Journal of College Reading and Learning, 42*(1), 24–44. doi:10.1080/10790195.2011.10850346

Troxler, H., Vann, J. C., & Oermann, M. H. (2011). How baccalaureate nursing programs teach writing. *Nursing Forum, 46,* 280–288. doi:10.1111/j.1744-6198.2011.00242.x

Wanda, D., Fowler, C., & Wilson, V. (2016). Using flash cards to engage Indonesian nursing students in reflection on their practice. *Nurse Education Today, 38,* 132–137. doi:10.1016/j.nedt.2015.11.029

Weimer, M. (2010). *Inspired college teaching: A career-long resource for professional growth.* San Francisco, CA: Jossey-Bass.

Williams, J., O'Connor, M., Windle, R., & Wharrad, H. (2015). Using reusable learning objects (rlos) in injection skills teaching: Evaluations from multiple user types. *Nurse Education Today, 35,* 1275–1282. doi:10.1016/j.nedt.2015.06.001

Wilson, A., Blake, B., Taylor, G., & Hannings, G. (2013). Cinemeducation: Teaching family assessment skills using full-length movies. *Public Health Nursing, 30,* 239–245. doi:10.111/phn.12025

Zazkis, R., & Nejad, M. (2014). What students need: Exploring teachers' views via imagined role-playing. *Teacher Education Quarterly, 41*(3), 67–86.

Zhang, Y. (2011). Supporting adult learners' use of reading strategies through effective literacy scaffolding. *International Forum of Teaching and Studies, 7*(2), 20–31.

Zipp, G., & Maher, C. (2013). Prevalence of mind mapping as a teaching and learning strategy in physical therapy curricula. *Journal of the Scholarship of Teaching and Learning, 13*(5), 21–32.

⑤

Integrating Technology in Education

JENNIE C. DE GAGNE, HELEN B. CONNORS, AND KATHY TALLY

OBJECTIVES

- Examine technology integration and technology tools to support teaching and student learning outcomes
- Give an overview of selected instructional technologies useful in nursing education and their application to the teaching-learning environment
- Evaluate infrastructure needs when considering technology integration that supports the teaching–learning process with attention to pedagogy and classroom alignment

Technology permeates every aspect of our lives, including education. The rapid advances and constant pace of change in technology create challenges and opportunities for teaching and learning. Nationally and internationally, education leaders and policymakers are promoting efforts to transform education to improve student achievements and readiness for lifelong learning and career options. Education leaders, policymakers, parents, teachers, and students all seem to agree that technology is an essential component of education. The more educators use technology, the more they recognize and value its strong positive effects on student learning and engagement and its connection to 21st-century skills. This means that educators need to be prepared to adopt existing technologies and explore emerging technology tools; they should be collaborators in learning, constantly seeking new knowledge and skills along with their students as the technology evolves. Technology is helping teachers to expand beyond linear, text-based learning, and to engage students who have a variety of learning styles. Successful integration of technology in the curriculum requires a paradigm shift and new set of necessary competencies as technology continues to evolve.

The ability to use and evaluate technology is a critical competency for nurse educators. Technology is increasingly being integrated into today's classrooms, nursing laboratories, and clinical sites in an effort to enhance learning outcomes, promote quality patient care, and incorporate evidence-based practice. Thus, nurse educators should understand use of a theoretical model or framework to select and incorporate new technologies into instruction so the innovation can be evaluated for use and implementation by others. This chapter focuses on technology integration that supports achievement of learning outcomes with attention to curriculum and classroom alignment that increases rigor, relevance, and relationships. This chapter also provides an overview of a wide range of instructional technologies useful in nursing education settings and their application in a teaching-learning environment. In addition, processes for evaluating and selecting technology that supports course processes such as tracking student assignments, participation, outcomes assessment, and grading are discussed.

BACKGROUND

Technology is commonly thought of as gadgets, instruments, machines, and devices; however, in today's world, most educators refer to technology for the classroom as equipment, particularly electronic equipment. Educational technology, especially computers and computer-related peripherals, have expanded rapidly over the past few decades. The continued development and expansion of the Internet in the 1980s laid the foundation for networking capabilities. Then, with the availability of the web in the 1990s, followed by Web 2.0 tools in the early 2000s, digitalized communication and networking in education exploded, taking on many forms and changing the face of education. In addition, the more recent emergence of mobile devices and ubiquitous technology gave new meaning to teaching and learning and challenged educators to look at new education paradigms. It also challenged faculty, administrators, and policymakers to question the quality, evaluate outcomes, and establish standards for technology-based education.

These emerging technologies are examples of disruptive innovations that have changed the education marketplace over the past decade, pushing the boundaries of higher education, and providing new and disruptive pathways to offer higher education. The increasing number of pathways has not only created greater education market competition, but also emphasized the development of quality programs and the need for standards to evaluate and guide continuous improvement processes that reflect ongoing changes in technology-based education.

THE INTERNET AND THE WEB

The terms *Internet* and *the web* are frequently used interchangeably, although they are not one and the same. The Internet is the hardware: It is a collection of computer networks connected through either copper wires, fiber optic cables, or wireless connections. The web is considered the software: It is a collection of web pages connected through hyperlinks and universal resource locators (URLs) or addresses to specific locations so that information that is sent or retrieved is located and delivered to the requesting computer or end user. The web depends on the Internet to make it work. The web is a complex and highly organized set of electronic pathways similar to highways and interstate systems used by people to travel from one point to another in search of information. A request for information travels across the Internet to reach resources that are located in different sites on the web. Once those resources are located, that information, which may include files or media, is sent to the requesting computer/user.

Educators using technology to teach need to have a basic understanding of how information travels along these pathways. This is particularly important as we explore more robust teaching technologies including virtual worlds (VWs), web-conferencing, and content delivery using different types of media such as podcasts (audio files) and vodcasts (video files). Text-based information transfers to the requesting computer/user at a much faster rate than larger files like audio and video, or rich media found in VWs. All this information travels in packets; the larger the file, the greater number of packets required for travel from one location to another. Having the right Internet connection and hardware are essential for students to be successful in accessing the teaching technologies and content used in media-rich online learning environments. It is recommended that the teacher include guidelines in the course syllabi and program description about the type of Internet connection that is needed. The statement in Exhibit 5.1 is an example of the information the teacher might include in the syllabus. It can be modified to reflect the specific teaching technologies.

EXHIBIT 5.1 Sample Statement on Internet Connection

General technology requirements include the use of a broadband Internet connection for all online or hybrid courses. The most reliable broadband connections are cable and DSL. Although satellite, which is often used in rural areas where cable or DSL are not available, and wireless cards purchased through mobile Internet providers are also broadband connections, these two broadband connections can be less reliable, producing intermittent connections and slower Internet speed. That can interfere with successful web-conferencing session, robust information transfer of course content, and connections during online assessments delivered via an LMS.

Additionally, we recommend that you do not use a wireless connection when taking online assessments or participating in high-stakes web-conferencing events such as applied demonstrations. Instead, connect your computer directly to the router with an Ethernet (Internet connection) cable.

DSL, digital subscriber line; LMS, learning management system.

The web is considered one of several services provided by the Internet. Other services over the Internet include e-mail, chat, and file transfer services. All of these services are readily available to consumers for use by businesses, educational institutions, governments, and individuals creating their own networks or platforms. The Internet is a huge network that is available to anyone and most anywhere around the world.

Over the past decade, the education community has worked with Web 2.0 technologies. Web 2.0 is an umbrella term for a host of recent Internet applications such as social networking, wikis, folksonomies (or social tagging), virtual societies, blogging, and multiplayer online gaming. These applications differ in form and function; however, all these applications share a common characteristic of supporting Internet-based interaction between and within groups, which is why the term "social software" is often used to describe Web 2.0 tools and services.

In addition to the Internet, many other technologies, such as simulation and VWs, tablet devices, smartphones, gaming, and learner response systems, among others, are transforming education. These technologies are evolving quickly, and the pace seems to increase each year. Educators need to keep current with the emerging instructional technologies to ensure they are adopting the best tools to support active learning, use student and faculty time productively, improve learning outcomes, and prepare students for lifelong learning and successful careers. Technology implementations in schools and classrooms, no matter how big or small, will benefit from thoughtful strategic planning and evaluation.

TECHNOLOGY TOOLS: PRESENT AND FUTURE

LEARNING MANAGEMENT SYSTEMS

One of the most common tools used to support technology integration in education today is a learning management system (LMS). The International Forum of Educational Technology & Society (IFETS) defines an LMS as a collection of e-learning tools available through a shared administrative interface (Avgeriou, Papasalouros, Retalis, & Skordalakis, 2003). LMS interface technologies vary from simple to complex in how they are used and what tools support and deliver online content. LMSs have been adopted widely by educational institutions across the globe to meet specific needs and requirements of increasing education demands. Educators and instructional designers working together can effectively use LMS tools to develop and deliver online course components that maximize the technology inherent in most LMSs. The outcome can result in high-quality courses that reduce faculty workload and provide students with access to information and learning tools that facilitate the highest levels of learning in a completely online environment, blended courses (integrating face-to-face and online activities), or a web component that reinforces content delivered in a face-to-face classroom (Avgeriou et al., 2003). A few examples of proprietary LMSs include Blackboard, Desire2Learn, and Canvas. Examples of open source systems available include Sakai and Moodle. New systems are being developed as demand continues to increase with the expansion of online course offerings and programs.

WEB 2.0 TOOLS

Web 2.0 is a second generation of the web that provides users the opportunity to interact and collaborate with each other, as opposed to websites that limit them to passive viewing of the content. Web 2.0 and similar emerging technologies are new tools and ways of creating, collaborating, editing, and sharing user-generated content online. Some basic examples of Web 2.0 tools are weblogs, wikis, video casting, social bookmarking, social networking, podcasts, and picture sharing tools. There is a growing abundance of Web 2.0 applications that are readily available, making technology easier to use and more accessible to faculty and students.

Many of these applications are free and can be integrated into a course to support all levels of Bloom's digital taxonomy (Churches, 2016). The digital taxonomy follows the learning process on a continuum of lower order thinking skills (LOTS) to higher order thinking skills (HOTS). It is not about the tools but about integrating the tools to engage students and enhance the learning outcomes. Over the years, Bloom's taxonomy of educational objectives has been revised to address new behaviors and learning opportunities that have been enriched by technologies (Churches, 2016). Examples of Bloom's and Churches's digital taxonomy and potential technologies to support the desired learning outcomes are available at http://edorigami.wikispaces.com. An infographic of the digital taxonomy verbs is downloadable at https://globaldigitalcitizen.org/blooms-digital-taxonomy-verbs.

WEB 3.0

Imagine what will happen as the web "gets smarter" and can assist in organizing, integrating, and evaluating the information it provides? This is currently referred to as the semantic web or Web 3.0 (World Wide Web Consortium [W3C], 2015). Internet experts believe this next generation of the web will be similar to having a personal assistant: The more you use the web, the more your browser will learn about you and bring you specific information from a variety of sources that meets your needs. It will personalize learning and provide richer and more significant information based on your individual profile.

The semantic web will have profound implications for nursing education. When a user searches the web, it will bring the learner more than a list of websites to explore to find the most relevant information. Instead, it will provide a multimedia report integrating many sources, including websites, scientific repositories, textbook chapters, blogs, speeches, videos, and others. The multimedia report will focus on knowledge areas that emerge from the individual's research (Ohler, 2008). Currently, much of faculty time is spent teaching students to identify legitimate information, organize and synthesize it, integrate it with other information from multiple sources, and ultimately produce new knowledge. This is the essence of critical thinking. With the technology doing much of this work for the learner, students can spend more time making sense of the synthesis, creating new knowledge, and applying the learning to real-world situations. Teachers will need new skills in the near future with a shift to Web 3.0.

CLOUD COMPUTING

Advances in hardware, software, and networking have pushed academic institutions to seek out alternative sources of information technology (IT) services such as cloud computing. Although there are many definitions, the National Institute of Standards and Technology (NIST) defines cloud computing as "a model for enabling ubiquitous, convenient, on-demand network access to a shared pool of configurable computing resources (e.g., networks, servers, storage, applications, and services) that can be rapidly provisioned and released with minimal management effort or service provider interaction" (Mell & Grance, 2011, p. 2). These evolving cloud-based services are purported to increase institutional flexibility and reduce operating costs, thus offering attractive alternatives to traditional IT services on campus (Tamarkin & Rodrigo, 2011). The most gains have been with institutions moving e-mail, LMS, and customer relationship management operations to the cloud. Although there are performance benefits and cost savings to be realized in migrating to the cloud, the challenges faced by academic institutions are related to risk, trust, and control. The cloud computing space is an emerging paradigm with many promising opportunities. Therefore, developing a campus-wide cloud strategy will continue to be important for academic institutions (Grajek & Pirani, 2012).

MASSIVE OPEN ONLINE COURSES

With Internet access, Web 2.0 technologies, open-access (unrestricted access to scholarly publications), and cloud-based services, a new phenomenon in learning has occurred in higher education in the past few years. The original concept of a massive open online course (MOOC) was a web course developed by experts in a specific field that people from all over the world could take for free and offered no course credit. Some MOOCs, however, have a fee and can be taken for credit. Most MOOCs typically have massive enrollments. With this kind of support for anywhere, anytime, and no-cost online learning, MOOCs have evolved at an unprecedented pace and moved to the center of a national discussion about the future of higher education. MOOCs have attracted millions of learners from all over the world to learn from top professors at elite universities. MOOC List (www.mooc-list.com) is an open-access aggregator or directory of

MOOCs offered by different providers. At this point, it remains debatable as to how to determine the impact of MOOCs in higher education.

SIMULATION, VWs, AND GAMING

The use of simulators as teaching tools in health professions education has grown rapidly as a mechanism to improve the quality and safety of health care, much like airline simulators have improved the safety of air travel. As with other teaching tools, using simulation to improve patient safety requires full integration of its applications into the routine structure of the curriculum. The best outcomes occur when simulation is integrated across the curriculum rather than added on top of an already overcrowded curriculum.

Integrating simulation in the curriculum starts with a roadmap. This involves all faculty teaching across the curriculum and embeds simulation where it appropriately matches learning objectives instead of viewing simulation exercises as independent learning experiences. The process of mapping simulation to the curriculum allows educators to develop unfolding cases where each successive simulation builds on preceding ones. As the curriculum progresses, the learner is expected to demonstrate increased knowledge and competencies. Mapping simulation to the curriculum creates efficiencies and develops an evidence-based simulation curriculum that engages both students and faculty across the academic program or programs.

For the most part, the word *simulator* in nursing and health professions education brings to mind the human patient simulator (HPS). This type of simulator is probably the most widely used; however, it is only one aspect of re-creating a realistic clinical environment for teaching patient care skills without harming patients. Today, emerging information and communication technologies, such as electronic health records (EHRs), telehealth technologies, mobile home healthcare, personal health records (PHRs), patient portals, geographical positioning systems (GPSs), and Radiofrequency Identification (RFID), are changing health care delivery (Bajwa, 2014). Those changes need to be reflected in our education practices in order to prepare students with the health IT competencies needed for practice.

The clinical simulation environment provides an excellent opportunity to integrate health IT competencies with the curriculum. Merging EHR technology with laboratory simulation provides students with virtual clinical experiences that closely represent the increasingly automated practice environments (Warren, Manos, Meyer, & Roche, 2013). Just as the HPS can be programmed to simulate patient care experiences, a simulated EHR can be used to simulate patient data and clinical decision-making scenarios to accompany the virtual case studies enacted through the HPS. In other words, the simulated patients have their own EHR-like environments, with access to clinical data to enable students to develop critical thinking skills and make data-driven decisions in a safe environment. An example of an academic EHR integrated into the simulation curriculum is the Simulated E-hEalth Delivery System (SEEDS) at the University of Kansas (www.kumc.edu/health-informatics/seeds). In 2000, through a partnership with a leading EHR software supplier, the company's well-established clinical information system was adapted to fit the education workflow of the academic environment and led to the creation of a virtual care delivery system supported with the EHR. The virtual care delivery system includes an acute care hospital, as well as outpatient environments such as school-based clinics, public health clinics, ambulatory care clinics, and home settings. The virtual care environments reflect all aspects of nursing and other health professions curriculum, and each simulated patient has his or her own EHR within the virtual environment (Warren et al., 2013). The product adapted for use with the

SEEDS program is called the Academic Education Solution (AES©). Several other vendors developed academic EHRs that are similar to the AES, thus providing schools with vendor choices to help simulate more closely the reality of practice in a technology-rich health care environment.

VWs, such as Second Life© (secondlife.com), There (there.com), ActiveWorlds (activeworlds.com), and Twinity (twinity.com), add another dimension to simulation. VWs are part of Web 2.0 and future Web 3.0. For example, hundreds of colleges and universities across the globe are using Second Life as supplemental learning experiences in health-related disciplines such as nursing, medicine, and allied health (De Gagne, Oh, Kang, Voderstrasse, & Johnson, 2013). In a VW, existing educational tools such as a PowerPoint presentations, images, and links to websites, course material, and three-dimensional objects can be aggregated into a dynamic learning hub. The uses of VWs are varied and can be adapted to different needs. Exhibit 5.2 displays some common applications for VWs.

EXHIBIT 5.2 Common Applications for Virtual Worlds

Communication Scenarios. VWs are being used to teach specific communication skills and working together as a team. For example, a health informatics class may meet virtually with different key individuals from a health facility to negotiate the terms and conditions for developing a database for the facility.

Collaboration. Second Life© gives students a common place to interact regardless of their physical location.

Staging an Exhibit. Students can present their final course project in a virtual auditorium or exhibit hall created in Second Life to display these projects to faculty and peers.

Virtual Campuses. Many colleges and universities are building a virtual presence to focus on learning resources, student centers, and marketing efforts.

Virtual Classrooms. Some nursing faculty are using the VW platform to deliver lectures embedded with PowerPoint, videos, links to websites and other virtual spaces, e-books, and three-dimensional models to create a dynamic learning hub.

Virtual Centers. Several research laboratories and centers, such as the Ames Research Center, the Jet Propulsion Lab, and NASA, have partnered to create a virtual presence in Second Life to provide a space to try out new ideas and host meetings and talks.

Conference Facilities. Second Life can be used to offer conferences (for example, to host seminars on health problems and treatments).

Technical Training. Nurse anesthesia faculty have developed a VW operating room simulation to assist first-year students with learning the basic induction procedure. This activity builds confidence and emphasizes important safety techniques.

Virtual Field Trip. These can provide experiences for learning to navigate VWs or as a final project. For example, a nursing student might visit the Virtual Ability Island to learn more about living with a disability or to address a problem area.

Simulated Experiences. Through simulated experiences, occupational, physical therapy, and nursing students can develop skills in home assessment and recommending modifications in the home through a series of virtual home environments.

Research Studies. VWs are the subject of much academic research. In addition, researchers are exploring how VWs can help to practice and promote healthy behaviors such as activities involved in weight loss programs or managing posttraumatic stress disorders.

VWs, virtual worlds.

Game-based learning (GBL) is in the early stages of adoption in higher education. While there are many examples of simulation-based learning in nursing education in both real and virtual environments, few edugames have been used successfully in higher education so far. Edugames are expanding, driven largely by growing consumer fascination with games and the abundance of mobile technology making gaming techniques readily available (Epper, Derryberry, & Jackson, 2012). In the health care sector, the University of Minnesota School of Nursing has partnered with the Minnesota Hospital Association and VitalSims™ to develop a series of interactive web-based games that engage nursing and other health professions students (www.vitalsims.com). These games, coupled with classroom and simulation laboratories, will be another valuable tool to better equip future nursing and health professionals. Some experts have projected widespread adoption of serious GBL in upcoming years (Johnson et al., 2016). Serious gaming in education is gaining additional support among researchers and educators who recognize that GBL engages students and stimulates critical inquiry among them. Examples of universities exploring GBL are in Table 5.1.

MOBILE DEVICES

The pervasiveness of mobile devices such as smartphones, tablets, e-book readers, and other emerging mobile technologies used in everyday personal and work life is making its way into the classroom. Today, many students, faculty, and staff members arrive on campus with one or more mobile devices and expect to use these personal devices to access the network and its resources. They expect institutions to provide reliable wireless connectivity. This is known as the "Bring Your Own Device" (BYOD) or more recently as "Bring Your Own Everything" (BYOE) phenomena. This move to mobile

TABLE 5.1 University Research Centers Exploring Game-Based Learning

Research Center	Website
The Education Arcade at Massachusetts Institute of Technology	www.educationarcade.org
Games + Learning + Society at University of Wisconsin-Madison	www.gameslearningsociety.org
Center for Game Science at University of Washington	http://centerforgamescience.org
The Games for Learning Institute at New York University	www.g4li.nyu.edu/about
Institute for Simulation & Training at University of Central Florida	www.ist.ucf.edu
Center for Transformational Media at Parsons The New School for Design	http://ctm.parsons.edu
Interactive Communications & Simulations at University of Michigan	http://ics.soe.umich.edu
Center for Games & Impact at Arizona State University	https://gamesandimpact.org
Serious Games Center at Purdue University	www.education.purdue.edu/research-and -engagement/centers-and-institutes/ serious-gaming-center

computing on campus coincides with a push among educational publishers toward digital content, such as electronic textbooks, multimedia-rich applications, online videos, and other online tools for faculty and students. Schools of nursing programs and colleges and universities are struggling to meet these expectations and are finding that they need to rethink their IT strategies in order to enhance learning.

To successfully implement a campus-wide mobile computing initiative, there needs to be an institutional commitment to support these devices through the campus infrastructure as well as the pedagogical approaches in the classroom. Many institutions need to increase bandwidth, add access points and sufficient power, boost their network management capabilities, address security concerns, and hire or develop IT personnel who are familiar with a common variety of mobile device operating systems. The meaningful use of mobile devices and applications in the curriculum gives users instant access to information and encourages student engagement, participation, and collaboration, while fostering a personal learning network. As nursing faculty members more fully integrate technology into the curriculum, improved learning outcomes may result. According to a survey by the Pew Research Center that explored learning and technology in the United States, 82% of individuals surveyed had smartphones and home Internet service, and did some personal learning activity in the past year, which indicates that technology assets are strongly related to the likelihood that adults engage in personal learning (Horrigan, 2016).

The rapid expansion of BYOD complements other trends in higher education, such as virtualization and technology-enriched classrooms. As with these other trends, faculty buy-in and support is critical to successful implementation. According to the 21st-Century Campus Report, the top challenge to increased classroom technology, as rated by faculty, administrators, and students, is the faculty's lack of technology knowledge and skill (CDW, 2011). Although 81% of the institutions surveyed provided technology-specific professional development, faculty members perceived that this approach did not meet their needs. Faculty suggested that the institutions offer discipline-specific faculty development and that tech-savvy faculty members lead the sessions. This same strategy could be used for preparing nurse educators.

LEARNING ANALYTICS

Learning analytics is the collection and analysis of data about learners to better understand and optimize learning (Siemens, 2013). The Horizon Report indicated that learning analytics was associated with deciphering trends and patterns from educational large datasets, huge sets of student-related data, to further the advancement of a personalized, supportive system of higher education (Johnson et al., 2016). Traditionally, learning has been measured by student evaluation, analysis of grades, and attrition rates, as well as the faculty member's perception of the student. As more educational activities move online, an extraordinary amount of data about these learning activities is becoming captured and available.

Recent interest in how this unique information can be used to improve teaching and learning has emerged as the field of learning analytics. Initially, uses of student data were focused on at-risk students to improve outcomes. However, with advances in technology and its powerful tools, it is possible to use the data to personalize learning and provide student-specific coaching to yield more productive learning habits and improved outcomes. A report from the U.S. Department of Education Office of Educational Technology (2013) focuses on using these data to examine how people learn and create learning systems that support these best practices. As the field of learning analytics develops over the next few years, the goal is for the data and tools to provide a better understanding of learning outcomes and assessment in higher education including nursing education.

RETHINKING THE EDUCATION PARADIGM

Technology enhances active learning, accommodates a variety of learning styles, and allows for communication, collaboration, and sharing among students. A technology-oriented strategy should support and facilitate learning, including critical thinking, problem solving, creativity, and innovation. The specific technology is chosen not because it is available and exciting but because it is a good fit with the learning pedagogy and goals of the nursing course or program. The pedagogy and goals provide the framework for nurse educators to decide on the best technology for their courses. When a school of nursing decides to offer technology-based courses or programs, a significant amount of attention should focus on the infrastructure, resources, and support. Lack of attention to any of these will result in foreseeable and preventable challenges (Hartman, 2008).

INFRASTRUCTURE

Investment in infrastructure is of utmost importance to a successful online program. Schools must support their evolving technological demands. This infrastructure must be secure, available 24/7, able to handle a wide range of applications, and adaptable to new technologies. To accomplish these goals, campuses must develop and implement strategic technology plans that align with the institution's mission and goals. These plans should not be static because new technologies are competing for infrastructure resources almost on a daily basis. The key to success is a commitment from institutional and nursing program leadership to support IT and to use technology to improve and maintain institutional performance.

Alignment With Institution and School of Nursing Mission and Goals

Over the past three decades, colleges and universities have made substantial investments in technological infrastructure such as course management systems, wireless networks, multimedia classrooms, and a wide array of technology tools to transform teaching and learning. There are many technologies available and ways to implement them, making it difficult for faculty members, including nurse educators, to keep pace and know whether the use of the technology is having an impact on learning outcomes (Hartman, 2008). Questions about technology integration persist, even after more than half a century of research documenting the use of technologies from television to mobile devices and the benefits of technologies for learning.

Reviews of the literature reveal that the emphasis of teaching and learning with technology has been on the technology itself. However, the technology alone does not transform education. In fact, there is a large body of research demonstrating no significant difference when the focus of the research is on the technology and not on the teaching practices (Means, Toyama, Murphy, Bakia, & Jones, 2010). As cited in Hartman's (2008) article, all too often teachers "bolt on" the technology rather than redesign the teaching and learning process supported and enhanced by it. Because there are so many technologies for teachers to choose and ways to use them, and many faculty members with diverse pedagogical approaches, most institutions have been unable to determine on an enterprise level whether the introduction of technologies is having a positive impact on student learning outcomes (Hartman, 2008). The same is true at the level of the school of nursing or nursing department.

What is needed is an institutional approach to teaching and learning with technology to determine efficiency, effectiveness, sustainability, and quality. A systematic approach may not be appropriate for all technology, but this approach is ideal for those technologies that have a broad applicability across the institution. A more individualized approach may be appropriate for specific technologies and for use in a specialized area of study such as nursing. However, to truly transform education with technology, technology integration needs to be part of the mission and goals of the institution, not used arbitrarily by a few educators across the institution. Unless the culture and structure of a school are compatible with and supportive of specific uses of technology, technology integration is not likely to succeed. When technology-enhanced education is part of the mission and goals of the institution, it is evident in all aspects of the program and should create an innovative culture that is necessary for truly transforming education.

Innovation is frequently defined as the introduction of something new that leads to a positive change: a new idea, method, or device. It can also be viewed as productivity and quality improvement (Malloch & Porter-O'Grady, 2011). An innovative culture establishes innovation as a central theme in the organization's vision and purpose. With innovation as an integral part of the framework, the organization will not only embrace creative thinking, teaching, and learning that is outside the traditional processes, but it also will encourage and support such creativity through established practices such as hiring, coaching, mentoring, and rewarding faculty and staff. A culture of innovation provides a framework to assist institutions and nursing programs to turn disruptive innovation into productive innovation.

Pedagogy

Pedagogy is the study of the art and science of teaching and includes multiple theories of behavior that are based on the learning process or the observation and scientific study of how individuals learn. Most nursing faculty members were in school when the teacher-centered model of instruction was popular. This model emphasized the presentation of knowledge or a skill set that teachers believed students needed to learn. In these settings, teachers are active and students are passive. Over the past several decades, however, new learning theories have emerged, such as social constructivism and other student-centered pedagogical practices, which support new paradigms for learning. These new learning pedagogies recommend that to best prepare 21st-century learners for the increasingly complex and interconnected global society in which they live and work, teachers should implement practices that involve interactive, problem-based, and technology-enriched teaching and learning.

Constructivism is a theory of learning founded on the premise that learners are actively involved and create their own learning through interaction with others and with the environment. They construct their own understanding of the world through experiential learning and reflection on their past experiences to build new knowledge (Bruner, 1966). In Bruner's (1996) more recent work, he expanded his theoretical framework to include the social and cultural aspects of learning. Modern constructivists believe that learning is a social process and is more active and self-directed than either Behaviorism or Cognitive Theory. Much of today's instructional technologies promote constructivist principles of learning by creating learning environments that challenge students to work collaboratively and to become actively engaged, self-directed lifelong learners inside and outside of formal learning spaces.

A goal for nurse educators is to use Learning Theory and best practice teaching strategies to guide technology integration and derive quality outcomes. Although technology has expanded the educational paradigm, good teaching has not changed. What has changed is the availability of technology tools to support teaching. Just as curriculum and pedagogy must be assessed and rethought, so must teaching and learning strategies. For example, Chickering and Gamson's (1987) Seven Principles for Good Practice in Undergraduate Education continue to be applicable in today's digital enabled classrooms and web-based learning environments. Chickering and Ehrmann (1996) provided further evidence that technology integration encourages and supports each of the seven principles. Exhibit 5.3 displays the Seven Principles as applied to teaching and learning with technology.

EXHIBIT 5.3 Seven Principles for Good Practice in Education Applied to Teaching With Technology

1. Contacts between student and faculty (before, during, and after class)
2. Develops reciprocity and cooperation among students (team-based learning in web-enabled collaboration rooms via web conferencing, Skype, FaceTime, and social media outlets)
3. Uses active learning techniques (simulation, VWs, student applied demonstrations, and standardized patient interviews, all conducted in a virtual environment)
4. Gives prompt feedback (using LMSs for formative evaluations via quizzes that provide immediate feedback and multiple learning opportunities)
5. Emphasizes time on task (knowledge and comprehension tasks that are done as preparatory work to allow time on task to be directed to higher order learning, such as application and creation)
6. Communicates high expectations (knowledge acquisition occurs first in self-directed learning with high expectations for student–student and faculty–student interactions that are rich and engaging)
7. Respects diverse talent and ways of learning (teaching technology tools provide multiple modalities for the learner and allow rehearsal and repetition of content for all learning paces and learning styles)

LMSs, learning management systems; VWs, virtual worlds.
Source: From Chickering and Ehrmann (1996) and Chickering and Gamson (1987).

Decision-Making Framework for Technology Selection

Successful use of technology is closely related to the appropriate selection of tools and their utilization. Educators must examine various tools within the context of the learning outcomes, considering content, format, interface design, and completeness of application (Smaldino, Lowther, & Russell, 2011). The SECTIONS Model (Bates & Poole, 2003) allows teachers to systematically answer a series of questions when choosing technologies for their teaching. The purpose of this model is to provide educators with technology to integrate into their courses. The SECTIONS Model can be used "in the initial choice of technologies for course, program, or institution (strategic) and in making decisions during the actual course design process with respect to appropriate media (tactical)" (Bates & Poole, 2003, p. 105). SECTIONS stands for:

- Students
- Ease of use and reliability

- Cost
- Teaching and learning
- Interaction
- Organizational issues
- Networking and novelty
- Speed and security

Technology will expand education offerings to a broader range of the population, including those with less access to higher education, including individuals with disabilities. As there is no single technology that suits all educational environments, experienced educators and skilled developers must plan carefully, strategically choosing instructional and delivery media components. It is also critical to understand how to match the mechanisms of education technology with learning environments.

Classroom Redesign

As technology and learning theories change, so does the design of the classroom. Across the country, many educational institutions and schools of nursing are renovating existing learning space or constructing new learning environments. A key impetus in classroom space renovation or new construction is the need to accommodate new technologies and teaching strategies (Lippincott, 2009). Technology-enhanced education calls for a redesign of the traditional learning space and new pedagogical approaches to learning. The recent widespread adoption of technology and technology tools along with the availability of wireless access has challenged nurse educators to change pedagogical approaches to learning, which in turn has brought about a rethinking of classroom space.

New learning spaces such as the active learning classroom are designed to facilitate a more active, student-centered pedagogy and take advantage of the room's potential. Typically, students bring their own computers to class and use the building's wireless capability to collaborate with peers in small groups to build new ideas and applications. The faculty member becomes a facilitator of learning by answering questions and making suggestions. Active learning classrooms are designed to facilitate hands-on activities and to require students to interact with each other to reach a solution to a problem. Students can display their work on large LCD (liquid crystal display) screens mounted around the room to promote small- and large-group discussions. A clear goal in the redesign of learning spaces is to promote a change in pedagogy; therefore, the nurse educator's interest and motivation for making change in the curriculum and pedagogy through the use of technology must be taken into consideration during the redesign phase, or the active learning classroom may not be successful (Lippincott, 2009). Figure 5.1 is a photograph of an active learning classroom.

Although the literature on learning space suggests that design features have an impact on learning outcomes, there is little evidence-based research to support this assertion. Whiteside, Brooks, and Walker (2010) found that students attending classes in active learning classrooms had a significant positive effect on learning outcomes as measured by grades. The active learning classroom also had a positive influence on teaching and learning activities employed by faculty members and students in terms of lecture, discussion, coaching, and group activities. Further research is needed to explore the connections among learning spaces, pedagogical approaches, and student learning outcomes. As active learning classroom environments become more common in nursing education, it will be possible to conduct longitudinal studies of the impact of taking multiple courses in new learning spaces on broad strategic outcomes such as student enrollment, retention, and failure rates.

FIGURE 5.1 Active learning classroom.

Source: Image provided courtesy of Duke University School of Nursing. Reprinted by permission of Duke University School of Nursing.

Flipping the Classroom

A recent teaching revolution referred to as "flipping the classroom" is a good example of how technology and redesigned learning space can be used to structure learning. Flipping the classroom is a pedagogical approach that uses technology integration to provide students with knowledge- and comprehension-based learning activities that are provided via the web prior to coming to class in either a face-to-face, blended, or virtual learning environment. Flipping the classroom refers to swapping lecture time for active or applied learning in the classroom. This technique allows for more focused learning to take place in the classroom and engages students in a more active learning process (Honeycutt & Warren, 2014). It makes sense because why should nursing faculty members use valuable class time for content delivery when there are other more efficient ways of doing that outside of class? Why should nursing students engage with the material alone and without the benefit of the faculty member's expertise? It would be better to do that during class time.

In a flipped classroom, students are accountable for prelearning activities that prepare them to discuss, apply, and assimilate what they have learned outside of class when they meet in a synchronous learning environment, either the traditional classroom or in a virtual classroom via the web. It is in the classroom environment (traditional or virtual) where they share and collaborate with their peers and work in teams to expand their knowledge and incorporate their ideas with others. The teacher guides and facilitates higher learning, remediating, and scaffolding (providing instructional support to promote learning when first introduced to a new concept). Flipping the classroom requires flipping the minds of students and faculty. The concept of flipping the classroom is not new; it is the way the concept is applied and the use of assistive technology that is gaining attention. Flipping uses technology to replace passive learning such as lecture for a more active teacher–learner, student-centered interaction in the classroom. Flipping the classroom, however, does not guarantee student success. The nurse educator needs to embrace the concept and use effective teaching strategies that guide learning. Some examples of a Flipped Classroom Model are included in Exhibit 5.4.

EXHIBIT 5.4 Examples of Flipping the Classroom

1. Students assume the teaching role via applied demonstrations of knowledge and assignments and present during the face-to-face or synchronous online web-conferencing sessions. The faculty member becomes the facilitator; the student becomes the educator.

2. Team-based learning approaches that help ensure students come to class prepared for learning include the use of individual quizzes with immediate feedback provided via an LMS assessment. In class, students are placed in teams, and they retake the quiz as a group, using discussion and collaboration to arrive at the correct answers.

3. Case studies that are embedded in the academic EHR can be reviewed by students prior to class and then presented in class. Students can be placed in teams to navigate the EHR and problem-solve the case.

4. Educational games (e.g., ones based on formats such as *scavenger hunts*) can be used to review content to create a collaborative and competitive learning atmosphere.

5. Chat rooms can be used in large classrooms to solicit feedback after mini-lectures or group discussion, allowing all students to have a voice.

6. Role-playing scenarios, with preassigned roles, can be performed during class.

7. Individual students or teams can be assigned topics to research in preparation for in-class debates on topics in health care, health care reform, patient safety, or other topics.

EHR, electronic health record; LMS, learning management system.

DEVELOPING FACULTY COMPETENCIES AND MENTORING

Nursing faculty have been cited as a barrier to IT integration in nursing education programs because they lack knowledge and skills about new technologies (Institute of Medicine, 2010). Many faculty members are overwhelmed by the various technologies and challenged by the need to keep up with the ever-changing LMSs, Web 2.0 technologies, and various software applications for classroom and clinical teaching. Although 81% of colleges and universities are providing technology-specific professional development, faculty members report that the approaches used most frequently, such as group meetings, seminars, online tutorials, one-to-one meetings, and peer mentoring, are not meeting their needs (CDW, 2011). Faculty suggested that professional development sessions would be more effective if the individuals who actually used the technology in the classroom led the training, and if the sessions were targeted to the unique needs of specific academics. Most faculty members need to work with others to implement new pedagogical approaches and learn how to use technology.

The aim of faculty development should not focus on teaching nurse educators how to use the technology; rather, the aim should be to understand what learning outcomes the teacher is attempting to achieve and suggest innovative technology and strategies to effectively reach those outcomes (Lippincott, 2009). For example, the University of Kansas School of Nursing joined with the schools of nursing at the University of Colorado, Indiana University-Purdue University Indianapolis, and Johns Hopkins University and the National League for Nursing to develop and implement the Health Information Technology Scholars (HITS) Program (www.hits-colab.org). The overall aim of the HITS program was to educate a cadre of well-informed nursing faculty to focus on real-world applications of technologies in their education practices. The 1-year program consists of online modules with discussion, webinars, a 3-day face-to-face workshop, and mentoring. Faculty applied for the program with a project that they intended to implement at their respective institutions. The faculty scholars engaged in active learning strategies by discussing their projects with their groups and receiving feedback from peer groups as well as mentors.

The success of this faculty development program can be attributed to targeting the learning to nurse educators' specific needs, thus ensuring intrinsic motivation and personal relevance; using faculty experts and instructional designers to model pedagogies associated with new technologies; providing sustained mentorship and peer support through the group-mentoring process; and fostering collaboration among faculty and institutions, which for many continued well after the faculty development program ended.

QUALITY FIRST, THEN TECHNOLOGY

Any nursing program, school of nursing, or institution that incorporates technology-based education should consider standards of quality equivalent to those for traditional educational approaches. Several comprehensive approaches to evaluating quality have been established. These various approaches use differing terminology to present evaluation criteria, including use of benchmarks, pillars, indicators, dimensions, best practices, and paradigms. Quality frameworks that exist for online, hybrid or blended, and face-to-face approaches to education include: (a) the International Association for K-12 Online Learning (iNACOL) standards; (b) the Online Learning Consortium (OLC) Scorecard; and (c) Quality Matters (QM). Although originally designed to assess online programs for quality indicators, for the most part the standards can be applied to courses and curricula that integrate technology. The three frameworks focus on indicators based on best practice standards for teaching and learning, sound instructional design principles, and research findings. They also include tools to evaluate, create, and improve student learning environments through a Continuous Improvement Process Model.

International Association for K-12 Online Learning

In 2006, the North American Council for Online Learning conducted a review of course standards and adopted the Southern Regional Education Board (SREB) Standards for Quality Online Courses (SREB, 2006). The iNACOL has continued the development of these standards. The standards for quality online courses are categorized into five areas:

1. Content
2. Instructional Design
3. Student Assessment
4. Technology
5. Course Evaluation and Support (iNACOL, 2011)

A scoring guide is available to rate the effectiveness of each standard using a 0 to 4 scale, with 0 indicating absent and 4 very satisfactory.

The OLC Quality Scorecard

The OLC Quality Scorecard for the Administration of Online Programs and the Quality Scorecard for Blended Learning Programs provide a comprehensive framework to evaluate the quality of a program or institutional approach to online or blended learning (Online Learning Consortium, 2016). The scorecard for online programs includes 75 indicators in nine categories, while the blended learning scorecard consists of 70 indicators in eight categories. A handbook is available to support each scorecard. It includes detailed information on the specific indicators, examples of evidence that can be used to show compliance with the standard, and a rubric to facilitate overall scoring. The completed scorecard can be submitted for an independent review by a team of experts, which could lead to program endorsement by OLC. The categories found on the scorecards include:

1. Institutional Support
2. Technology Support
3. Course Development and Instructional Design
4. Course Structure
5. Teaching and Learning
6. Social and Student Engagement (only in the Quality Scorecard for the Administration of Online Programs)
7. Faculty Support
8. Student Support
9. Evaluation and Assessment

The strength of these scorecards is that institutions complete an in-depth and overarching review of the institution's online or blended program based on standards established by industry experts. Using the results of the scorecard, an institution is then able to identify areas for improvement (Online Learning Consortium, 2016).

Quality Matters

QM provides a robust rubric used to evaluate online, hybrid or blended, and technology-integrated courses. The QM Rubric 5th Edition has eight General Standards with 43 Specific Review Standards and is complete with Annotations that explain the application of the standards and relationships among them (Quality Matters Program, 2014). The QM toolset and process are:

- Based on national standards of best practices, research findings, and instructional design principles
- Designed to promote student learning
- Integral to continuous quality improvement
- Part of an inter-institutional, faculty-driven peer review process

Courses are submitted for review to a team of experienced faculty trained to use the rubric to evaluate them. There is a scoring system and set of online tools to facilitate the review. The goal of the review team is to provide constructive, specific, measurable, sensitive, and balanced feedback that guides faculty and course developers to implement changes based on the standards to improve course design. The eight standards are:

1. Course Overview and Introduction
2. Learning Objectives (Competencies)
3. Assessment and Measurement
4. Instructional Materials

5. Course Activities and Learner Interaction
6. Course Technology
7. Learner Support
8. Accessibility and Usability

An integral part of the QM Rubric is the focus on alignment. During a course review, evaluators examine the Specific Review Alignment Standards to ensure that critical course components align with the course objectives and/or competencies, so learners can be successful in achieving course outcomes.

CHALLENGES AND OPPORTUNITIES

Creating effective learning environments with technology poses ongoing challenges as the technology and infrastructure for its use continue to evolve. When thinking about the next level of teaching with technology, academic leaders of nursing programs and nurse educators should reflect on how their students currently use technology and how increased use of social media, mobile applications, and emerging technologies might influence the technology classroom of the future. Nursing faculty need to keep current with the rapidly changing technology trends to ensure that the preparation of today's graduates is always focused on educating them for the world in which they live and work. Assisting nursing and other faculty in higher education with the instructional integration of IT continues to be a top priority. Despite the widespread agreement on the importance of digital media literacy, training in developing skills and techniques is lacking in formal and informal preparation for faculty (Johnson et al., 2016). According to the 2016 Campus Computing™ Project, the top five campus IT priorities for the next 2 to 3 years are: (a) hiring/retaining qualified IT staff (82%); (b) assisting faculty with instructional integration of IT (81%); (c) upgrading/enhancing network and data security (81%); (d) providing adequate user support services (78%); and (e) leveraging IT resources to support student success (76%) (Green, 2016).

SUMMARY

The rapid advances and constant pace of change in technology create challenges and opportunities for teaching in nursing. The more nurse educators use technology, the more they recognize its positive effects on student learning and engagement and its connection to 21st-century skills. Nurse educators need to be prepared to adopt existing technologies and explore emerging technology tools. Technology is helping teachers to expand beyond linear, text-based learning and engage students who have a variety of learning styles. The role of technology in nursing education has evolved from a contained "computer class" into versatile learning tools that change how faculty demonstrate concepts, guide students' learning, assess progress, and increase access to nursing education.

Nurse educators should not use technology just because they can, but rather should integrate appropriate technology in their courses based on quality standards and pedagogical approaches that support best practices and improve students' ability to learn. This chapter explored technology integration and technology tools such as LMS, Web 2.0, Web 3.0, VWs and gaming, and others, to support student achievement of learning outcomes with attention to curriculum and classroom alignment that increase rigor, relevance, and relationships. Classroom redesign, including flipping the classroom, was also discussed in this chapter. When a nursing program and faculty decide to offer technology-based courses or programs, a significant amount of attention should focus on the infrastructure, resources, and support.

Technology is the tool—pedagogy and quality promote its use in nursing education. Technology will continue to disrupt nursing education, and the disruption will change as technology evolves over time. The goal is to explore and embrace technology tools that support good teaching practices.

REFERENCES

Avgeriou, P., Papasalouros, A., Retalis, S., & Skordalakis, M. (2003). Towards a pattern language for learning management systems. *Educational Technology & Society, 6*(2), 11–24.

Bajwa, M. (2014). Emerging 21st century medical technologies. *Pakistan Journal of Medical Sciences, 30*(3), 649–655. doi:10.12669/pjms.303.5211

Bates, A. W., & Poole, G. (2003). *Effective teaching with technology in higher education: Foundations for success* (1st ed.). San Francisco, CA: Jossey-Bass.

Bruner, J. (1966). *Towards a theory of instruction.* Cambridge, MA: Harvard University Press.

Bruner, J. (1996). *The culture of education.* Cambridge, MA: Harvard University Press.

CDW. (2011). *2011 CDW-G 21st-Century Campus Report.* Retrieved from http://www.cdwnewsroom.com/2011-cdw-g-21st-century-campus-report

Chickering, A. W., & Ehrmann, S. C. (1996). Imprementing the seven principles: Technology as Lever. *AAHE Bulletin, 49*(2), 3–6. Retrieved from http://www.tltgroup.org/programs/seven

Chickering, A. W., & Gamson, Z. F. (1987). Seven principles for good practice in undergraduate education. *AAHE Bulletin, 39*(7), 3–6.

Churches, A. (2016). Bloom's digital taxonomy. Retrieved http://edorigami.wikispaces.com/Bloom%27s+Digital+Taxonomy

De Gagne, J. C., Oh, J., Kang, J., Voderstrasse, A., & Johnson, C. M. (2013). Virtual worlds in nursing education: A synthesis of the literature. *Journal of Nursing Education, 52*(7), 391–396. doi:10.3928/01484834-20130610-03

Epper, R. M., Derryberry, A., & Jackson, S. (2012, August 9). *Game-based learning: Developing an institutional strategy* (Research Bulletin). Louisville, CO: EDUCAUSE Center for Applied Research.

Grajek, S., & Pirani, J. A. (2012). The top-ten IT issues, 2012. *EDUCAUSE Review, 47*(3). Retrieved from http://er.educause.edu/articles/2012/6/topten-it-issues-2012

Green, K. (2016). The 2016 campus computing survey. Retrieved from http://www.campuscomputing.net/cc2016

Hartman, J. L. (2008). Moving teaching and learning with technology. *EDUCAUSE Review, 43*(6), 24–25.

Honeycutt, B., & Warren, S. E. (2014). *What are 5 FAQ's about faculty roles in the flipped class?* Madison, WI: Magna Publications.

Horrigan, J. B. (2016). *Lifelong learning and technology.* Pew Research Center. Retrieved from http://www.pewinternet.org/2016/03/22/lifelong-learning-and-technology

Institute of Medicine. (2010). *The future of nursing leading change, advancing health.* Washington, DC: National Academy of Sciences.

International Association for K-12 Online Learning. (2011). *National standards for quality online courses: Version 2.* Vienna, VA: Author.

Johnson, L., Adams Becker, S., Cummins, M., Estrada, V., Freeman, A., & Hall, C. (2016). *The NMC horizon report: 2016 higher education edition.* Austin, TX: The New Media Consortium.

Lippincott, J. K. (2009). Learning spaces involving faculty to improve pedagogy. *EDUCAUSE Review, 44*(2), 17–24.

Malloch, K., & Porter-O'Grady, T. (2011). Innovations in academic and practice partnerships: New collaborations within existing models. *Nursing Administration Quarterly, 35*(4), 300–305. doi:10.1097/NAQ.0b013e31822f8cc0

Means, B., Toyama, Y., Murphy, R., Bakia, M., & Jones, K. (2010). *Evaluation of evidence-based practices in online learning: A meta-analysis and review of online learning studies.* Washington, DC: United States Department of Education Office of Planning, Evaluation, and Policy Development.

Mell, P., & Grance, T. (2011). *The NIST definition of cloud computing.* The National Institute of Standards and Technology, United States Department of Commerce. Special Publication 800-145. Gaithersburg, MD: National Institute of Standards and Technology.

Ohler, J. (2008). The semantic web in education. *EDUCAUSE Quarterly, 31*(4), 7–9.

Online Learning Consortium. (2016). OLC quality scorecard. Retrieved from http://onlinelearningconsortium.org/consult/quality-scorecard

Quality Matters Program. (2014). *Quality Matters™ Rubric Standards Fifth Edition with Assigned Point Values.* Annapolis, MD: MarylandOnline. Retrieved from https://www.qualitymatters.org/qa-resources/rubric-standards

Siemens, G. (2013). Learning analytics: The emergence of a discipline. *American Behavioral Scientist, 57*(10), 1380–1400.

Smaldino, S. E., Lowther, D. L., & Russell, J. D. (2011). *Instructional technology and media for learning* (10th ed.). Upper Saddle River, NJ: Pearson.

Southern Regional Education Board. (2006). Standards for quality online courses. Atlanta, GA: Author. Retrieved from http://publications.sreb.org/2006/06T05_Standards_quality_online_courses.pdf

Tamarkin, M., & Rodrigo, S. (2011). Evolving technologies: A view to tomorrow. *EDUCAUSE Review, 46*(6), 63–80.

U.S. Department of Education Office of Educational Technology. (2013). *Expanding evidence approaches for learning in a digital world.* Retrieved from http://tech.ed.gov/files/2013/02/Expanding-Evidence-Approaches.pdf

Warren, J. J., Manos, E. L., Meyer, M., & Roche, A. (2013). Integrating an academic electronic health record into simulations. In S. Campbell & K. Daley (Eds.), *Simulation scenarios for nursing educators: Making it real* (2nd ed., pp. 519–528). New York, NY: Springer Publishing.

Whiteside, A., Brooks, D. C., & Walker, J. D. (2010). Making the case for space: Three years of empirical research on formal and informal learning environments. *EDUCAUSE Quarterly, 33*(3). Retrieved from https://er.educause.edu/articles/2010/9/making-the-case-for-space-three-years-of-empirical-research-on-learning-environments

World Wide Web Consortium. (2015). Semantic web. Retrieved from https://www.w3.org/standards/semanticweb

6

Teaching in Online Learning Environments

JENNIE C. DE GAGNE

OBJECTIVES

- Describe the roles and responsibilities of educators as facilitators in the online learning environment
- Examine instructional technologies and resources that can help nurse educators select and incorporate new strategies into their online teaching
- Evaluate the process of reconceptualizing to design and evaluate online courses and modules

Teaching online is not the same as teaching in a classroom. Nurse educators must be knowledgeable about how online teaching affects their learners and their profession. The original purpose of the web was to communicate and to share information, and thus using the web to teach was a natural progression of its original purpose. Web-based, or online, teaching and learning means using the web to impart information and to learn. The web, when effectively used, can reduce time and space barriers to learning by reaching individuals for whom traditional systems are inaccessible due to geographical distance from traditional classrooms or busy lives with families, professions, and other responsibilities.

Addressing a wide range of challenges affecting today's students, online education continues to grow in popularity and to evolve at a rapid pace. Many higher education institutions, including nursing schools and programs, now offer hybrid or all-online courses and programs. The focus of this chapter is on the differences between teaching in the traditional classroom and teaching online. The role of the facilitator and the student are discussed in relation to pedagogy, course content, teaching strategies, reconceptualizing and designing online learning environments, interacting online, and using technology to teach and learn.

This chapter was prepared based on work by Carol O'Neil, PhD, RN, CNE, in the first edition of this book.

DEFINITIONS

Several definitions need clarification. *Distance learning* is the term used to describe any learning environment in which the teacher and student are separated by time and geography (M. L. Williams, Paprock, & Covington, 1999). Distance learning is not new; it has been around at least 100 years. It started out as correspondence (independent study) delivered by mail. Since its inception, correspondence education only grew in popularity. Many innovations emerged along the way, one of which was electronic learning (e-learning). *E-learning* is a combination of content and instructional methods delivered via words, sound, and video on a computer or mobile device (R. C. Clark & Mayer, 2016). Interchangeably used, *online learning* or *web-based learning* takes place over the Internet or web. If part of the learning opportunity is online and part is face to face, it is called *hybrid* or *blended learning*. The content material can be presented in a variety of media including text, videotapes, audiotapes, films, links to websites, charts, graphs, statistics data, and case studies. Interaction takes place online, and this happens in three ways: from the instructor to the student, from the student to the student, and from the student to the content. Interaction can be *synchronous* (real time or scheduled time) or *asynchronous* (delayed or at any time of the student's choosing). Allowing students to complete their work at their own pace, asynchronous interaction entails leaving messages at a specific posting site that others in the learning environment can read and respond to at their convenience. By contrast, synchronous interaction requires students to participate in learning activities at a predetermined time (Miller, 2014).

ADVANTAGES AND DISADVANTAGES OF ONLINE LEARNING

The advantages of online learning environments are that course material and activities are accessible 24 hours a day and 7 days a week anywhere with Internet access. The use of the Internet allows for an access to resources and links on the web. Learning is student centered, and there are opportunities for high-quality dialogue. Some considerations are that learners need to be computer literate in an online course, they need hardware and software that are compatible with the online learning systems, and there may be failures that prevent the system from functioning properly (Table 6.1).

TABLE 6.1 Advantages and Disadvantages of Online Learning

Advantages	Disadvantages
• Time barrier is reduced • Space barriers are reduced • Learning takes place anytime and anywhere • Learning is flexible	• Computer literacy is required, including word-processing and file management • Students need to be motivated and self-disciplined • Students have limited face-to-face time with peers and the instructor

PREVALENCE OF ONLINE COURSES

The Sloan Consortium® conducts an annual survey of online education. While the number of students not taking any online courses continues to decrease, the growth rate from 2013 to 2014 of the number of students taking at least one online course was 3.9%, up from the 3.7% rate for the previous year. The 2015 Survey of Online Learning estimated that a total of 5.9 million students took all of their courses online and 2.97 million took some online in the fall 2014 term (Allen & Seaman, 2016). Other key findings include:

- The growth rate in online course enrollment was markedly different between private not-for-profit institutions (11.3%) and private for-profit institutions (2.8%) for the second year in a row.
- Institutions with online courses offerings remain steadfast in their belief that it is critical for their long-term strategy (77.2% in 2014 and 77.1% in 2015).
- Academic leaders remain far more positive about the learning outcomes for blended instruction than they are for online education (Allen & Seaman, 2016).

Online courses and programs are offered by colleges and universities as part of their curriculum. For example, the University of Maryland School of Nursing offers core undergraduate and graduate courses both online and face-to-face. In addition to online courses, there also are online universities, such as Penn State Online (www .worldcampus.psu.edu), and virtual universities, such as the California Virtual Campus (www.cvc.edu). There are online professional organizations and journals such as EDUCAUSE® (www.educause.edu), The Sloan Consortium (www.sloanconsortium .org), and MERLOT (www.merlot.org). Faculty can learn best practices in teaching online through courses, certificates, and programs offered through these organizations and others.

Massive open online courses (MOOCs) are bringing another layer of complexity to online education. MOOC courses offered by more than 500 universities around the world served more than 35 million students (ICEF Monitor, 2016). Examples of these courses can be found at Coursera® (www.coursera.org) and edX (www.edx.org) websites. In the most recent Sloan Consortium survey, still a small segment of higher education institutions was experimenting with MOOCs while most institutions were against a MOOC or remained undecided (Allen & Seaman, 2016). The impact of MOOCs on teaching and learning remains unclear and debatable in many universities and colleges.

SUCCESSFUL ONLINE COURSES

The American Association for Higher Education (AAHE) created the Principles of Good Practice in Undergraduate Education for teaching in the classroom in 1987. Chickering and Ehrmann (1996) used the AAHE principles and developed a new set of principles for incorporating technology into teaching. The principles for good online teaching practice are listed in Exhibit 6.1, and examples of each follow:

1. *Good practice encourages contact between students and faculty.* Teachers can contact students before the course starts with a welcoming text or video greeting sent by e-mail to each student and begin the course with a warm welcome. Teachers as facilitators conference with students via media chat or Skype and by asynchronous communication in a discussion board. Having a question-and-answer forum allows for interaction of students and faculty.
2. *Good practice develops reciprocity and cooperation among students.* Students interact with each other via postings on the discussion board. Students enter a course and are directed to a forum to introduce themselves. They are assigned to chat rooms where they can complete assignments in discussion groups and have asynchronous or synchronous discussions with their teacher and peers.

3. *Good practice uses active learning techniques.* Students need to be actively involved in their learning through the use of active teaching strategies. Some of the strategies that can be used online are discussions, debates, concept maps, and case studies. Using these strategies, the instructor must be able to assist students in developing ideas and learning how to link theory and practice.

4. *Good practice gives prompt feedback.* Timely, meaningful, and detailed feedback is an important element of effective online teaching (De Gagne & Walters, 2010). Feedback provides students with specific information about how they are doing in the course. The teacher develops a schedule for feedback, communicates it to the students, and follows it. Feedback should be standardized, and this can be accomplished by using rubrics. Quizzes or games can help students identify how they are mastering the content and expected outcomes.

5. *Good practice emphasizes time on task.* Taking a course online does not necessarily mean more or less work. Coursework in an online class should be comparable to that assigned in a traditional class. It can be estimated that the student will spend a minimum of 3 hours per week for a traditional 14-week undergraduate course. A three-credit course, therefore, would suggest that students spend a minimum of 9 hours weekly on the course. Sharing this rule of thumb with students will help them plan and organize their coursework load.

6. *Good practice communicates high expectations.* At the beginning of the course, teachers should provide students with a list of rules and policies for online learning. This information is usually found in the course syllabus. For courses with face-to-face and online sections, and for which the syllabus cannot be changed, the teacher should create a manual for the online section of the course that includes the policies. For example, the manual might include a definition of the items on menus, netiquette, the day of the week that the modules start, and expectations for the student and teacher. Expectations for participation and posts should be clearly delineated, and students should be held accountable for following the policies. If they are not followed, the student should obtain feedback detailing expected changes in behavior.

7. *Good practice respects diverse talents and ways of learning.* Each person in the course is an individual with unique knowledge, experience, and strengths. The course should include experiences that engage all students. Strategies include: asking broad and open-ended questions; developing evaluation methods that use different formats, such as a paper, video, or presentation; and considering group assignments that have several components and allow each student to choose the component most suited for him or her.

EXHIBIT 6.1 Principles of Good Practice in Online Teaching

1. Encourage contact between students and teachers.
2. Develop reciprocity and cooperation among students.
3. Use active learning techniques.
4. Give prompt feedback.
5. Emphasize time on task.
6. Communicate high expectations.
7. Respect diverse talents and ways of learning.

Source: Adapted from Chickering and Ehrmann (1996).

SUCCESSFUL ONLINE STUDENTS

There are many assessment tools that are available online to guide students in deciding if online learning is a good option for them. Questions focus on the need and time for online learning, learning style, self-motivation, and experience with technologies. Results of the self-assessment indicate if distance education would work for the student and whether changes in schedule and study habits might be needed for success. Another resource is YouTube, which has videos available to help students decide whether online courses are appropriate for them, considering their learning styles and circumstances. Some of these videos present student views of online courses and include information about time management, motivation, writing skills, computer skills, and learning style. These videos are a resource for students when making the decision about whether to take an online nursing course or program. The Illinois Online Network (ION) identified strategies for students learning online to be successful (ION, 2015b). These are described in Exhibit 6.2.

EXHIBIT 6.2 Strategies for Students' Success When Learning Online

1. Online students should be open minded about sharing life, work, and educational experiences as part of the learning process.
2. Online students need to communicate by writing and typing, and it is helpful to enjoy engaging in these activities.
3. Online students need to be self-motivated and self-disciplined and develop a set schedule and keep to it.
4. Online students need to be willing to "speak up" if problems arise. If the student believes there is a problem, the sooner the teacher knows about it, the faster it can be resolved.
5. There is a weekly time commitment, and online students need to schedule this into their lives.
6. Online students need to meet the requirements for the course.
7. Students should acknowledge that learning online will include high-level thinking and decision making.
8. Online students need to have the required hardware and software.
9. Online students should be willing to think through ideas before responding.
10. Online students should value online learning.

Source: Adapted from Illinois Online Network (2015b). Reprinted by permission of Illinois Online Network, University of Illinois, www.ion.uillinois.edu.

Personal reasons also come into play. Compared to traditional students who enter directly after high school, online students typically work fulltime and have families. They must plan a learning environment that includes life, work, and educational experience. Online learners should be ready to commit time every day to their course material online and for additional study offline. It is important for students to keep track of their assignments and complete them on time. Knowing how to access journal databases for articles and how to distinguish academically credible websites are important skills for them to succeed in their learning.

As peers, they should understand that their participation and contributions are vital to online learning. For students to learn collaboratively, the group should create a supportive environment. They should post supportive comments and share personal anecdotes and information with mutual respect and trust. This kind of communication builds the sense of friendship and belonging that can motivate fellow learners if they find it hard to manage their studies along with their busy lives. Such emotional support plays a major role in learning at a distance; it takes away the isolation of online education. The group should understand that although they do not see each other, they must be sensitive to their peers' feelings whenever sending e-mails, chatting, or making comments about assignments. In other words, students should not alienate their peers or instructor. The more the group strives to establish an effective learning environment, the more they become familiar, secure, and supportive.

SUCCESSFUL ONLINE FACILITATORS

Compared with teaching in traditional classrooms, in online learning environments, the instructor acts as a moderator and facilitates learning. This change of roles calls for educators to consider how their interactions with students affect the teaching and learning process. For the teacher, it is critical to gain knowledge of effective teaching strategies. The teacher must understand the nature and philosophy of online education and be able to organize instructional resources suitable to students' learning needs. Unlike traditional education, online learning casts the teacher in the role of resource person rather than a dispenser of knowledge. The ION describes the role of the teacher in an online course as an educator who facilitates learning (ION, 2015a). This role requires a unique set of characteristics, which include the need for:

- Broad-based knowledge, not only of the content, but of the real world
- An online presence characterized by "openness, concern, flexibility, and sincerity"
- Clear written communications
- An ability to guide students in the critical thinking process so they can relate knowledge to real-world experiences
- An expertise in the subject matter, and skills and know-how in teaching online

Table 6.2 summarizes the characteristics of successful online students and teachers.

TABLE 6.2 Characteristics of Successful Online Students and Faculty

Characteristics of Successful Online Students	Characteristics of Successful Online Faculty
• Is self-motivated • Is self-directed • Is open-minded • Likes to communicate in writing • Meets minimum online requirements	• Is a facilitator of learning • Communicates clearly in writing • Has broad knowledge base • Has an area of clinical expertise (if practice-related course) • Is skilled in teaching online

EFFECTIVE FACILITATION OF ONLINE FORUM

Facilitation of discussion can be an art: where to add input, what to add, and how to direct the discussion are all areas facilitators approach in different ways. Some approaches might work better than others, and facilitators often refine their practices over time. Good facilitation posts identify a relevant idea or question from a participant and add ideas or perspectives to help "flesh out" the topic and examine it more critically. Including a follow-up question at the end of a facilitation post is also helpful for stimulating additional discussion. As facilitators, online teachers should actively interact with their students in the discussion and consistently guide them toward the learning objectives. When choosing where to add input as facilitator of the discussion, online teachers should look for opportunities to highlight and build upon ideas from the week's topics and learning objectives. Students may mention a course topic but not explore it in as much depth or as critically as possible. As facilitators and guides, teachers have the opportunity to "push" students gently to consider portions of the week's readings or other sources they may have overlooked or not read at all. They can ask follow-up questions that entice critical thinking (e.g., why, how, give an example).

The following A-B-C approach might be considered to facilitate effective online discussions:

- Acknowledge the student's input
- Build on the input by adding relevant thoughts, integration of the text, and/or alternate perspectives
- Conclude the message with a pointed follow-up question to move the discussion forward

When facilitating online discussions, it is critical to create a warm tone yet maintain a professional approach through "leading by example." By exerting a careful and positive attitude in their writing, teachers not only set the tone for the students, but they also improve their own practice.

CYBERCIVILITY AND CYBERINCIVILITY

When interacting in the online learning environment, all participants are expected to be as civil as they would be in the face-to-face classroom setting. Evidence has shown that the online environment is vulnerable to incivility or bullying (C. M. Clark, Ahten, & Werth, 2012; C. M. Clark, Werth, & Ahten, 2012; De Gagne, Choi, Ledbetter, Kang, & Clark, 2016, De Gagne, Yamane, & Conklin, 2016). Defined as the disrespectful, insensitive, or disruptive behavior of a user in cyberspace, *cyberincivility* is a pervasive issue that negatively affects one's personal, professional, and social well-being, as well as learning outcomes (De Gagne, Choi, et al., 2016). This phenomenon is evident in e-mail, texts, instant messages, and on social networking sites, as well as online discussion boards (De Gagne, Choi, et al., 2016; De Gagne, Yamane, & Conklin, 2016). That is why the role of online facilitators as gatekeepers is important in terms of creating a safe learning environment.

If a student's tone is coming across as uncivil in an online discussion, the teacher should send a private e-mail as soon as possible. In the message, the teacher would say that the student's experience of frustration in the online discussion was noted, but that the code of conduct must be observed at all times to ensure that every member of the learning community feels respected and valued. When students fear becoming the target of negative attention, they feel unsafe, may participate less, and lose interest in the class. In a worst-case scenario, they might withdraw from the course. To avoid such a situation, the teacher and students involved should identify the problem, talk about their feelings, and brainstorm and implement possible solutions. When put forth by students, solutions tend to be better accepted, thereby showing more positive outcomes and maintaining civility in the online learning environment. A key success factor in online teaching is the effective utilization of communication technology to build a trusting relationship. When used appropriately, students and the teacher can create a constructivist environment in which learning and teaching settings are facilitated and enhanced.

LEARNING THEORY

The pedagogy associated with online learning is Social Learning Theory related to constructivism. Constructivism allows for the construction of meaning by using a process of action and reflection. New knowledge is built on past experiences, and thus, learning is authentic and represents real life. Learning is active and interactive: the active component is enhanced with technology, and the interactive component is enhanced by the use of discussion boards and videoconferencing. Figure 6.1 provides a model of the stages and process of creating an online learning environment, which includes Learning Theory and technology as components.

FIGURE 6.1 Stages and process of creating an online learning environment.

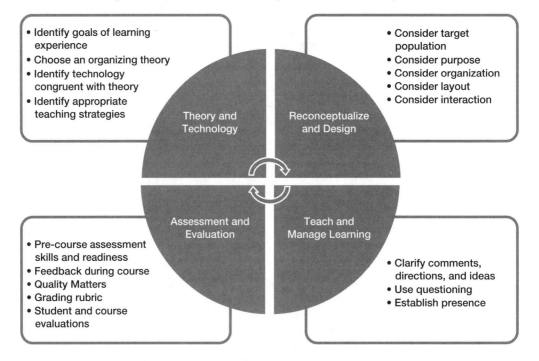

TECHNOLOGY IN ONLINE LEARNING

Technology supports learning through active strategies, such as simulations and case studies, so students can encounter real-world problems in a safe and supportive environment (O'Neil, Fisher, & Newbold, 2013). Content is delivered to students through course management systems such as Blackboard (2017) and Moodle (2017), among others. A course management system has management capability, such as student enrollment monitoring. In addition, it has a set of tools that can be used to create and manage the course. The tools can include discussion boards, announcements, quizzes and tests, videoconferencing, and learning modules. An online learning environment needs a set of specific components. It needs places for the syllabus and course content and the ability to submit and retrieve assignments and to share ideas about the content in synchronous or asynchronous ways. These places are organized to form a course learning platform.

One example of a course management system is Blackboard (2017), which has an assortment of software within its package that the school or teacher can choose to use. Because the software is within the package, Blackboard is called a closed-source system. Some of the features of Blackboard include tools for course management, assessment and grading, and collaboration and student engagement. Moodle (2017) is another example of a course management system; Moodle can be accessed online for free. It is modular, allowing the faculty member to add to and modify the software. When using Moodle, the teacher may need assistance with instructional design and technology. Moodle has an open advocacy forum where its comparisons with other learning management systems are available to assist the instructor in making a decision about which course management system to use. There are other course management systems that can be used in nursing education programs.

TECHNOLOGY REPORTS

There are two important reports on the use of technology in teaching. One of these is the Campus Computing Survey, which is conducted annually. These surveys and others are part of the Campus Computing Project™, a continuing study of the role of information technology in American higher education (www.campuscomputing.net). The second source of information is the New Media Consortium Horizon Report, which is an annual report about emerging technologies that will most likely have an impact on teaching (Johnson et al., 2016). The technologies are grouped into three categories: (a) those that will have an impact on teaching in the next 12 months or less, such as bring your own device (BYOD) and learning analytics and adaptive learning, (b) technologies to watch over the next 2 to 3 years, such as augmented and virtual reality, and (c) those to watch over the next 4 to 5 years, such as affective computing and robotics.

The 2016 Horizon Report explored the use of BYOD (practice of students bringing their own laptops, tablets, or other portable devices with them to school), learning analytics (gathering and analyzing details of individual student interactions), and adaptive learning (applying learning analytics through software and online platforms while adjusting to individual students' needs) (Johnson et al., 2016). In the next 5 years, augmented reality (layering of data over 3D spaces to produce a new learning experience), virtual reality (computer-generated environments to simulate the physical presence of students and objects), and robotics also will expand for use in online teaching and learning.

OVERVIEW OF ACCESSIBLE TECHNOLOGY

Online learning needs to be active, and technology should actively involve the student in the learning process. When determining whether to adopt certain instructional technologies, faculty have to find a balance between their benefits and risks while keeping in mind that not all students have the same number and types of technological preferences. Many technologies have the potential to improve learning and teaching, but they depend on the appropriate pedagogy and instructional design to implement. Among the tools that enhance active learning in the online learning environment are blogs, wikis, podcasts, and videocasts.

A blog or weblog is an online journal that is useful for an individual student or groups of students. Blogs can be public or private. Entries are saved in reverse chronological order, and students can view their peers' entries. Interaction can be enhanced by using the blog for case study discussions or answering discussion questions (Grassley & Bartoletti, 2009). When video content is involved, a weblog becomes a vlog, a form of web television.

Unlike a blog, which allows an individual voice, a wiki overwrites individuality. A wiki is a space on the web that allows individuals to share and collaborate. New ideas are added, and old ideas are saved, thus collecting and expanding on ideas. Grassley and Bartoletti (2009) developed ways to enhance student collaboration using blogs and wikis. They used blogs for discussion boards, and a group of students used wikis to develop thematic analysis. Each student had a journal blog and a research proposal wiki. They concluded that these technologies were useful in enhancing active and collaborative learning online.

A mixture of the words *iPod* and the word *broadcasting*, podcasting is the process of capturing audio sounds and posting their digital files on a website. Similar to podcasting, vodcasting delivers or displays content but in video format instead of audio only. The most frequent use of podcasting and videocasting is in the form of recorded lectures; faculty members record and publish them for students to access whenever and as often as desired. Podcasting and videocasting allow for repeated viewing at the student's convenience. Disseminating lectures through podcasting or vodcasting can be an effective instructional option, especially for independent and highly motivated students.

Communication is a necessary part of an online course. It is enhanced by technology. Interaction is between the teacher and student, among the students, and between the student and the content. Interaction between the teacher and student can be enhanced by using e-mail, online office hours via videoconferencing, and question-and-answer forums on the discussion board. Student-to-student interaction can be facilitated by using blogs and wikis, and student-to-content can be enhanced with podcasting and videocasting.

HOW TO CREATE ONLINE LEARNING ENVIRONMENTS

If you have taught a course in the traditional classroom and now want to offer that course online, how do you do that? Classroom material cannot simply be placed online. Online is a different learning environment, and content must be reconceptualized because what works in the classroom may not work online. The teacher first reconceptualizes the course and then designs the learning materials.

RECONCEPTUALIZATION

To reconceptualize means that the content is reviewed in the context of the goals of the institution, available technology, and expertise of the faculty and students. The end products of the reconceptualization process are the decisions about how the course, and modules (or units) within, will be organized and how the content will be presented.

One consideration is the projected reach of the course, for example, in terms of where students are located. The larger the reach, the more likely the content should be placed online. A statewide program with potential students who live at a great distance from the school would be better online than delivered in a traditional classroom setting. Another variable is how long the information will be offered. The longer it is offered to students, the more amenable it is to online access. For example, a statewide program repeated throughout the year is best provided online.

Many schools of nursing offer large classroom courses with 100 or more students. Online courses, however, are most successful when there are a smaller number of students. This emphasizes the need for the support of administration. Do online learning environments fit into the mission and vision of the school? Does the administration view online learning as important? Online courses typically have fewer students enrolled than large lecture-type courses; will the school of nursing support one faculty member for 25 or 30 students rather than or in addition to one faculty member for 100 students in a face to face? If the administration and the budget support online learning, these courses can be successful. The last institutional variable is resources. Nursing faculty considering online courses should assess the school's resources and support, both instructors and course content. Some resources include a course management system such as Blackboard, technical support, instructional designers, faculty who are technologically competent, and the school's ability to successfully market online courses and programs. It is important for nursing faculty to build resources before developing online courses.

The second variable in reconceptualizing a course is assessing the available technology. What hardware and software are available? How will the online courses be maintained? Having appropriate technology and support is important in creating an environment for success in online teaching. To effectively use technology in academia, various stakeholders have to make considerable investments in hardware, software, infrastructure, and support services, and researchers and educators have to justify these investments with regard to efficacy and cost-effectiveness.

The third variable is faculty. Faculty members in the school of nursing need to learn how to teach online. Preparing educators to deal with this new experience is essential to create successful online learning communities. Faculty should be mentored and provided with the instruction they need to become successful online facilitators. They should know about pedagogy, online theory, learning and managing online courses, evaluation of students and the course, and ethical and legal issues surrounding online education. One method of faculty development is to place the orientation material and learning activities online and provide an orientation similar to what a student would receive. As part of faculty development, teachers should learn to use teaching methods such as PowerPoint with voiceover narration, video clips, and methods for online group work. They should have an opportunity to discuss with each other the advantages and disadvantages of each for their own courses. Faculty should participate in synchronous and asynchronous learning activities and be guided in assessing and grading assignments in an online environment. For ongoing development, faculty members who are teaching online can form a group to meet regularly to discuss issues and explore alternate approaches to use.

The next consideration is students. Do they have the hardware and software essential for online learning, and do they have the support needed to take a course online? While ongoing technical help is necessary for students, it is particularly important the first week of class. Librarians should be accessible for students who need additional resources to complete their assignments. Online tutoring for certain subjects, such as writing and statistics, should be made available for all online students. Students also need an orientation to online learning, advice to help them determine if an online course is best for them, and support services. Exhibit 6.3 provides the A-to-F tips and guidelines for successful online learning.

Reconceptualizing means making decisions about the type and structure of the course as well as thinking about the mental models that connect the course and modules. Reconceptualizing results in a course that is organized and logical to the learner, so the objectives, content, interaction, and assessments work well with one another.

EXHIBIT 6.3 The A-to-F Tips and Guidelines for Successful Online Learning

A: Avoid self-doubt phrases. The use of phrases such as "Do I really belong here," "I'm too old to learn new technology," or "I'll never succeed," increases your anxiety or fear of failure and interferes with motivation and confidence in learning. Negative thoughts and feelings inhibit the morale and interfere with your learning progress.

B: Be self-disciplined. The flexibility and convenience of online learning come with more responsibility. You must set a plan for your work time and rigorously follow it. You must be self-disciplined enough to access your course assiduously and to invest sufficient time in offline reading and writing.

C: Communicate effectively. Because of lack or absence of face-to-face encounter, your message may lead to misinterpretation or misunderstanding. Not only should you be competent in expressing yourselves in writing, but you must also be vigilant about your written tones, building effective e-communication skills to avoid any misunderstanding or distrust.

D: Develop time management skills. Procrastination is one of the biggest enemies for your productivity. You must know how to prioritize tasks and avoid distraction, making sure your surroundings are conducive to studying.

E: Engage in the learning process. Engagement is the heart of online learning. You may feel more comfortable being a passive learner at the beginning of the learning process, but you must understand that your participation and contribution are vital to your success in any online courses.

F: Find practical support. You need to seek out all the help and support you can get. There may be designated academic counselors, advisors, or technical concierges for you. It is much easier to accomplish goals when you have support from peers, colleagues, and family members. A good source of support can be an experienced peer with online learning.

After the first set of decisions is made, the next decisions relate to how the course will be organized. The teacher should develop a course that will meet the needs of most of the learners and for which the teacher has skills (O'Neil et al., 2013).

HOW TO DESIGN ONLINE COURSES AND MODULES

Design means how the teacher develops the course and its components to achieve its objectives or outcomes. The component parts of an online course are the target population, purpose and objectives, course organization, navigation, page layout, and interaction (O'Neil et al., 2013).

The target population is the learner. An assessment of students' knowledge and learning styles is needed. What do the learners know and not know about the topic, and how will they best learn? When designing a module, the teacher should consider students' different learning styles and preferences and include multiple strategies. In addition to learning styles and preferences, students may differ in age, computer experience, socioeconomic status, motivation, and other characteristics. When planning technology, the teacher should consider using technology that meets the students' needs and is appropriate for the majority of students in the course.

The purpose and objectives of the course must be considered in the design. If this is a didactic learning environment, it would be designed differently than a seminar course. If there are skills to be learned, the laboratory experience might need to be arranged differently from a traditional classroom experience. If the course has a clinical component, this component needs to be organized with considerations that might differ from a more traditional laboratory experiment.

The organization of the course is its flow. Can the student get from one section of the online course to another with ease? Students should locate what they need within three clicks of the mouse. Each module should appear the same in terms of structure, so students know from module to module where to find information.

In creating the page layout, lines should be clean and crisp. The font size should be considered based on the needs of the target population. There should be headers that divide the material, which are different fonts and colors from that of the general content. The teacher should use colors that facilitate reading and are pleasing to look at. Well-known to graphic designers, the Big 4 (CRAP) principle can be useful and applied when creating an appealing layout; CRAP stands for Contrast, Repetition, Alignment, and Proximity (R. Williams, 2014). More information about the use of CRAP principles in online learning is found at https://elearningindustry.com/using-crap-web-design-for-elearning.

Online interactions can be designed with either synchronously or asynchronously. Synchronous can include videoconferencing, which can be used for office hours, student conferences, student group or individual projects, and seminars. As this type of interaction is live, the day and time need to be scheduled so students can attend. There should be a purpose and an agenda for each session. The purpose is for face-to-face communication; synchronous interaction can be used for sharing, teaching, or evaluation. Asynchronous interaction strategies include the discussion board, blogs, and wikis. The purpose of these is to share ideas and provide feedback to students. There can be open or closed discussions for individual students or groups.

Quality Matters Rubric and Its Use in Designing Online Course

Quality Matters (QM) is a faculty-centered and peer review process designed to assess and certify the quality of online and blended courses (MarylandOnline, 2017). QM has three components: the QM rubric, peer review process, and professional development. When designing a course, the teacher should begin by reviewing the QM rubric. The rubric is a table of characteristics that high-quality online courses have. The rubric, which was presented in Chapter 5, has eight standards: a course overview and introduction, learning objectives and competencies, assessment and measurement, instructional materials, learner interaction and engagement, course technology, learner support, and accessibility.

Although the QM rubric is used for assessment of an online course, the standards should be considered when designing the course. For example, the first standard in the rubric indicates that the instructions are clear as to how to get started and where to locate the course components. One way of accomplishing this clarity is to include a welcome message for students as they enter the course. A sample welcome message is in Exhibit 6.4.

If all of the courses in a nursing program are taught online, the faculty can include the QM rubric in the course syllabus. When a course is taught both online and in a traditional classroom setting, it would not be appropriate to include online specifications in the syllabus. By following the standards in the rubric, the teacher can identify information that should be included in the syllabus and as part of the online material.

Meeting the QM standards is a measure of the course structure, not of the teacher's effectiveness. Faculty peer review within the school of nursing determines the quality of teaching. This means that instructions are present, and the purpose of the course

EXHIBIT 6.4 Sample Welcome for Students in an Online Course

Welcome to the introduction to this course, and I am glad that you found us. This is the place to start, and your beginning steps will be outlined here. Go to the Course Information section and find the course syllabus and online material. Open and read them. The syllabus will tell you about the content, and the online material will tell you about the technology. Remember to print both because if there is a power outage and a paper is due, it will be too late to look for my phone number. After completing this task, go to the discussion board and type "I did it" in the "I did it" forum. Then go to the Introduction section and tell us about yourself.

is clear. There are learning objectives that match the purpose, and the assessment and measurement to validate whether students have met the objectives, and the instructional materials are accessible. How students interact with each other, with the content, and with the faculty, and the technology used to facilitate the learning process are described for students. The students need to know where to go for support, and the course needs to be accessible to all students (Quality Matters Program, 2014).

HOW TO TEACH AND MANAGE ONLINE LEARNING ENVIRONMENTS

Faculty members are facilitators of learning, and thus managing learning is the process of guiding the student to achieve learning objectives. Prior to beginning the course, the syllabus and online expectations should be available to students, so they can read them and become familiar with the course. One strategy is to make the course available to students—"open the course"—a few days before the first module. A scavenger hunt is a way of encouraging students to access different parts of the course and become familiar with them. For example, the teacher can ask how many students are enrolled in the course, and students can navigate to the roster to locate this information. Orientation to the course management system should be included as a reference for students who may be taking an online course in the nursing program for the first time. Netiquette should be discussed, and acceptable online behavior should be stated clearly for students.

Ragan (2007) identified the principles of best practice for online teachers. These include:

- Show up and teach (interact with students and guide them through the learning experience)
- Practice proactive course management strategies (such as monitoring assignment submissions and reminding students of upcoming deadlines)
- Establish patterns of course activities (establish and communicate a course pace and pattern of work)
- Plan for the "unplanned" (have a strategy in place for informing students of unexpected situations)
- Expect and require responses (provide timely feedback to students and respond promptly)
- Think before you write (be clear and concise in written responses to students to avoid misinterpretation)
- Help maintain forward progress of students (ensure timely return of assignments and test scores)

- Maintain a safe and secure learning environment (use the institutionally supported course management system, which provides security and confidentiality)
- Remember that quality counts (establish strategies for addressing the quality of the online course)
- Confirm the technological infrastructure for offering the online course

There are several functions of the online teacher during the course, and the first and foremost is to correct errors. For example, when the discussion board opens, the teacher should enter the course and review what is posted. If the first student who posts a comment in the discussion board has not understood the assignment, other students might continue to make the same error. Or, a student may provide inaccurate information on a discussion board, which the teacher should correct immediately. Students need to know that faculty members are reading the postings and assessing the accuracy of the information posted.

A second function of the online teacher is to clarify the points a student makes and relate them to the module objectives or outcomes. To do this, the teacher can start a reply with the phrase, "I think you are saying that . . ." and then summarize the key points in the post. Students can provide examples from clinical practice, or the teacher can include scenarios that apply the concepts learned in the module to practice.

Questioning is an effective technique to raise the level of student thinking. One technique is called the "sandwich," which starts with positive reinforcement of the student's answer, followed by another question to extend thinking about other possibilities. For example, the teacher might pose this series of questions using the "sandwich" approach: "You have made some valid and important points. What might be the impact of this idea on the budget? I appreciate your rethinking this." Asking "what if" questions is another way of encouraging higher level thinking among students.

Presence is a concept that means the students know that the instructor is in the course and actively involved in their learning. One way is through posting to the discussion board, but this is not the only way. Other ways of letting students know that the instructor is present is through announcements, the addition of a humorous comment related to the content being learned, or change in the order of the modules on the course site. For example, if students are working on Module 8, the teacher might move modules 1 to 7 to the bottom of the list, indicating he or she is present in the course. Telling a story is another strategy for enhancing the instructor's online personality. One idea is to create a folder for the course with stories that relate to modules. In the appropriate module, the instructor can copy and paste that story into the module discussion.

ASSESSMENT AND EVALUATION

Traditional classroom evaluation measures are neither comprehensive nor appropriate for online learning. Some reasons are that students need to assess their skills and that they desire to enroll in an online course. Students need continued feedback about how they are progressing through the course. An online course should be created and ready to be implemented before the students enter it. The course needs to be reviewed before it goes live, and links need to be tested and updated. To accommodate the differences in evaluation, O'Neil et al. (2013) developed a model of evaluation for online courses. The model is based on student assessment and course evaluation, each conducted in three phases. Students should be assessed before the course begins, during the learning experience, and at the end of the learning experience. The course should be evaluated before it goes live, during the learning experience, and at the end of the learning experience.

Examples of student assessment before the course begins include surveys of computer skills, pretests, and readiness surveys. During the learning experience, students can keep logs or journals, take formative quizzes, and post answers to the discussion board. Student learning at the end of selected modules and the course itself can be assessed by examinations, presentations, or papers.

Similar to traditional courses, online courses should use grading rubrics for the assessment and grading of students' assignments to provide them with a clear understanding of what is expected of them. Nursing faculty members can create their own rubrics or can use rubrics posted in a public gallery (Rcampus™, 2017). In the Rubric Gallery, faculty can develop, assess, and share rubrics with others. Further discussion and examples of rubrics for assessment in nursing courses are in Chapter 12.

Courses should be evaluated before they go live, allowing the teacher to resolve any problems or issues with the course before the students begin. An excellent tool for evaluating an online course is the QM rubric, discussed earlier in the chapter (MarylandOnline, 2017). Schools can join the QM organization and learn about evaluating their courses through workshops and consultations.

Continuous feedback is necessary throughout the course because with most online courses, the teacher does not "see students" and take attendance. One example of formative evaluation is the "pulse check." This should be done several times during the course. In an announcement, the teacher can ask students to "Stop a moment and take your pulse. Is it strong and bounding, weak and thready, or another combination? E-mail me your assessment and tell me what I can do to help you be successful." The teacher can post a summary announcement if the feedback will assist the group (O'Neil et al., 2013). Summative evaluation is assessment of the modules and course, typically at the end. Surveys may be sent to students and faculty members, asking questions pertinent to course evaluation such as student satisfaction with the course content, instructional methods, assignments, and other areas (O'Neil et al., 2013).

SUMMARY

Online teaching, a vehicle that uses technology to enhance a traditional approach to learning, has attracted tremendous interest and gained popularity in nursing education. Yet, teaching online is different from teaching in a classroom because the students cannot be seen and different technology is used. The advantage of learning online is the flexibility of learning anytime and anywhere. The disadvantage is often the technology and learning alone. The pedagogy differs in that students learn from each other. Interaction with the teacher as facilitator, the content, and other students is essential. Learning in an online environment is reflective and active. Online learning requires administrative support for the technology, and choices need to be made about course management systems. Learning modules are designed before the students enter the online course. A module includes objectives, content, learning activities, strategies for interaction, and resources for learning. After the students begin, the role of the teacher is to guide them through the learning experience, assess the outcomes of student learning, and evaluate the course.

Learning in online environments plays an important role in nursing education, and the learning environment must be of high quality. Technology continues to influence online courses and programs, and teaching online will continue to evolve and improve over time.

REFERENCES

Allen, E., & Seaman, J. (2016). *Online report card: Tracking online education in the United States.* Retrieved from http://onlinelearningsurvey.com/reports/onlinereportcard.pdf

Blackboard Inc. (2017). Blackboard. Retrieved from http://www.blackboard.com

Chickering, A. W., & Ehrmann, S. C. (1996). Implementing the seven principles: Technology as Lever. *AAHE Bulletin, 49*(2), 3–6. Retrieved from http://www.tltgroup.org/programs/seven

Clark, C. M., Ahten, S., & Werth, L. (2012). Cyber-bullying and incivility in an online learning environment, part 2: Promoting student success in the virtual classroom. *Nurse Educator, 37*(5), 192–197. doi:10.1097/NNE.0b013e318262eb2b

Clark, C. M., Werth, L., & Ahten, S. (2012). Cyber-bullying and incivility in the online learning environment, part 1: Addressing faculty and student perceptions. *Nurse Educator, 37*(4), 150–156. doi:10.1097/NNE.0b013e31825a87e5

Clark, R. C., & Mayer, R. E. (2016). *E-learning and the science of instruction: Proven guidelines for consumers and designers of multimedia learning* (4th ed.). San Francisco, CA: Pfeiffer.

De Gagne, J. C., Choi, M., Ledbetter, L., Kang, H., & Clark, C. M. (2016). An integrative review of cybercivility in health professions education. *Nurse Educator, 41*(5), 239–245. doi:10.1097/NNE.0000000000000264

De Gagne, J. C., & Walters, K. (2010). The lived experience of online educators: Hermeneutic phenomenology. *Journal of Online Learning and Teaching, 6*(2), 357–366.

De Gagne, J. C., Yamane, S. S., & Conklin, J. L. (2016). Evidence-based strategies to create a culture of cybercivility in health professions education. *Nurse Education Today, 45,* 138–141. doi:10.1016/j.nedt.2016.07.007

Grassley, J. S., & Bartoletti, T. (2009). Wikis and blogs: Tools for online interaction. *Nurse Educator, 34,* 209–213. doi:10.1097/NNE.0b013e3181b2b59b

ICEF Monitor. (2016). MOOC enrolment surpassed 35 million in 2015. Retrieved from http://monitor.icef.com/2016/01/mooc-enrolment-surpassed-35-million-in-2015

Illinois Online Network. (2015a). What makes a successful online facilitator? Retrieved from http://www.ion.uillinois.edu/resources/tutorials/pedagogy/instructorProfile.asp

Illinois Online Network. (2015b). What makes a successful online student? Retrieved from http://www.ion.uillinois.edu/resources/tutorials/pedagogy/StudentProfile.asp

Johnson, L., Adams Becker, S., Cummins, M., Estrada, V., Freeman, A., & Hall, C. (2016). *The NMC horizon report: 2016 higher education edition.* Austin, TX: The New Media Consortium.

MarylandOnline. (2017). Quality matters program. Retrieved from https://www.qualitymatters.org

Miller, M. D. (2014). *Minds online: Teaching effectively with technology.* Cambridge, MA: Harvard University Press.

Moodle. (2017). Moodle. Retrieved from https://moodle.org

O'Neil, C. A., Fisher, C., & Newbold, S. (2013). *Developing online learning environments in nursing education* (3rd ed.). New York, NY: Springer Publishing.

Quality Matters Program. (2014). *Quality matters™ rubric standards fifth edition with assigned point values.* Annapolis, MD: MarylandOnline. Retrieved from https://www.qualitymatters.org/qa-resources/rubric-standards

Ragan, L. C. (2007, May 15). The 10 commandments of effective online teaching. *Distance Education Report, 11*(10), 3.

Rcampus. (2017). Rubric gallery. Retrieved from http://www.rcampus.com/rubricshellc.cfm

Williams, R. (2014). *The non-designer's design book* (4th ed.). Berkeley, CA: Peachpit Press.

Williams, M. L., Paprock, K. E., & Covington, B. (1999). *Distance learning: The essential guide.* Thousand Oaks, CA: Sage.

7

Clinical Simulations in Nursing Education: Overview, Essentials, and the Evidence

PAMELA R. JEFFRIES, KRISTINA T. DREIFUERST, AND
KATIE A. HAERLING

OBJECTIVES

- Describe types of clinical simulations in nursing and how to integrate and implement them into a nursing curriculum
- Identify strategies for creating realism and suspending disbelief in simulations
- Critique various debriefing approaches and their use in nursing education
- Describe evaluation processes to use when developing and implementing clinical simulations

Traditionally, simulations have been used to provide opportunities for students to practice patient care in a "safe" environment before going into the clinical setting. However, in the current environment of increasing patient acuity and limited clinical placements, simulation may serve a broader role as an adjunct or replacement for traditional clinical hours. Moreover, the Institute of Medicine (Committee on the Robert Wood Johnson Foundation Initiative on the Future of Nursing at the Institute of Medicine, 2011) recently cited simulation as a critical ingredient for producing an adequate numbers of competent nurses, and the National Council of State Boards of Nursing (2012) has findings from a landmark, national study exploring substituting simulations for real clinical time that is impacting nursing education today (Hayden, Smiley, Alexander, Kardong-Edgren, & Jeffries, 2014). As simulation pedagogy progresses, it also will play an increasingly important role in both formative and summative student and graduate evaluation.

This chapter provides an overview of types of clinical simulations in nursing, as well as how to integrate and implement them into a nursing curriculum. The importance of how to create realism and suspend disbelief in the simulations is also discussed. In addition, debriefing approaches and evaluation processes to use when developing and implementing clinical simulations are presented. Finally, the evidence regarding the use of clinical simulations, beyond the point of asking if the pedagogy actually works, but also how to make it work best, is highlighted.

DIFFERENT TYPES OF SIMULATION

There are several different types of simulations that vary in the degree of fidelity, or the ability of the simulation environment to best replicate the actual clinical environment (Jeffries & Rogers, 2007). This fidelity, or realism, allows the learner to become engaged within the simulation on a physical, conceptual, emotional, and experiential level (Bauchat, Seropian, & Jeffries, 2016; Rudolph, Simon, & Raemer, 2007).

MANIKIN-BASED SIMULATION

Manikin-based simulation has been used for hundreds of years, including both the bronze acupuncture teaching statues from the Song Dynasty in China as well as "Mrs. Chase," the classic nursing manikin used for task training since 1922 (Herrmann, 2008; Owen, 2012). Manikins, as human patient simulators (HPSs), vary in the amount and degree of technology and fidelity built into the device. Simulation fidelity is defined as the extent to which a simulated experience is real or believable to the participants (International Nursing Association for Clinical Simulation and Learning [INACSL] Standards Committee, 2016). It can be thought of on two dimensions: "engineering fidelity," or how authentic the simulation looks and feels; and "psychological fidelity," or how realistic the behaviors and actions required mimic what is anticipated or expected (Norman, Dore, & Grierson, 2012). Hayden et al. (2014) suggested using an appropriate level of fidelity to help learners achieve the objectives of the simulation activity. Some learning objectives require very simple resources, such as performing an intramuscular injection on an orange, while other learning objectives require higher levels of fidelity to create a realistic experience. Fidelity is important to consider when developing simulations for students because it reflects the level of engagement that will be expected of participants as they are involved in the experience (Feinstein & Cannon, 2002) and the extent to which the nurse educator and simulation personnel will go in creating it.

Manikins that are life-sized, have realistic anatomical structures, and contain technology that dynamically mimics changes in human physiology are called high-fidelity HPSs, whereas other full-sized manikins that may only partially or not as rapidly mimic physiologic changes are called medium-fidelity manikins (Lapkin, Levett-Jones, Bellchambers, & Fernandez, 2010). Low-fidelity HPSs are task trainers that are static and typically represent one function of the human body, such as an arm model used to practice venipuncture. These are particularly useful for novice students learning basic skills and general principles of patient care (Kardong-Edgren, Anderson, & Michaels, 2007).

High-fidelity HPSs are best used when learners are expected to successfully care for a patient with multiple abnormal physiologic findings within the simulation scenario. These manikins allow for changes of physiologic parameters within the simulation, either by programming ahead of the simulation or by changing the parameters within the simulation. This allows faculty to evaluate the learner's ability to rapidly respond to changes in the patient's condition or demonstrate the physiologic effects of any given treatment (medications or interventions). Multiple physiologic parameters, including pupil dilation/constriction, respiratory and cardiac (breath and heart sounds, pulses, blood pressure, pulse oxygenation), and abdominal (bowel sounds) signs may be programmed, depending on the type of high-fidelity HPS. High-fidelity HPSs also allow learners to practice and refine psychomotor skills, such as basic and advanced life support. When the simulation scenario requires only a limited number of physiologic changes or complex task training, using a medium-fidelity HPS may be sufficient.

The decision about what level of fidelity to select is determined by what is available, the objectives of the experience, and the intended learner outcomes. Fidelity can also involve a variety of dimensions, including (a) physical factors such as environment, equipment, and related tools; (b) psychological factors such as emotions, beliefs, and self-awareness of participants; (c) social factors such as participant and instructor motivation and goals; (d) culture of the group; and (e) degree of openness and trust, as well as participants' modes of thinking (Dieckmann, Gaba, & Rall, 2007; Vincent, Sheriff, & Mellott, 2015). The level of fidelity is an important consideration for nurse educators during the process of selecting or designing simulations. The patient's story in the scenario and objectives for the simulation become part of the fidelity or realism of the experience and help to socialize the student to the role of the nurse.

Moulage is another aspect of fidelity that nurse educators can consider for simulation learning with manikins and other simulation modalities. Moulage incorporates the use of makeup, dress, and wigs to enhance the patient story, and wax, latex, artificial fluids, and simulation enhancers to simulate injury, disease, aging, and other physical enhancements to the manikin (Smith-Stoner, 2011). Adding moulage to the simulation increases the realism for the student and can make the simulation experience more authentic for holistic learning.

Fidelity in simulation is intended to immerse the student in a realistic learning experience that represents a clinical setting or client care situation. Attention to having realistic equipment and creating a representative physical environment impacts the believability of the simulation experience for many students and may impact clinical learning. Low-, moderate-, and high-fidelity simulations can all be valuable learning environments when they are incorporated into the curriculum and learning objectives for nursing students.

STANDARDIZED PATIENTS

A standardized patient (SP) is an individual who is trained to portray a patient with specific condition. Standardized patients are able to play their role the same way during every encounter. During a simulation, an SP will provide a consistent answer to questions asked by the learner and has been trained prior to the simulation not to go off script, embellish the response, or provide additional information that was not asked by the learner. To do this, the SP rehearses the role with the faculty member to ensure that each learner experiences the same patient portrayal in each and every simulation. Sometimes an individual is enlisted to "role-play" a part in a simulation with little or no training. In this case, this individual is not an SP, as there is no assurance that the role will be played in the same manner for each simulation.

Standardized patients may be further subdivided according to the objective of the simulation and the role that they play. Within the simulation, they can portray patients, but also may function as the teacher, evaluator, or both. Standardized patients are often used to teach and evaluate other physical examination skills, such as a head-to-toe assessment. Certain SPs obtain further education and training to evaluate the student in either formative evaluation or summative evaluation, including high-stakes simulation. Objective structured clinical examinations (OSCEs) are a series of stations where students care for a variety of patients according to a predetermined time-limited schedule for each station.

Standardized patients are used to portray these patients and may participate in the evaluation of the student as well.

Simulations may be enhanced by the use of SPs, particularly in simulation scenarios that teach and evaluate communication skills (Ryan et al., 2010). Many prelicensure nursing programs use SPs for a variety of psychiatric mental-health simulations, whereas advanced practice nursing programs use SPs to teach and evaluate history-taking skills. Other uses of SPs include simulations involving interprofessional education teams, ethical and cultural competencies, safety, and patient education. Standardized patients also are used as "unannounced" patients to evaluate providers, similar to "secret shoppers" who evaluate customer service.

Incorporating SPs within a simulation program requires planning and sufficient funds to hire and train them. They can be trained actors, students in other programs, or community members. Additional manpower may be required to coordinate the SP program within the school; however, most programs that use SPs believed that the experience is valuable (May, Park, & Lee, 2009).

AUGMENTED REALITY, VIRTUAL SIMULATION, AND GAMING

Augmented reality and virtual simulations provide seemingly endless possibilities for innovative teaching and learning in nursing (Foronda et al., 2017). Augmented reality refers to a variety of two- or three-dimensional applications where digital images merge with the real environment (Carlson & Gagnon, 2016). Foronda et al. (2017) provide several examples of augmented reality applications, including a flight simulator and Microsoft's Hololens, where learners can interact with holograms representing the human anatomy. Virtual reality applications allow learners to access Internet-based, two- or three-dimensional simulated environments for an educational experience (LeFlore et al., 2012). Some virtual simulations also have been built on Second Life® and may be used for teaching and learning or for evaluation. Although expensive to develop, there is some evidence that suggests this type of simulation may be superior when compared with traditional lecture method or interaction with an SP (Irwin & Coutts, 2015; LeFlore et al., 2012; Wendling et al., 2011).

Gaming also has been incorporated within simulation. One of the primary benefits of gaming as a teaching and learning strategy is that it engages learners in a way that they are highly motivated to achieve a goal or solve a problem (Verkuyl, Atack, Mastrilli, & Romaniuk, 2016). One nursing program found that high-fidelity simulation along with a gaming experience enhanced the curriculum on end-of-life care (Kopp & Hanson, 2012). Another innovative simulation experience involved the use of a fictitious registered nurse blog to describe challenges during her first year of practice (Thomas, Bertram, & Allen, 2012). Depending on the objectives of the learning experience, games may be designed to allow learners to interact with the content independently or to collaborate with a facilitator or other learners.

The simulation learning objectives should dictate the type of simulation that will allow the student to accomplish the desired clinical outcomes. Regardless of the type of simulation selected, it is important to identify clearly how it will provide the realism necessary for the learner to fully engage in the simulation. To do this, a detailed simulation scenario should include the type of HPS to be used, along with the patient condition and corresponding physiologic parameters throughout the simulation. Any additional equipment needed to either more accurately replicate the clinical setting or that will be used by the learner to accomplish the objectives of the simulation must also be included in the experience.

INTEGRATION OF SIMULATION INTO CURRICULUM

High-fidelity simulations offer a rich opportunity to improve student learning and achieve desired outcomes throughout a nursing curriculum. Simulations can be used in a variety of ways by faculty to meet different learning goals, ranging from knowledge acquisition to application of a theoretical concept, professional role development, and evaluation of student competency.

Perhaps the most obvious use of high-fidelity simulation is creating a clinical experience for a student. This experience may supplement or replace clinical hours or a clinical day for any type of experience in a nursing curriculum.

Simulation allows all students in a program to experience patient care situations deemed critical for professional practice which cannot be guaranteed in a clinical setting. For example, it might be considered critical for all new nurses to know how to assess and care for a diabetic patient with significant hypoglycemia. While all students could be assigned a diabetic patient in a clinical setting, there is no guarantee that they would all provide care for a patient with hypoglycemia. Yet, this experience can be granted to every student using simulation. Simulations also can create clinical experiences that are rare in clinical practice, but potentially life threatening and require prompt recognition and intervention. Clinical simulations can be developed to provide students with a practice setting or a type of experience that is difficult to offer because of a variety of factors such as limited clinical sites, lack of qualified faculty in a specialty area, or geographic remoteness. For example, it may be difficult to place all of the students in labor and delivery, and there may be limited inpatient pediatric units. In those cases, simulation can be used to meet the learning needs of students to care for mothers during childbirth and children of all ages.

There are several possible ways to provide simulation experiences for students in remote locations where significant travel is needed to reach the school or an appropriate clinical agency. For example, a live simulation with a small group of students could be broadcast to a satellite location where there is not a simulation lab. Simulations could also be integrated completely online where a recording of the simulation is posted and then debriefing occurs via an asynchronous discussion. Or, students could be assigned to view an online video clip of a simulation or interact with a live telehealth simulation followed by synchronous or asynchronous discussions. Simulations encourage students to develop critical thinking, clinical reasoning, team building, and communication skills, and other professional attributes needed in a graduate nurse. Through simulation the student acts in the role of the nurse caring for patients, interacting with other health care providers, acting independently on physician orders, and documenting care, because it is a safe learning environment.

Simulations should be leveled throughout the curriculum, building in complexity and ambiguity. When selecting or writing simulations, faculty should create experiences that help students develop competencies to meet national goals for professional practice, such as patient safety or quality goals. Faculty should also consider what content and skills students have found difficult to master and incorporate these into simulations.

High-fidelity simulation, in addition to its use in clinical courses, can also be incorporated into traditional theory courses. This assists students in linking the content between theory and practice. For example, a didactic presentation could present the facts about a myocardial infarction and standard care of these patients. Following this classroom presentation, students could participate in a simulation that allowed them to apply those facts to assessment and care for a simulated patient with a myocardial infarction. Using another approach, the content could be presented via the simulation, with students given materials to prepare for the experience with the goal that knowledge would be attained through the simulation.

A mechanism of introducing increasingly complex simulations into a curriculum is to use an unfolding case. In an unfolding case, students are introduced to a particular patient repeatedly at different points in the care continuum within a simulation, throughout a course or throughout the curriculum. The patient scenario becomes more complex and requires different assessment skills or interventions on the part of the nurse. For example, in a psychiatric mental health class, the students could be introduced to a patient with depression. Later in the semester the students may "meet" the same patient, but this time the patient is suicidal. The students interact with the same patient again at a later date in a different course, such as community health, when they are making a home health visit. During the home visit, the students can observe the patient interacting with his or her family.

Another way to add complexity to a simulation is to repeat the same case but use a modified version. This could occur in one course where, after debriefing a simulation, the students switch roles and repeat the simulation. This time, the scenario progresses in a slightly different way. For example, the first scenario might have the postpartum patient with normal vaginal discharge after delivery. When the simulation is repeated, the patient develops signs and symptoms of a postpartum hemorrhage, and the nurse needs to identify the difference as well as the appropriate nursing actions. Each of these simulations offers different opportunities for teaching and learning.

Simulation can play an important role in developing professional roles and behaviors in nursing students. In addition to learning to think and act like a nurse, students need to learn how to work with other health care professions. Interprofessional education (IPE) has been nationally promoted as critical to providing high-quality and safe patient care (Greiner & Knebel, 2003). Interdisciplinary simulations can represent basic to complex interactions in patient care. For example, beginning students might be involved in a simulation where a patient has an abnormal laboratory value. The nurse would be responsible for identifying the problem, contacting the physician, and receiving and acting on new medical orders. The physician would be responsible for evaluating the data presented by the nurse, making a diagnosis, and providing appropriate medical orders. With more advanced students, the interdisciplinary simulation might reflect a difference of opinion as to best care or an ethical dilemma related to possible care and treatment options. Other team members that should be incorporated include physical therapists, respiratory therapists, nutritionists, social workers, and pharmacists, among others.

In IPE simulations, students typically portray roles within their own profession. They learn about other professions by observing others portray their role in the simulation and through the discussion in debriefing. There may be occasions when it is valuable to switch roles. A variety of simulation experiences may be used to help students understand other health care provider roles and responsibilities and to create some empathy for what the other professions experience.

Simulation can be used as a method to evaluate student knowledge and abilities. In introductory courses, students might have to identify normal or abnormal heart or breath sounds; in more advanced courses they might be required to demonstrate competency, for example, by recognizing deterioration of a patient's status and taking appropriate action. Faculty need to reach a philosophical consensus when using simulation as an evaluation tool. Is the desired outcome to bring all students to a certain level of ability prior to allowing them to progress in the curriculum? This would typically indicate that students would have multiple opportunities to attempt the simulation, with assistance to improve as needed. Or, is the intent of the graded simulation to prevent progression of students unable to demonstrate a certain level of ability? This might mean that students would have only one opportunity to pass the simulation. Is there a grade associated with the simulation? If the simulation contributes to a grade in a course, a grading rubric is needed. Faculty also should reach a curricular consensus as to how to evaluate a simulation. At this time there is no standard recommendation as to how to most effectively evaluate student performance in a simulation; however, many options exist in the literature.

When students must achieve a certain level of performance during a simulation or else they fail a course or cannot graduate, the simulation is termed "high stakes." Cordeau (2010), in her study of students' perceptions of clinical simulation, provides several insights relevant to high-stakes simulations, which should be considered by faculty. First, students will have increased anxiety when simulation is used as a testing or evaluation criteria. Second, anxiety is experienced at all phases of the simulation from presimulation to the debriefing process. While a small amount of anxiety can sharpen performance, high anxiety will impair performance. Faculty should make efforts to maintain student anxiety at a manageable level so that students can be successful in meeting the outcomes of the clinical simulation.

Third, adequate student preparation is needed to overcome anxiety and to foster success. Students should be oriented to the simulation environment and given adequate information about the simulation experience prior to the start. Prebriefing should include information about the simulated patient, similar to the nursing report that is shared before a nurse assumes the care of a patient. In addition, practice sessions, appropriate cues, and fidelity in a simulation can help students to be successful and demonstrate their best performance during the simulation. Finally, one of the most important issues related to using simulation for high-stakes testing is the need to use multiple evaluators who have had preparation and then establish interrater reliability prior to initiating this form of assessment. Finally, educators need to be prepared to legally defend the scenarios and the evaluation rubrics used for high-stakes testing with simulation (Rutherford-Hemming, Kardong-Edgren, Gore, Ravert, & Rizzolo, 2014).

The National League for Nursing (NLN, 2012) has developed competency assessments using standardized simulations to assess postlicensure competence (Hinton et al., 2012; Rizzolo, Kardong-Edgren, Oermann, & Jeffries, 2015). Decker, Utterback, Thomas, Mitchell, and Sportsman (2011) contended that assessment of continued competency must be considered a responsibility shared by the individual nurse, professional organizations, regulatory agencies, and employers. As these assessment simulations are developed, it is likely that they will be added as a component for determining prelicensure competency.

IMPLEMENTATION OF SIMULATIONS

Once simulation experiences that are needed in the curriculum and the best methodology of presenting them have been identified by faculty, implementation can begin (Exhibit 7.1). To create an effective learning experience, faculty should carefully plan all aspects relevant to running the simulation. Using simulation as a teaching strategy cannot be done successfully as a spur-of-the-moment decision.

The first step is the creation or selection of the simulation scenario. This might be done with several content experts writing and reviewing a draft of the simulation after consulting the literature to ensure that current guidelines for evidence-based practice are met. A template is helpful to provide a standardized structure for the simulation and to guarantee that key aspects are not overlooked; resources for faculty are available

EXHIBIT 7.1 Checklist for Implementation of a Simulation

- Create or select the simulation scenario and objectives
- Determine your resources
  - Number of manikins or standardized patients available
  - Number of simulation rooms available
  - Number of faculty available to assist in running simulation
- Determine the time needed to run scenario and debriefing
- Determine the time needed to allow all students to participate in simulation
  - Number of student groups
  - Include time to rotate groups
- Determine the date(s) and time(s) the simulation will run

at the NLN Simulation Innovation Research Center (SIRC; sirc.nln.org). Specific learning objectives and student outcomes should be identified. They should accurately reflect what students can actually accomplish in the allotted time given their skills and abilities. A detailed description related to staging the scene should include factors such as how the manikin or patient will "look," what equipment needs to be in the room, what supplies the student will need to perform in the simulation, what props will add realism, what information needs to be in the patient's medical record, and how the patient will respond (verbally, physiologically) to interventions made by the nurse. All of these details must be considered, planned, and directly written into the simulation scenario.

An alternative to writing simulations is using premade or purchased scenarios. These have the advantage that the content has, in most circumstances, been reviewed by experts and determined to accurately reflect current standards of practice. Premade or purchased simulations may be adjusted to meet local differences in care practices or to level the simulation to meet the learner's abilities at a given point in the curriculum. For faculty just learning to use simulation, this simplifies the process of incorporating simulation into the curriculum.

The remainder of planning and implementing simulations into a course involves practical issues of running a simulation. A primary consideration is how much time will be needed for the simulation and debriefing. Many times, scenarios run 10 to 30 minutes, and historically the debriefing has taken at least twice the time of the scenario or longer, but these are generalizations. Many factors go into the timing decisions of simulation planning, including the complexity of the simulation, the level and roles of the learners, and the outcomes of the experience. It also is important to take into account the total number of students participating in simulation and the amount of time that is available.

Consider this example. A basic simulation of 10 minutes also has 20 minutes of debriefing time. It will therefore take 30 minutes for each group of students to complete the simulation. If you have 50 students, and you want them to participate in the simulation in groups of five, and each group needs 30 minutes for the simulation and debriefing, it will take at least 5 hours to run the simulation if you only have one manikin or SP to use at a time. Next consider how much time you have available. Are you using class time (for example, a 50-minute time slot)? This amount of time is not sufficient to run the simulation twice. At least 60 minutes is needed to run it twice, plus the additional time that is needed to rotate students and reset the room for the next group.

In addition to time, there are other resources that should be considered. The number of simulation rooms and manikins or SPs that can be used at a single time is an important variable. Also important to consider is how many faculty members and simulation staff are familiar with the pedagogy and technology and can be available to assist with facilitating the simulation. Faculty need to plan thoroughly for a simulation experience and consider all aspects needed to run the simulation smoothly. Attention to detail is important. Sufficient time has to be allotted to design, plan, and implement simulations into the curriculum. When the simulation day runs smoothly, faculty and staff are less stressed, and students receive a more positive learning experience.

DEBRIEFING

Debriefing is an important component of student learning in simulation. Typically, debriefing immediately follows a simulation as an opportunity for the nursing students and teachers to review the experience and learn from what happened (Arafeh, Hansen, & Nichlos, 2010; Dreifuerst, 2009; Fanning & Gaba, 2007; Waznonis, 2014). During debriefing, teachers can guide students to discuss, analyze, and synthesize their thoughts and feelings about the experience. It is also a time to carefully review the actions and clinical decisions that occurred during the simulation (Dreifuerst, 2012; Lusk & Fater, 2013) and discuss options and alternatives to improve the nursing care or patient outcomes. Because of the sensitive nature of the discussion, holding debriefing in a comfortable private area, away from the actual simulated patient environment, is an important consideration (Wickers, 2010). There are many ways to debrief; however, it is common for teachers and students to focus the discussion on what went right, what went wrong, and what should be done differently during the next simulation experience or similar patient encounter (Dismukes, Gaba, & Howard, 2006; Dreifuerst & Decker, 2012).

Because debriefing is a constructivist, reflective teaching strategy (Cantrell, 2008; Dufrene & Young, 2014; Shinnick, Woo, Horwich, & Steadman, 2011), it commonly involves an interactive discussion between the students who were directly involved in the simulation scenario, the students who observed the simulation, and the teacher. These lively discussions should use the learning objectives or outcomes as a guide. Debriefing using this format becomes a type of formative feedback, which is intended to change thinking and behaviors when the student encounters similar issues in clinical practice (Fey, Scrandis, Daniels, & Haut, 2014; Rudolph, Simon, Raemer, & Eppich, 2008).

Providing feedback is only one component of the role of the teacher as debriefer. The debriefer typically guides the debriefing experience by acting as a mentor, coach, or teacher depending on the situation, students, and simulation outcomes. The debriefer's role in the debriefing process can vary because it is dependent on the skill level of the participants, how much guidance is needed to keep the discussion flowing, and the outcome of the simulation. Teachers generally are more active debriefing facilitators when the students are novices and new to simulation and when there has been an emotional experience by one or more of the participants. Likewise, the teacher can guide the discussion to provide additional support when negative simulation outcomes or poor student performance have occurred (Dreifuerst, 2015; Fanning & Gaba, 2007). As the students gain experience and knowledge, they assume a more active role in the discussion and the debriefer can become more of a guide and less of a facilitator.

Guiding the discussion can involve the use of many communication strategies by the teacher doing the debriefing. These include incorporation of open-ended questions, active listening, Socratic questioning, re-stating, re-phrasing, and leading questions. These techniques may require training and practice by the teacher prior to the actual simulation experience (Cheng et al., 2016; Dreifuerst, 2015; Dufrene & Young, 2014).

Continuing education opportunities to learn evidence-based debriefing practices and strategies are available from a variety of venues, including formal education sessions and informal peer coaching. These are also opportunities to learn new ways and methods that can be used to debrief students. Recent studies have shown the importance of faculty development and training in debriefing for consistent outcomes (Jeffries, Dreifuerst, & Kardong-Edgren, 2015; Waznonis, 2014).

There are many debriefing methods that are used in health care simulations (Exhibit 7.2). While many of these methods share similar practices, each has unique attributes that support different learners and environments (Husebo, Dieckmann, Rystedt, Soreide, & Friberg, 2013; Overstreet, 2010). Reflection is an essential component of debriefing regardless of the method used (Dreifuerst, 2009; Shinnick et al., 2011). Revisiting the events of the simulation is important to understand the student's behaviors, decision making, and impact on patient outcomes. Reflecting also solidifies learning from the experience, particularly when attention is paid to reflecting-in-action, reflecting-on-action, and reflecting-beyond-action (Dreifuerst, 2009; Schön, 1983). There are many debriefing methods that can be used to guide the reflective process. Some of the more common debriefing methods include Plus Delta, Debriefing for

EXHIBIT 7.2 Debriefing Methods

Plus Delta
- What went right
- What would you change

DML
- Reflection-in-action
- Reflection-on-action
- Reflection-beyond-action
- Clinical reasoning and thinking like a nurse
- Relationship between thinking and actions

Advocacy-Inquiry
- Statement of advocacy or assertion
- Request for clarification

GAS
- Pull together pertinent information
- Discuss details of what went well and what did not
- Review all aspects of the experience in the context of the debriefing discussion

PEARLS
- Reaction Phase
- Description Phase
- Analysis Phase
- Learner Self-Assessment
- Feedback and Teaching
- Summary Phase

DML, Debriefing for Meaningful Learning; GAS, Gather-Analyze-Summarize; PEARLS, Promoting Excellence and Reflective Learning in Simulation.

Meaningful Learning© (DML), Advocacy-Inquiry, Gather-Analyze-Summarize (GAS), and Promoting Excellence and Reflective Learning in Simulation (PEARLS).

Variations of the Plus Delta debriefing method are popular in interdisciplinary health care simulations. This method emphasizes what went well (plus) and what could be done better or differently (delta, which is the Greek symbol for change), by soliciting reflective responses from the students involved in the simulation (Fanning & Gaba, 2007). This method is not difficult and is easily adapted to many different types of simulations and learners.

DML is a structured method that incorporates clinical teaching with debriefing to emphasize reflection-in-action, reflection-on-action, and reflection-beyond-action; clinical reasoning; and thinking like a nurse (Dreifuerst, 2009, 2015; Schön, 1983; Tanner, 2006). A premise of this method is that the facilitator must be a clinician or a clinical teacher with knowledge about the patient population. The facilitator guides the reflective process of uncovering the students' thinking that underpinned their actions and decisions during the simulation (Dreifuerst, 2015).

In the Advocacy-Inquiry debriefing method, which comes from the Debriefing with Good Judgment Model (Rudolph, Simon, Rivard, Dufresne, & Raemer, 2007), the teacher focuses the debriefing on a particular component of the simulation because the student involved in the experience has done something unexpected or unanticipated. The discussion begins with a statement of advocacy or assertion about what was observed from the teacher's perspective, followed by a question or request for clarification about their thinking and actions from the students in a nonthreatening way (Rudolph et al., 2007).

The GAS method uses a three-step debriefing process (American Heart Association, 2010). Teachers guide the students to integrate or gather all of the pertinent information about the simulation experience, including what occurred, the decisions that were made, and outcomes. Next, the participants and facilitator analyze the information that has been gathered using the objectives for the simulation as well as what went right and what did not. Finally, everything that has been discussed is summarized to reinforce learning. PEARLS represents a method of debriefing that advocates educators' intentional use of a variety of debriefing strategies to individualize the discussion to meet particular learner needs and unique learning environments (Cheng et al., 2016).

Regardless of the method used, debriefing that includes reflection and revisiting of the events and actions to understand behaviors, decision making, and the impact on patient outcomes is an essential part of simulation learning (Decker & Dreifuerst, 2012; Dreifuerst, 2009; Shinnick et al., 2011). Additionally, debriefing should include the objectives of the experience and an intentional method of recalling the events of the simulation. Students should be actively involved in the discussion and have an opportunity to clarify anything that is uncertain during debriefing. Teachers who use simulation should feel comfortable facilitating debriefing as an important component of student learning.

SIMULATION EVALUATION

Simulation activities offer educators and researchers unique opportunities for evaluation. Similar to clinical evaluation, simulation evaluations often focus on participant performance. However, many view simulation as a highly adaptable alternative to traditional clinical experiences and consequently may hold simulation to higher evaluation standards. This is because when there was no alternative to clinical practice for students, there was little reason to question how well it worked. However, with the advent of simulation, it became necessary to examine the efficacy of teaching in both the clinical and simulation environments more carefully. Simulation evaluations, therefore, focus not only on participant performance, but also on design characteristics, educational practices, participant satisfaction, how learning that takes place in simulation occurs and subsequently transfers to the clinical area, and ultimately the impact of simulation on patient outcomes.

The first step in planning an effective simulation participant evaluation is to identify the purpose and focus of the evaluation. Questions to ask at this stage include: What type of data will be gathered and what will it be used for? Should the evaluation reflect individual or group performance? At this stage, it is also important to decide whether the evaluation is formative or summative. Next, it is important to identify the ideal simulation modality for the evaluation. For example, if the evaluation is meant to reflect participants' IV insertion skills, a task-trainer may be the most efficient simulation modality. However, if interpersonal communication skills are to be evaluated, an SP may offer the most realism and opportunities for valid evaluation.

Selecting or developing an appropriate evaluation instrument is the next key step in the evaluation process. From this point, carefully selecting and training raters to complete the evaluation helps ensure valid and reliable results. This may be as simple as identifying an individual or as complex as selecting and training a group of raters and assessing important criteria such as interrater reliability. With these decisions made, it is finally time for collecting, interpreting, and reporting evaluation data. Additional guidelines on assessment are provided in Chapter 12 and on clinical evaluation in Chapter 14. These guidelines are relevant to the evaluation process using simulation.

CATEGORIZING SIMULATION EVALUATION STRATEGIES

Recent years have seen a proliferation of published simulation evaluation instruments (Kardong-Edgren, Adamson, & Fitzgerald, 2010) and articles about simulation evaluation in nursing (Ball & Kilger, 2016; Benbenek et al., 2016; Oermann, Kardong-Edgren, & Rizzolo, 2016; Stayt, Merriman, Ricketts, Morton, & Simpson, 2015; Trail Ross, Otto, & Stewart Helton, 2017), and the health sciences (Bray, Schwartz, Odegard, Hammer, & Seybert, 2011; Kogan, Holmboe, & Hauer, 2009). Simulation evaluation can be categorized into three basic phases: pre-implementation, implementation, and outcomes. The Simulation Design Scale (SDS) and Educational Practices Simulation Scale (EPSS; Jeffries, 2012) are examples of resources that may be used for evaluation during the pre-implementation and implementation phases to evaluate the quality of simulation activities. The quality of simulation activities, in turn, influences the outcomes of the activities. Most simulation evaluations focus on learners' outcomes.

Kirkpatrick (1998) described four levels of outcomes that are helpful for categorizing evaluation strategies (Table 7.1). These levels, as they apply to simulation evaluation, are:

- Level 1: participants' reactions to the simulation activity
- Level 2: participants' learning from the simulation activity
- Level 3: changes in participants' behavior as a result of the simulation activity
- Level 4: long-term results in practice that take place because of the simulation activity

The category of learning (Level 2) may be further divided using the three domains of learning: cognitive, affective, and psychomotor. While many simulation evaluations seek to cover multiple levels and learning domains, using Kirkpatrick's language helps to describe the focus (or foci) of the particular strategy.

Evaluations become increasingly more difficult, but potentially more meaningful, as learners progress from Level 1 (reaction) to Level 4 (results). For example, it is

TABLE 7.1 Different Levels of Evaluation According to the Kirkpatrick Model (1998)

Level of Evaluation	Example	Reference
Level 1: Reaction	National League for Nursing Participant Satisfaction and Self-Confidence in Learning Instruments	National League for Nursing www.nln.org
	Emergency Response Confidence Tool	Arnold et al. (2009)
Level 2: Learning *Cognitive*	Paper-and-pencil exam questions	Hoffman, O'Donnell, and Kim (2007)
	Observation-based simulation evaluation instruments such as the Sweeny-Clark Simulation Performance Evaluation Rubric	Clark (2006)
Level 2: Learning *Affective*	Interpersonal Communication Assessment Scale (ICAS)	Klakovich and de la Cruz (2006)
Level 2: Learning *Psychomotor*	Skills checklists such as the American Heart Association performance evaluation rubrics for CPR, ACLS, PALS, etc.	American Heart Association (2010)
Level 3: Behavior	Clinical performance of students who attended simulations and students who did not	Meyer, Connors, Hou, and Gajewski (2012)
	Multiple measures to investigate thinking and behaviors related to care of patient with heart failure	Shinnick and Woo (2013)
Level 4: Results	Measure of cost savings resulting from simulation-based training on central venous catheters and blood infections	Cohen et al. (2010)
	Measures related to improved management of neonatal shoulder dystocia that resulted from simulation-based training	Draycott et al. (2008)

ACLS, advanced cardiac life support; CPR, cardiopulmonary resuscitation; PALS, pediatric advanced life support.

much easier to ask participants to rate their level of satisfaction with a simulation activity (Level 1: reaction) or assess participant knowledge before and after a simulation activity (Level 2: learning [cognitive]) than it is to determine whether a simulation activity impacts how participants performed in the clinical environment (Level 3: behavior) or changes patient outcomes (Level 4: results). However, the effort to produce such evaluations is commensurate with their potential impact. The information provided by Level 3 and 4 evaluations has much greater impact than the information provided by the lower levels of evaluation (Levels 1 and 2).

PARTICIPANT PERFORMANCE EVALUATION

Many of the characteristics of clinical evaluation discussed in Chapter 14 are relevant to simulation participant evaluation. However, simulation offers evaluation opportunities that may not exist in traditional clinical environments. These include, but are not limited to, the ability to (a) create and standardize scenarios to isolate and elicit specific participant skills and behaviors, (b) allow multiple participants to engage in a given scenario or an individual participant to engage in a given scenario multiple times, and (c) allow a participant to make errors without endangering a patient.

Simulation holds enormous promise for participant evaluation (Benner, Sutphen, Leonard, & Day, 2010) beyond augmenting assessment in the clinical environment. In the future, these evaluations may be implemented as an alternative or adjunct to the current multiple-choice examinations used for academic progression and licensure, or may simply be employed to reflect formative evaluations of participant performance. Thoughtful planning and a focus on higher levels of evaluation that reflect learning, behavior, and results from simulation training are important to the development of simulation pedagogy.

BEST EVIDENCE AND RESEARCH IN SIMULATION

Simulation has been shown to be an effective educational method. Some recent meta-analyses examined learning outcomes from simulation and showed positive effects of simulation (Cook, 2014; Lee & Oh, 2015). Over the past decade, researchers have been able to identify 12 best practices that lead to effective learning in simulation (McGaghie, Isenberg, Petrusa, & Scalese, 2010). The most important practice for simulation learning is to provide feedback. In most cases, feedback is provided within the debriefing period to identify and correct performance gaps observed during the simulation. Although further research is needed to identify specific models for feedback, one method, DML, has shown to improve clinical reasoning and judgment scores when compared with usual debriefing methods (Dreifuerst, 2012; Mariani, Cantrell, Meakim, Prieto, & Dreifuerst, 2012). Further research is needed on evidence-based strategies for debriefing methods that address the structure of debriefing, faculty demeanor, environment, types of probing and cueing questions, and the timeliness of debriefing (Neill & Wotton, 2011).

Deliberate practice, another best practice within simulation, is a method used to assist the learner to master a clinical skill or behavior (Ericsson, 2008). This method requires well-defined objectives that guide engaged learners to improve their ability to perform a skill through repetitive practice with feedback, error correction, mastery, and advancement to the next level. Simulation that incorporates deliberate practice is associated with a large effect size (ES = 0.71) when compared with traditional clinical education, and has been shown to be superior to traditional education in achieving acquisition of clinical skills such as advanced cardiac life support, cardiac auscultation, and central venous catheter insertion (McGaghie, Issenberg, Petrusa, & Scalese, 2010).

Although simulation as an educational method has been shown to have a positive effect on learning when compared with other educational modalities, more research is needed in several areas. First, there is a lack of valid and reliable evaluation instruments to measure simulation outcomes (Kardong-Edgren, Adamson, & Fitzgerald, 2010). Evaluation tools must be developed and tested to ensure that the tool measures the outcomes of simulation, whether for formative or summative evaluation, and that improved patient outcomes may be attributed to simulation learning. Next, if simulation is to be used for high-stakes, end-of-program evaluation, further research is needed to determine the type of simulation scenarios as well as reliable and valid tools that best measure these outcomes (Bensfield, Olech, & Horsley, 2012; Oermann, Kardong-Edgren, & Rizzolo, 2016). Finally, there is much interest in determining whether using simulation in an educational program has a positive effect on quality and safety in the health care setting. To that end, there is a move to use simulation as a method to evaluate continued competence of health care providers on the public's behalf (Decker et al., 2011; Hinton et al., 2012).

Nurse educators who are interested in simulation research should seek opportunities to work collaboratively with other nursing and health care colleagues to build on current knowledge and expand the scholarship of simulation. There is a call for more large-scale multisite national studies to better evaluate the effect of simulation in nursing and health care.

Simulation will play an increasingly important role in shaping the future of nursing education (Committee on the Robert Wood Johnson Foundation Initiative on the Future of Nursing at the Institute of Medicine, 2011). In response to widespread questions about the use of simulation as an adjunct or replacement to traditional clinical experiences, the National Council of State Boards of Nursing (2012) completed a national, multiyear study to guide the current and future use of simulation in nursing education (Hayden, 2010; Hayden et al., 2014; Kardong-Edgren, Willhaus, Bennett, & Hayden, 2012). This landmark study explored the amount of real clinical time that could be substituted for clinical simulations in a controlled, nonthreatening environment. There were three groups of participants ($N = 666$) across 10 different schools of nursing (five baccalaureate and five associate degree programs in the United States). One group, serving as the control, had less than 10% of clinical time substituted by clinical simulations, another group had 25% of the clinical time substituted with simulations, and a third group had up to 50% of clinical time across seven different courses. The clinical practice time was substituted with controlled, immersive clinical simulations in four semesters of a generic baccalaureate and an associate degree nursing program.

Findings from this national study included:

1. Up to 50% simulation can be effectively substituted for traditional clinical experience in all core courses across the prelicensure nursing curriculum.
2. Fifty percent simulation can be effectively used in various program types, in different geographic areas in urban and rural settings with good educational outcomes.
3. NCLEX-RN® pass rates were unaffected by the substitution of simulation throughout the curriculum.
4. All three groups were equally prepared for entry into practice as a new graduate RNs.
5. Policy decisions about the use and amount of simulation in nursing should depend on the use of best practices in simulation.

This study in nursing education has made an impact on how teachers are using and integrating simulations into the nursing curricula. In addition, guidelines for state boards of nursing regulators and for leaders in schools of nursing have been developed, with variance across states and programs (Alexander et al., 2015).

The science of simulation also continues to develop. The NLN Jeffries Simulation Framework has now been labeled as a mid-range theory called the NLN Jeffries Simulation Theory, as shown in Figure 7.1. The variables within the theory remain similar to the framework with the theory guiding and providing a roadmap for simulation development, integration, evaluation, and research (Jeffries, 2015). The INACSL Standards of Best Practice Simulation[SM] (www.inacsl.org/i4a/pages/index.cfm?pageID=3407) and certifications in simulation education have become more mature and operationalized in simulation work and development.

FIGURE 7.1 Diagram of NLN Jeffries Simulation Theory©.

NLN, National League for Nursing.

Source: Copyright 2015 by the National League for Nursing (2012). Reprinted with permission.

There are two types of certification offered by the international organization Society for Simulation in Healthcare (SSH; www.ssih.org/Certification). These include certified health simulation educator (CHSE) and advanced certification for health simulation educators (CHSE-A). The purposes for which health professionals might seek these certifications include to: (a) improve health care simulation education through the identification of best practices and recognition of practice; (b) improve health care simulation by providing standardizations and a pool of knowledge of best practices; (c) provide external validation of individual educator knowledge, skills, and attitudes; and (d) strengthen the organizational community and learner confidence in the quality of education provided in simulation (Society for Simulation in Healthcare [SSH], 2017a). These credentials define and recognize achievement of best practices in simulation pedagogy. Simulation holds great promise for increasing the validity of nursing licensure and credentialing processes through incorporation of standardized testing practices involving simulation. Internationally, simulation is used for inter-disciplinary health care professional licensure examinations and may play a role in such processes within the United States in the future (Holmboe, Rizzolo, Sachdeva, Rosenberg, & Ziv, 2011).

Simulation centers, local and global, can now be accredited through the SSH. Certification of simulation centers, or simulation programs in health care, is possible when there is evidence of an organizational group with dedicated resources (person-nel and equipment) whose mission is specifically targeted toward improving patient safety and outcomes through assessment, research, advocacy, and education using simulation. Centers and programs can seek SSH accreditation in three areas of simula-tion: (a) assessment, (b) research, and (c) teaching/education (Society for Simulation in Healthcare [SSH], 2017b).

SUMMARY

The importance of the development of simulation pedagogy in nursing education can-not be underestimated. The rapid infusion of the innovative technology associated with high-fidelity manikins, sophistication of gaming, and impact of the use of SPs have all contributed to the rise in simulation use in nursing education today. Despite this increased use, there is continued need for research into best practices for further inte-gration into the nursing curriculum and evaluation of simulation use and impact on health care practices of the future.

REFERENCES

Alexander, M. A., Durham, C. F., Hooper, J. I., Jeffries, P. R, Goldman, N., Kardong-Edgren, S., . . . Tillman, C. (2015). The NCSBN simulation guidelines for prelicensure nursing programs. *Journal of Nursing Regulation, 6*(3), 39–42.

American Heart Association. (2010). Structured and supported debriefing. Retrieved from http://members.nata.org/education/f/ATEC2015/GAS-Model-of-Debriefing.pdf

Arafeh, J. M., Hansen, S. S., & Nichols, A. (2010). Debriefing in simulated-based learning: Facilitat-ing a reflective discussion. *Journal of Perinatal & Neonatal Nursing, 24*, 302–309. doi:10.1097/JPN.0b013e3181f6b5ec

Arnold, J. J., Johnson, L. M., Tucker, S. J., Malec, J. F., Henrickson, S. E., & Dunn, W. F. (2009). Evaluation tools in simulation learning: Performance and self-efficacy in emergency response. *Clinical Simula-tion in Nursing, 5*(1), e35–e45. doi:10.1016/j.ecns.2008.10.003

Ball, L. S., & Kilger, L. (2016). Analyzing nursing student learning over time in simulation. *Nursing Education Perspectives, 37*, 328–330.

Bauchat, J. R., Seropian, M., & Jeffries, P. R. (2016). Communication and empathy in the patient-centered care model: Why simulation-based training is not optional. *Clinical Simulation in Nursing, 12*(8), 356–359. doi:10.1016/j.ecns.2016.04.003

Benbenek, M., Dierich, M., Wyman, J., Avery, M., Juve, C., & Miller, J. (2016). Development and imple-mentation of a capstone objective structured clinical examination in nurse practitioner and nurse-midwifery programs. *Nurse Educator, 41*, 288–293. doi:10.1097/NNE.0000000000000283

Benner, P. E., Sutphen, M., Leonard, V., & Day, L. (2010). *Educating nurses: A call for radical transformation.* San Francisco, CA: Jossey-Bass.

Bensfield, L., Olech, M., & Horsley, T. (2012). Simulation for high-stakes evaluation in nursing. *Nurse Educator, 37*, 71–74. doi:10.1097/NNE.0b013e3182461b8c

Bray, B. S., Schwartz, C. R., Odegard, P. S., Hammer, D. P., & Seybert, A. L. (2011). Assessment of human patient simulation-based learning. *American Journal of Pharmaceutical Education, 75*(10), Article 208. doi:10.5688/ajpe7510208

Cantrell, M. A. (2008). The importance of debriefing in clinical simulations. *Clinical Simulation in Nursing, 4*(2), e19–e23. doi:10.1016/j.ecns.2008.06.006

Carlson, K. J., & Gagnon, D. J. (2016, April). Augmented reality integrated simulation education in health care. *Clinical Simulation in Nursing, 12*(4), 123–127. doi:10.1016/j.ecns.2015.12.005

Cheng, A., Grant, V., Robinson, T., Catena, H., Lachapelle, K., Kim, J., . . . Eppich, W. (2016). The promoting excellence and reflective learning in simulation (PEARLS) approach to health care debriefing: A faculty development guide. *Clinical Simulation in Nursing, 12*(10), 419–428. doi:10.1016/j.ecns.2016.05.002

Clark, M. (2006). Evaluating an obstetric trauma scenario. *Clinical Simulation in Nursing, 2*(2), e75–e77. doi:10.1016/j.ecns.2009.05.028

Cohen, E. R., Feinglass, J., Barsuk, J. H., Bernard, C., O'Donnell, A., McGaghie, W. C., & Wayne, D. B. (2010). Cost savings from reduced catheter-related bloodstream infection after simulation-based education for residents in a medical intensive care unit. *Simulation in Healthcare, 5,* 98–102. doi:10.1097/SIH.0b013e3181bc8304

Committee on the Robert Wood Johnson Foundation Initiative on the Future of Nursing at the Institute of Medicine. (2011). *The future of nursing: Leading change, advancing health.* Washington, DC: National Academies Press.

Cook, D. A. (2014). How much evidence does it take? A cumulative meta-analysis of outcomes of simulation-based education. *Medical Education, 48,* 750–760. doi:10.1111/medu.12473

Cordeau, M. A. (2010). The lived experience of clinical simulation of novice nursing students. *International Journal for Human Caring, 14*(2), 9–15.

Decker, S., & Dreifuerst, K. T. (2012). Integrating guided reflection into simulated learning experiences. In P. Jeffries (Ed.), *Simulation in nursing from conceptualization to evaluation* (2nd ed., pp. 91–104). New York, NY: National League for Nursing.

Decker, S., Utterback, V., Thomas, M., Mitchell, M., & Sportsman, S. (2011). Assessing continued competency through simulation: A call for stringent action. *Nursing Education Perspectives, 32,* 120–125.

Dieckmann, P., Gaba, D., & Rall, M. (2007). Deepening the theoretical foundations of patient simulation as social practice. *Simulation in Healthcare, 2,* 183–193. doi:10.1097/SIH.0b013e3180f637f5

Dismukes, R. K., Gaba, D. M., & Howard, S. K. (2006). So many roads: Facilitated debriefing in healthcare. *Simulation in Healthcare, 1*(1), 23–25.

Draycott, T. J, Crofts, J. F., Ash, J. P., Wilson, L. V., Yard, E., Sibanda, T., & Whitelaw, A. (2008). Improving neonatal outcome through practical shoulder dystocia training. *Obstetrics and Gynecology, 112*(1), 14–20.

Dreifuerst, K. T. (2009). The essentials of debriefing in simulation learning: A concept analysis. *Nursing Education Perspectives, 30,* 109–114.

Dreifuerst, K. T. (2012). Using debriefing for meaningful learning to foster development of clinical reasoning in simulation. *Journal of Nursing Education, 51,* 326–333. doi:10.3928/01484834-20120409-02

Dreifuerst, K. T. (2015). Getting started with debriefing for meaningful learning. *Clinical Simulation in Nursing, 11*(5), 268–275. doi:10.1016/j.ecns.2015.01.005

Dreifuerst, K. T., & Decker, S. (2012). Debriefing: An essential component for learning in simulation pedagogy. In P. Jeffries (Ed.), *Simulation in nursing from conceptualization to evaluation* (2nd ed., pp. 105–130). New York, NY: National League for Nursing.

Dufrene, C., & Young, A. (2014). Successful debriefing: Best methods to achieve positive learning outcomes: A literature review. *Nurse Education Today, 34,* 372–376. doi:10.1016/j.nedt.2013.06.026

Ericsson, K. (2008). Deliberate practice and acquisition of expert performance: A general overview. *Academic Emergency Medicine, 15,* 988–994. doi:10.1111/j.1553-2712.2008.00227.x

Fanning, R. M., & Gaba, D. M. (2007). The role of debriefing in simulation-based learning. *Simulation in Healthcare, 2,* 115–125. doi:10.1097/SIH.0b013e3180315539

Feinstein, A. H., & Cannon, H. M. (2002). Constructs of simulation evaluation. *Simulation & Gaming, 33,* 425–440. doi:10.1177/1046878102238606

Fey, M. K., Scrandis, D., Daniels, A., & Haut, C. (2014). Learning through debriefing: Students' perspectives. *Clinical Simulation in Nursing, 10*(5), e249–e256. doi:10.1016/j.ecns.2013.12.009

Foronda, C. L., Alfes, C. M., Dev, P., Kleinheksel, A. J., Nelson, D. A., O'Donnell, J. M., & Samosky, J. T. (2017). Virtually nursing: Emerging technologies in nursing education. *Nurse Educator, 42,* 14–17. doi:10.1097/NNE.0000000000000295

Greiner, A. C., & Knebel, E. (2003). *Health professions education: A bridge to quality.* Washington, DC: National Academies Press.

Hayden, J. (2010). Use of simulation in nursing education: National survey results. *Journal of Nursing Regulation, 1*(3), 52–57. doi:10.1016/S2155–8256(15)30335-5

Hayden, J., Smiley, R., Alexander, M. A., Kardong-Edgren, S., & Jeffries, P. J. (2014). The NCSBN National simulation study: A longitudinal, randomized, controlled study replacing clinical hours with simulation in prelicensure nursing education. *Journal of Nursing Regulation, 5*(Suppl. 2), S3–S40.

Herrmann, E. K. (2008). Remembering Mrs. Chase. Before there were Smart Hospitals and Sim-Men, there was "Mrs. Chase". *Imprint, 55*(2), 52.

Hinton, J. E., Mays, M. Z., Hagler, D., Randolph, P., Brooks, R., DeFalco, N., . . . Weberg, D. (2012). Measuring postlicensure competence with simulation: The nursing performance profile. *Journal of Nursing Regulation, 3*(2), 45–53.

Hoffman, R., O'Donnell, J., & Kim, Y. (2007). The effects of human patient simulators on basic knowledge in critical care nursing with undergraduate senior nursing students. *Simulation in Healthcare, 2*, 110–114. doi:10.1097/SIH.0b013e318033abb5

Holmboe, E. M., Rizzolo, M. A., Sachdeva, A. K., Rosenberg, M. D., & Ziv, A. (2011). Simulation-based assessment and the regulation of healthcare professionals. *Simulation in Healthcare, 6*(Suppl. 7), S58–S62.

Husebo, S. E., Dieckmann, P., Rystedt, H., Soreide, E., & Friberg, F. (2013). The relationship between facilitators' questions and the level of reflection in post simulation debriefing. *Simulation in Healthcare, 8*, 135–142. doi:10.1097/SIH.0b013e31827cbb5c

International Nursing Association for Clinical Simulation and Learning Standards Committee. (2016). INACSL standards of best practice: Simulation℠ Simulation glossary. *Clinical Simulation in Nursing, 12* (Suppl.), S39–S47. doi:10.1016/j.ecns.2016.09.012

Irwin, P., & Coutts, R. (2015). A systematic review of the experience of using second life in the education of undergraduate nurses. *Journal of Nursing Education, 54*, 572–577. doi:10.3928/01484834-20150916-05

Jeffries P. R. (2012). Designing simulation scenarios to promote learning. In P. R. Jeffries (Ed.), *Simulation in nursing education: From conceptualization to evaluation* (2nd ed., pp. 43–76). New York, NY: National League for Nursing.

Jeffries, P. R. (2015). *The NLN Jeffries simulation theory: A monograph.* Philadelphia, PA: Wolters Kluwer.

Jeffries, P. R., Dreifuerst, K. T., & Kardong-Edgren, S. (2015). Faculty development when initiating simulation programs: Lessons learned from the NCSBN simulation study. *Journal of Nursing Regulation, 5*(3), 1–8.

Jeffries, P. R., & Rogers, K. (2007). Theoretical framework for simulation design. In P. R. Jeffries (Ed.), *Simulation in Nursing Education from conceptualization to evaluation* (pp. 21–33). New York, NY: National League for Nursing.

Kardong-Edgren, S., Adamson, K., & Fitzgerald, C. (2010). A review of currently published evaluation instruments for human patient simulation. *Clinical Simulation in Nursing, 6*(1), e25–e35. doi:10.1016/j.ecns.2009.08.004

Kardong-Edgren, S., Anderson, M., & Michaels, J. (2007). Does simulation fidelity improve student test scores? *Clinical Simulation in Nursing, 3*(1), e21–e24. doi:10.1016/j.ecns.2009.05.035

Kardong-Edgren, S., Willhaus, J., Bennett, D., & Hayden, J. (2012). Results of the National Council of State Boards of Nursing national simulation survey: Part II. *Clinical Simulation in Nursing, 8*(4), e117–e123. doi:10.1016/j.ecns.2012.01.003

Kirkpatrick, D. L. (1998). *Evaluating training programs: The four levels* (2nd ed.). San Francisco, CA: Berrett-Koehler.

Klakovich, M. D., & de la Cruz, F. A. (2006). Validating the interpersonal communication assessment scale. *Journal of Professional Nursing, 22*(1), 60–67. doi:10.1016/j.profnurs.2005.12.005

Kogan, J. R., Holmboes, H., & Hauer, K. E. (2009). Tools for direct observation and assessment of clinical skills of medical trainees. *Journal of the American Medical Association, 302*, 1316–1326. doi:10.1001/jama.2009.1365

Kopp, W., & Hanson, M. (2012). High-fidelity and gaming simulations enhance nursing education in end-of-life care. *Clinical Simulation in Nursing, 8*(3), e97–e102. doi:10.1016/j.ecns.2010.07.005

Lapkin, S., Levett-Jones, T., Bellchambers, H., & Fernandez, R. (2010). Effectiveness of patient simulation manikins in teaching clinical reasoning skills to undergraduate nursing students: A systematic review. *Clinical Simulation in Nursing, 6*(6), e207–e222. doi:10.1016/j.ecns.2010.05.005

Lee, J., & Oh, P. J. (2015). Effects of the use of high-fidelity human simulation in nursing education: A meta-analysis. *Journal of Nursing Education, 54*, 501–507. doi:10.3928/01484834-20150814-04

LeFlore, J., Anderson, M., Zielke, M., Nelson, K., Thomas, P., Hardee, G., & John, L. (2012). Can a virtual patient trainer teach student nurses how to save lives: Teaching nursing students about pediatric respiratory distress. *Simulation in Healthcare, 7*(1), 10–17. doi:10.1097/SIH.0b013e31823652de

Lusk, J. M., & Fater, K. (2013). Postsimulation debriefing to maximize clinical judgment development. *Nurse Educator, 38,* 16–19. doi:10.1097/NNE.0b013e318276df8b

Mariani, B., Cantrell, M. A., Meakim, C., Prieto, P., & Dreifuerst, K. T. (2012). Structured debriefing and students' clinical judgment abilities in simulation. *Clinical Simulation in Nursing, 9*(5), e147–155. doi:10.1016/j.ecns.2011.11.009

May, W., Park, J., & Lee, J. (2009). A ten-year review of the literature on the use of standardized patients in teaching and learning. *Medical Teacher, 31,* 487–492. doi:10.1080/01421590802530898

McGaghie, W., Issenberg, S., Petrusa, E., & Scalese, R. (2010). A critical review of simulation-based medical education research: 2003–2009. *Medical Educator, 44*(1), 50–63. doi:0.1111/j.1365-292009.03547.x

Meyer, M. N., Connors, H., Hou, Q., & Gajewski, B. (2011). The effect of simulation on clinical performance. *Simulation in Healthcare, 6,* 269–277. doi:10.1097/SIH.0b013e318223a048

National Council of State Boards of Nursing. (2012). NCSBN national simulation study. Retrieved from https://www.ncsbn.org/685.htm

National League for Nursing. (2012). A nursing perspective on simulation and interprofessional education (IPE): A report from the National League for Nursing's Think Tank on using simulation as an enabling strategy for IPE. Retrieved from http://www.nln.org/docs/default-source/professional-development-programs/a-nursing-perspective-on-simulation-(ipe-nln-invitational-think-tank-report,-2011)-pdf.pdf?sfvrsn=0

Neill, M., & Wotton, K. (2011). High-fidelity stimulation debriefing in nursing education: A literature review. *Clinical Simulation in Nursing, 7*(5), e161–e168. doi:10.1016/j.ecns.2011.02.001

Norman, G., Dore, K., & Grierson, L. (2012). The minimal relationship between simulation fidelity and transfer of learning. *Medical Education, 46,* 636–647. doi:10.1111/j.1365-2923.2012.04243.x

Oermann, M. H., Kardong-Edgren, S., & Rizzolo, M. A. (2016). Summative simulated-based assessment in nursing programs. *Journal of Nursing Education, 55,* 323–328. doi:10.3928/01484834-20160516-04

Overstreet, M. (2010). E-chats: The seven components of nursing debriefing. *Journal of Continuing Education in Nursing, 41*(12), 538–539. doi:10.3928/00220124-20101122-05

Owen, H. (2012). Early use of simulation in medical education. *Simulation in Healthcare, 7*(2), 102–116. doi:10.1097/SIH.0b013e3182415a91

Rizzolo, M. A., Kardong-Edgren, S., Oermann, M., & Jeffries, P. R. (2015). The National League for Nursing project to explore the use of simulation for high stakes assessment: Process, outcomes, and recommendations. *Nursing Education Perspectives, 36,* 299–303. doi:10.5480/15-1639

Rudolph, J. W., Simon, R., & Raemer, D. B. (2007). Which reality matters? Questions on the path to high engagement in healthcare simulation. *Simulation in Healthcare, 2,* 161–163. doi:10.1097/SIH.0b013e31813d1035

Rudolph, J. W., Simon, R., Raemer, D. B., & Eppich, W. J. (2008). Debriefing as formative assessment: Closing performance gaps in medical education. *Academic Emergency Medicine, 15,* 1010–1016. doi:10.1111/j.1553-2712.2008.00248.x

Rudolph, J. W., Simon, R., Rivard, P., Dufresne, R. L., & Raemer, D. B. (2007). Debriefing with good judgment: Combining rigorous feedback with genuine inquiry. *Anesthesiology Clinics, 25*(2), 361–376. doi:10.1016/j.anclin.2007.03.007

Rutherford-Hemming, T., Kardong-Edgren, S., Gore, T., Ravert, P., & Rizzolo, M. A. (2014). High-Stakes evaluation: Five years later. *Clinical Simulation in Nursing, 10*(12), 605–610. doi:10.1016/j.ecns.2014.09.009

Ryan, C., Walshe, N., Gaffney, R., Shanks, A., Burgoyne, L, & Wiskin, C. (2010). Using standardized patients to assess communication skills in medical and nursing students. *BMC Medical Educator, 10*(24), 1–8. doi:10.1186/1472-6920-10-24

Schön, D. A. (1983). *The reflective practitioner: How professionals think in action.* New York, NY: Basic Books.

Shinnick, M. A., & Woo, M. A. (2013). The effect of human patient simulation on critical thinking and its predictors in prelicensure nursing students. *Nurse Education Today, 33,* 1062–1067. doi:10.1016/j.nedt.2012.04.004

Shinnick, M. A., Woo, M. A., Horwich, T. B., & Steadman, R. (2011). Debriefing: The most important component in simulation. *Clinical Simulation in Nursing, 7*(3), e105–e111. doi:10.1016/j.ecns.2010.11.005

Smith-Stoner, M. (2011). Using moulage to enhance educational instruction. *Nurse Educator, 36,* 21–24. doi:10.1097/NNE.0b013e3182001e98

Society for Simulation in Healthcare. (2017a). CHSE. Retrieved from http://www.ssih.org/Certification/CHSE

Society for Simulation in Healthcare. (2017b). SSH accreditation of healthcare simulation programs. Retrieved from http://www.ssih.org/Accreditation

Stayt, L. C., Merriman, C., Ricketts, B., Morton, S., & Simpson, T. (2015). Recognizing and managing a deteriorating patient: A randomized controlled trial investigating the effectiveness of clinical simulation in improving clinical performance in undergraduate nursing students. *Journal of Advanced Nursing, 71*, 2563–2574. doi:10.1111/jan.12722

Tanner, C. A. (2006). Thinking like a nurse: A research-based model of clinical judgment in nursing. *Journal of Nursing Education, 45*, 204–211.

Thomas, C., Bertram, E., & Allen, R. (2012). Preparing for transition to professional practice: Creating a simulated blog and reflective journaling activity. *Clinical Simulation in Nursing, 8*(3), e87–e95. doi:10.1016/j.ecns.2010.07.004

Trail Ross, M. E., Otto, D. A., & Stewart Helton, A. (2017). Benefits of simulation and role-playing to teach performance of functional assessments. *Nursing Education Perspectives, 38*, 47–48.

Verkuyl, M., Atack, L., Mastrilli, P., & Romaniuk, D. (2016). Virtual gaming to develop students' pediatric nursing skills: A usability test. *Nurse Education Today, 46*, 81–85. doi:10.1016/j.nedt.2016.08.024

Vincent, M. A., Sheriff, S., & Mellott, S. (2015). The efficacy of high-fidelity simulation on psychomotor clinical performance improvement of undergraduate nursing students. *Computers, Informatics, Nursing, 33*(2), 78–84. doi:10.1097/CIN.0000000000000136

Waznonis, A. R. (2014). Methods and evaluations for simulation debriefing in nursing education. *Journal of Nursing Education, 53*, 459–465. doi:10.3928/01484834-20140722-13

Wendling, A., Halan, S., Tighe, P., Le, L., Euliano, T., & Lok, B. (2011). Virtual humans verses standardized patients: Which lead residents to more correct diagnosis? *Academic Medicine, 86*, 384–388. doi:10.1097/ACM.0b013e318208803f

Wickers, M. P. (2010). Establishing the climate for a successful debriefing. *Clinical Simulation in Nursing, 6*, e83–e86. doi:10.1016/j.ecns.2009.06.003

8

Weaving Interprofessional Education into Nursing Curricula

KAREN T. PARDUE, SHELLEY COHEN KONRAD, AND
DAWNE MARIE DUNBAR

OBJECTIVES

- Describe foundational frameworks for interprofessional education (IPE)
- Identify core competencies for IPE
- Examine the content and processes for integrating IPE into nursing curricula
- Describe teaching strategies for IPE in the classroom, simulation, and clinical learning environments

The transformation of health care, coupled with alarming patient care outcome data, is heralding a new mandate to prepare nurses for collaborative team-based models of care. The Institute of Medicine (IOM) has systematically examined the United States health care system for decades, noting concerns about care quality, patient safety, and astounding rates of medical error (Greiner & Knebel, 2003; IOM, 1972; IOM Committee on Quality of Health Care in America, 1999, 2001). Ineffective communication and poor collaboration are believed to be practices contributing to system failure and adverse patient care outcomes (Greiner & Knebel, 2003; IOM Committee on Quality of Health Care in America, 1999, 2001). The IOM calls on education to respond by reforming health profession curricula to include interprofessional (IP), collaborative team-based competencies as part of academic preparation (Greiner & Knebel, 2003).

The nursing profession has additionally been challenged through recommendations advanced in the IOM *Future of Nursing* report (Committee on the Robert Wood Johnson Foundation Initiative on the Future of Nursing at the Institute of Medicine, 2011). This report sets forth a blueprint for the profession to actively engage in leading health care reform and improving the nation's health.

To accomplish this, faculty need to prepare all nurses to function at the highest level commensurate with their degree, and this preparation should include education with other members of the health care team (Committee on the Robert Wood Johnson Foundation Initiative on the Future of Nursing at the Institute of Medicine, 2011). Such educational opportunities support the cultivation of nurses' abilities to contribute to and lead health care delivery.

This educational reform presents a daunting challenge, as the configuration of most nursing, medicine, and allied health programs reflects singular siloed programs of study. Such design results in nursing and health profession graduates who have little to no knowledge of what their respective colleagues do, and demonstrate little to no skill or experience in IP communication and ways of effectively working together on teams. This chapter examines the content and processes for weaving IPE into nursing curricula. Foundational frameworks are provided, along with examination of didactic, simulation, and clinical learning experiences that promote collaborative practice capabilities.

FOUNDATIONAL FRAMEWORKS

DEFINING INTERPROFESSIONAL EDUCATION

Interprofessional education is defined as involving two or more disciplines that "learn with, from, and about each other to improve collaboration and the quality of care and services" (Centre for the Advancement of Interprofessional Education [CAIPE], 2016). Based in the United Kingdom, CAIPE was established in 1987 and represents one of the initial organizations to formally propose a definition of IPE (Buring et al., 2009). The World Health Organization (WHO) augments the CAIPE definition, contending that IPE occurs when students "representing two or more professions learn about, from, and with each other to enable effective collaboration and improve health outcomes for patients and populations they serve" (WHO, 2010, p. 13). These perspectives and definitions are well accepted and frequently referenced in the IPE literature.

INTERPROFESSIONAL COLLABORATION

The word *collaboration* is derived from the Latin word *collaborare*, meaning "to labor, to work with and together" (LatDict, 2016). Collaboration requires active engagement between participants, characterized by a reciprocal giving and receiving of information, and mutuality of working relationship occurring within an environment of trust and respect. Interprofessional collaborative practice enables health professionals to engage and interact with one another, and with patients and their families, to render safe, high-quality care (WHO, 2010).

This collaborative practice imperative is advanced in the 2011 United States Interprofessional Education Collaborative (IPEC) core competency expert report. This landmark document instructs that the *way* health care is delivered is as important to the outcome as the *type* of care that is provided (IPEC Expert Panel, 2011, p.4). It reflects a new practice orientation, focusing on the contribution of communication, teamwork, problem solving, and conflict resolution in achieving optimal patient health outcomes. This renders a new nursing education directive, extending the curriculum beyond teaching what nurses do and including intentional learning experiences with other health disciplines to prepare a future collaborative workforce.

CORE COMPETENCIES FOR INTERPROFESSIONAL PRACTICE

In 2009, six national health profession associations established a collaborative to examine the nature and development of IPE. The initial membership included representatives from dentistry, nursing, medicine, osteopathic medicine, pharmacy, and public health. The collaborative issued an expert panel report in 2011, asserting that the goal of IP collaborative practice is the provision of safe, high-quality, patient- and family-centered care. The report identified four broad competency domains as characterizing IP collaborative practice:

- Values and Ethics for Interprofessional Practice
- Roles and Responsibilities for Collaborative Practice
- Interprofessional Communication Practices
- Interprofessional Teamwork and Team-Based Practice

Each of these broad competency domains is accompanied by eight to 11 specific sub-competency statements.

These four competency domains were reaffirmed in 2016 when IPEC issued an updated report. Membership in the collaborative has expanded since 2011, now including the additional disciplines of physical therapy, physician assistant, podiatric medicine, optometry, social work, and veterinary medicine (IPEC, 2016). The updated report reconceptualized IP collaboration as the primary central domain under which each of the four major competencies and associated subcompetencies are organized (IPEC, 2016, p. 4). Additionally, the updated version places greater emphasis on population health outcomes to realize health system quality and safety improvements (IPEC, 2016). These revisions reflect changes in the health care environment occurring through the enactment of the 2010 Patient Protection and Affordable Care Act. The integration of the Triple Aim (Berwick, Nolan, & Whittington, 2008), and associated goals for improving patient satisfaction with care, improving the health of populations, and reducing the cost of care has sharpened the focus toward aggregate health. Table 8.1 presents each of the four major IP competency domains and highlights sample subcompetency statements.

In addition to the United States competencies just discussed, the Canadian Interprofessional Health Collaborative (CIHC, 2010) identifies *collaborative leadership* as critical to best practice. The competency of collaborative leadership is grounded in relational strength, whereby the health care team jointly determines the member most equipped for leadership based upon the needs of a given situation (CIHC, 2010). Facilitation is at the heart of collaborative leadership, as are value and respect for every team member. Skills for collaborative leadership include soliciting input from all relevant members; listening to concerns, especially those that may affect patient safety; and modelling support for working together. Leaders are responsible for setting a culture of psychological safety in which all participants feel comfortable providing input. Collaborative leaders use good communication methods to assure that all members of the team know what is expected of them in their execution of patient care. As nurses commonly assume care coordination roles in both inpatient and outpatient settings, collaborative leadership presents a final important IP competency for inclusion in nursing education.

THEORETICAL FRAMEWORKS TO SUPPORT IPE

Interprofessional education differs from disciplinary education in that the primary focus is on dialogue and interaction among learners, as opposed to teachers imparting information and specific content. As such, IPE is grounded in social engagement within the context of learning, and numerous theories are useful for nurse educators when designing and implementing shared learning experiences.

TABLE 8.1 Four Interprofessional Core Competency Domains With Sample Subcompetency Statements

IPEC Competency Domain and Definition	Sample Subcompetency Statement
Values/Ethics for Interprofessional Practice: Work with individuals of other professions to maintain a climate of mutual respect and shared values. (p. 11)	Embrace the cultural diversity and individual differences that characterize patients, populations, and the health team. Act with honesty and integrity in relationships with patients, families, communities, and other team members. (p. 11)
Roles and Responsibilities for Collaborative Practice: Use knowledge of one's own role and those of other professions to appropriately assess and address the health care needs of patients and to promote and advance the health of populations. (p. 12)	Explain the roles and responsibilities of other providers and how the team works together to provide care, promote health, and prevent disease. Recognize one's limitations in skills, knowledge, and abilities. (p. 12)
Interprofessional Communication: Communicate with patients, families, communities, and professionals in health and other fields in a responsive and responsible manner that supports a team approach to the promotion and maintenance of health and the prevention and treatment of disease. (p. 13)	Choose effective communication tools and techniques, including information systems and communication technologies, to facilitate discussions and interactions that enhance team function. Listen actively, and encourage ideas and opinions of other team members. (p. 13)
Interprofessional Teamwork and Team-Based Practice: Apply relationship-building values and principles of team dynamics to perform effectively in different team roles to plan, deliver, and evaluate patient/population-centered care and population health programs and policies that are safe, timely, efficient, effective, and equitable. (p. 14)	Describe the process of team development and the roles and practices of effective teams. Engage self and others to constructively manage disagreements about values, roles, goals, and actions that arise among health and other professionals and with patients, families, and community members. (p. 14)

Source: From Interprofessional Education Collaborative (2016).

THEORIES FOR DESIGNING IPE LEARNING EXPERIENCES

No one theory is universally accepted for IPE; rather, most endeavors reflect a blend of Education and Social Engagement Theory to achieve collaborative learning outcomes. Principles of adult learning provide solid underpinning for IPE (Barr, 2013; Oandasan & Reeves, 2005). Knowles advanced the concept of andragogy and the belief that engaged adult learners are motivated and assume responsibility for their education experience (Bertrand, 2003). Adults seek relevant educational opportunities, making connections between new learning and their current and past life experience (Bertrand, 2003).

Mezirow (1998) builds on adult learning principles, asserting that critical reflection is an essential practice for transformative education. Critical reflection is founded on the premise that there are no simple solutions to complex problems, and this paradigm is particularly true in considering care for patients and families living with chronic health conditions. Faculty support critical reflection through incorporating introspective, contextual, and active learning strategies. Introspection challenges the student to think deeply and critically about personally held beliefs and assumptions (Mezirow, 1998). Interprofessional learning opportunities, which include building in a pause or an intentional time for students to engage in a free write (writing about their experiences for a set period of time without concern about format or grammar) are two ways faculty can foster introspection and critical reflection. Contextual thinking asks learners to consider people's health and wellness on a broader scale: for example, how economic, cultural, or social factors affect one's ability to access or adhere to care recommendations. Active learning strategies allow students to share their thoughts and reflections with one another, thereby rendering robust dialogue or discourse. When needed, faculty facilitators guide or steer students to elicit the views and knowledge of others, compare evidence, and test out arguments, thus promoting educational transformation (Mezirow, 1998). These constructs are consistent with IPE and are useful considerations for educators developing IPE programming.

Kolb (1984) advances the Theory of Experiential Learning, proposing that learning occurs when students move through four discrete domains in the learning cycle. Kolb defines these learning cycle phases as: concrete experience (new material is presented); reflective observation (observing, considering, and mentally reviewing the new material); abstract conceptualization (analysis and generation of questions about the material); and active experimentation (application or testing of new learning to the real- world situation). Creating IPE experiences that incorporate each stage of the cycle supports effective and lasting learning. Kolb's Experiential Learning Theory provides yet another helpful framework for nurse educators in designing IPE learning opportunities.

Social engagement models support Classic Education Theory in the development of IPE. Contact hypothesis, as proposed by Hewstone and Brown (1986), asserts that attitudinal change is fostered among individuals when participants have the opportunity to actively learn together. Learning with others cultivates new relationships and results in the questioning of negative stereotypes and assumptions as new associations are formed. Making connections supports the discovery of professional similarities and differences, thereby promoting mutuality and respect (Pettigrew, 1998). When integrating Contact Hypothesis Theory into the design of IPE, it is important that learners be of comparable stages of development, hold equal status in the learning experience, and be bound together via common educational goals (Hean & Dickinson, 2005).

Communities of practice reflect Constructivist Theory and the active role learners play in building new knowledge and capabilities together (Wenger-Trayner & Wenger-Trayner, 2015). Communities of practice involve three characteristics: the domain (common goal of learning), community (health profession students or clinicians), and practice (competencies and approaches for quality patient outcomes). This orientation advances collaborative problem solving to address "real-world" issues, where participants engage in peer-to-peer learning, active questioning, and robust discussion (Wenger-Trayner & Wenger-Trayner, 2015). This approach supports future IP collaborative practice, developing students' communication, teamwork, problem-solving, and critical thinking skills.

Model for Conceptualizing Process of IPE Student Learning

These theories provide a foundation for shaping and implementing collaborative learning. The University of British Columbia (UBC) offers a helpful model for conceptualizing the process of IPE student learning (Charles, Bainbridge, & Gilbert, 2010). The model serves as a guide to faculty in developing IP learning experiences across the curriculum. The initial stage in the UBC Model is *exposure*. Exposure learning is introductory and provides a foundation for success in future IP collaborations (Charles et al., 2010). Exposure learning is appropriate for novice prelicensure learners and involves bringing students together from diverse professions to begin to learn about collaborative practice. Sample topics reflective of the exposure stage of IPE might include:

- What is IP practice?
- Why does IP collaborative practice matter?
- What are the roles and responsibilities of various health profession disciplines?
- What are the myths and/or stereotypes associated with different health professions?
- What are critical elements inherent in high-functioning teams?
- What are communication tools and techniques that promote optimal team functioning?

Immersion represents the second stage in the UBC Model, involving more advanced learners with some experience from clinical practice settings (Charles et al., 2010). The immersion stage challenges students to work with each other, using their emerging professional knowledge and skills to determine how disciplinary roles and collaborative teamwork contribute to high-quality patient and family care delivery (Charles et al., 2010). Examples of immersion learning experiences include:

- Interprofessional teams of students analyzing a complex or unfolding case study.
- Interprofessional disciplines participating together in a shared high-fidelity simulation.
- Diverse health profession disciplines examining a standardized patient (patient actor).
- Interprofessional disciplines coordinating a clinical plan of care with a patient.

Mastery is the final stage of learning conceptualized in the UBC Model (Charles et al., 2010). The mastery phase represents advanced practice and is generally limited to postlicensure learners in graduate or doctoral education, or practicing clinicians engaged in continuing education. Mastery is realized through substantial clinical practice, and involves the ability to engage in high-level critical thinking and analysis, as well as deep self-reflection on one's own IP experiences (Charles et al., 2010).

CURRICULAR CONSIDERATIONS

Nurse educators often take the lead in championing IP learning opportunities, and such curricular integration requires significant planning and collaboration with disciplines outside of nursing. The following are a select number of pedagogical considerations essential for the successful design and implementation of IPE.

LEARNING OUTCOMES

A first step in successful curriculum design involves the identification of desired learning outcomes from collaborative experiences (Pardue, 2015). Nurse educators need to explicitly determine the knowledge, skills, abilities, and/or attitudinal changes students will demonstrate at the conclusion of IPE. These capabilities likely address the four IPEC competency domains (IPEC, 2016), including knowledge of disciplinary roles and responsibilities, effective communication, collaborative teamwork, and ethics for IP practice. For that reason, it is recommended that the subcompetencies as explicated in the IPEC competency report (2016) be used as a blueprint for identifying desired student learning outcomes (Pardue, 2015). Faculty planners need to engage in extensive collaboration to ensure collective affirmation of agreed-upon outcomes. Table 8.1 provides examples of outcomes-based learning achieved through IPE.

Nurse educators need to carefully plan and scaffold IPE learning to achieve desired outcomes. Consistent with any curriculum planning, IP knowledge, skills, and abilities should be formally introduced at an appropriate time for learning (exposure stage), and subsequently reinforced later on in the curriculum through experiential opportunities (immersion stage). Speakman (2017) advocates that nurse educators create a systematic plan for IPE, thereby formally mapping learner participation in IPE. Exhibit 8.1 provides a sample curriculum map addressing IPE.

EXHIBIT 8.1 Curriculum Mapping for Interprofessional Education: Sample Scaffolding of Exposure and Immersion Learning

| Professional Program Timeline (example) | IPE Competency | | | |
	Values and Ethics for Interprofessional Practice	Roles and Responsibilities for Collaborative Practice	Interprofessional Communication	Interprofessional Teamwork and Team-Based Practice
Fall, Year 1		Didactic/Exposure	Didactic/Exposure	Didactic/Exposure
Spring, Year 1	Didactic/Exposure	Immersion/Simulation Experience	Immersion/Simulation Experience	Immersion/Simulation Experience
Fall, Year 2	Immersion/Simulation Experience	Immersion/Adult Clinical Rotation	Immersion/Adult Clinical Rotation	Immersion/Adult Clinical Rotation
Spring, Year 2	Immersion/Clinical Rotation	Immersion/Specialty Clinical Rotation	Immersion/Specialty Clinical Rotation	Immersion/Specialty Clinical Rotation

IPE, interprofessional education.
Source: Based on the work of Charles et al. (2010).

LEARNER CONSIDERATIONS

Identifying potential programs and participants for collaborative education is a second early consideration in IP learning. This process can be challenging, as health profession education is disciplinarily nuanced, thereby reflecting diverse points in time for student readiness for IPE. Thibault (2011) referred to this mutual time for IPE readiness as curricular "sweet spots," requiring faculty to become well acquainted with their partnering program(s) in order to ascertain parallel points in time for student preparation.

This design also renders "asymmetrical" education encounters (Thibault, 2011), bringing together students from dissimilar academic years and even different degree levels (e.g., prelicensure nursing and doctoral physical therapy) for IPE. These learner considerations require intensive coordination between nursing faculty and other disciplines in planning and delivering effective IPE for all students.

Class size, disciplinary balance, and participant stability are other important learner considerations (Oandasan & Reeves, 2005; Reeves, Goldman, & Oandasan, 2007). Class size addresses the actual number of participants for collaborative education: How large are the disciplines being assembled, and is there space to accommodate shared learning? In planning for IPE, it is not necessary to include all professions in all events; such design becomes unwieldy and does not mirror actual clinical practice. To promote active student engagement, groups are generally divided into smaller subgroups or teams. There is disagreement in the IPE literature as to the appropriate size for optimal small group interaction, with scholars generally recommending that membership involve five to no more than ten participants (Oandasan & Reeves, 2005; Reeves et al., 2007).

Disciplinary balance presents a second consideration, as an equal mix of disciplines serves to foster equality of voice and equitable interaction. Ensuring a distributed composition of students supports team functioning and negates the opportunity for dominance by any one profession (Oandasan & Reeves, 2005; Reeves et al., 2007).

Participant stability is yet another important pedagogical aspect, as a one-time engagement in an IPE endeavor differs quite significantly from repeated collaborative learning with familiar peers (Oandasan & Reeves, 2005; Reeves et al., 2007). The opportunity for multiple interactions between learners supports team development and provides an authentic learning environment to achieve the goals of cross-disciplinary communication, knowledge of one another, professional respect, and teamwork.

Timing for IPE is another feature requiring attention by nurse faculty and their IP colleagues. In the IPE community, there is robust debate as to the best time to introduce collaborative learning. On the one hand, novice learners typically have limited clinical experience, rendering concepts such as team functioning, conflict resolution, and professional respect abstract and without meaningful context (Oandasan & Reeves, 2005). Alternatively, the early introduction of IPE can reduce disciplinary stereotyping and promote a culture of healthy dialogue and collaboration among all professions (Begley, 2009). Students respond favorably to IPE when they see the relevance of the experience to their current or future professional practice (Oandasan & Reeves, 2005). Pardue (2013) describes the introduction of IPE in the first semester of undergraduate study, whereby students begin to explore roles and responsibilities of various disciplines. This reflects introductory IPE learning with immediate relevance, as first-semester students may still be introspectively wrestling with their collegiate major selection. This introduction parallels the UBC Model of exposure, laying a foundation for future collaborative learning once students gain more knowledge about their own profession (Charles et al., 2010).

The process of helping students to learn with, from, and about each other requires active social learning pedagogical approaches (Begley, 2009; Oandasan & Reeves, 2005; Reeves et al., 2007). The key is promoting student interaction, reflecting an instructional strategy that may be unfamiliar to faculty. Faculty are typically well acquainted with lecture and the role of imparting information to students. In contrast, successful IPE relies on students interacting with each other; the focus in IPE centers on learner engagement and not on faculty transmitting content. Numerous active learning strategies foster the development of collaboration abilities, including small groups of students analyzing case studies, engaging in role-play, interacting with standardized patients, completing simulations, participating in web quests, and working together on a team activity.

FACULTY ROLE

The constructivist theories that underpin IPE inform the faculty role and associated approaches to instruction. As stated, faculty offer direction, not didactics, when engaged in collaborative learning. Faculty invite students to work and think together, during which time participants ask questions, examine multiple perspectives, and explore areas of similarities, differences, and potential conflict. Faculty use the skills of facilitation, paying close attention to team formation and group dynamics to anticipate and intervene with any issues that may arise (Oandasan & Reeves, 2005). Facilitators are responsible for creating a nonthreatening environment to support full engagement among all participants (Reeves et al., 2007). Most faculty are comfortable and familiar with traditional lecture and single-discipline teaching, and IP facilitation is not necessarily intuitive. For that reason, it is recommended that faculty be afforded additional training and support in IPE facilitation. Exhibit 8.2 offers select tips and techniques that support successful IPE facilitation.

EXHIBIT 8.2 Tips and Techniques for Successful Facilitation

Are there common, agreed-upon learning objectives?

Are two or more professions involved?

Are the sessions interactive?

Are contributions of different members encouraged?

Are learners, not teachers, doing most of the talking?

Are interprofessional (IP) communication strategies employed?

Is there time planned for a debrief?

Are faculty trained in IP facilitation?

In addition to facilitation, faculty model collaboration by interacting cross-professionally with colleagues during IPE instruction. The rationale for intentional faculty interaction is based on the observation that students regard IPE seriously when they see their own instructors actively engaged in communication, teamwork, and problem solving—the very behaviors targeted through IP learning. Conversely, when faculty are disengaged in IPE instruction, their students assume a similar posture and the experience is rendered "soft" and "unimportant." Opportunities for faculty role modeling are an important consideration in planning and implementing IPE.

The technique of debriefing reflects a constructivist method consistent with IP learning. Debriefing involves revisiting important conversations, examining changed assumptions, and discussing new insights gleaned from a given educational experience. Interprofessional education commonly culminates in a formal debriefing, and this may be conducted by instructors or alternatively by more senior students. Oftentimes, advanced students are well-equipped to debrief an IPE experience, providing powerful role modeling for learners. The practice of debriefing and summarizing all that transpired during an interactive IPE session reflects one method for successfully reinforcing new knowledge. The art of debriefing is discussed in more detail later in this chapter in the context of simulation.

CONCLUDING THOUGHTS

Nurse educators engaged in the design and implementation of IPE need to consider the structure for IP learning (Oandasan & Reeves, 2005). Will IPE experiences be a component of credit-bearing work, or is IPE extracurricular? Will IP learning involve all students in the major, or only those who have a special interest? Is IPE mandatory or elective in nature? The answers to these questions reflect departmental and institutional nuances, and highlight the current variability of IP learning across the health professions. The recent introduction of IP learning outcomes into discipline-specific accreditation requirements may serve, in time, to advance IPE learning as requisite in nursing and health profession education.

DIDACTIC LEARNING

Didactic learning is a common instructional format for introducing nursing students to IPE and reflects UBC exposure-level learning. A didactic approach supports a uniform educational experience for all participants and can be delivered in numerous ways. For example, some institutions require that all incoming students take part in an IPE session as part of their overall orientation. A mandatory session acknowledges the critical importance and integration of IPE, explicitly recognizing that collaborative competencies are essential to best practice and not, as previously mentioned, "soft" knowledge and skills. Sessions introduce core IP competencies and illustrate future IPE co-curricular and extracurricular activities in which students have an opportunity to apply their developing knowledge and skills.

Early learners are eager to gain knowledge of their own discipline; thus, integration of IPE must explicitly connect the dots between nursing education and collaborative competencies. Why is it important for nurses to know the skill set of an occupational therapist? What specialized skills are necessary for teamwork and how can nurses advance patient care when working on a team? In the classroom, faculty may use modules, videos, and interactive strategies to expose students to basic tenets of IPE competencies. Numerous low- or no-cost IPE resources exist to assist faculty, and some are depicted in Exhibit 8.3. Interactive instructional methods offer students a glimpse of the processes of team-based care in day-to-day practice.

Inviting cross-professional guest speakers is another approach that provides early exposure to the range of disciplinary skills and expertise that nursing students will work alongside in their future practices. Teachers are charged with prompting peer discussion that highlights similarities and differences in roles, examines communication and teamwork know-how, and imparts respect for the various roles professional and support staff play on the team.

Case-based learning (CBL) can be used to shed light on the advantages of IP collaboration. The most successful CBL scenarios involve situations familiar to students (for example, with foundational learners the case might depict a classmate struggling with homesickness or an eating disorder). Group projects bring students together to focus on a common health or social concern such as bullying or environmental hazards. Both of these assignments (CBL or group project) require students to reach out to and work with counterparts from another profession or, at the very least, study how another discipline might address the problem at hand. Presentation of findings from CBL and group projects reinforces what students have learned and invites input from other participants that can extend teachable moments.

Facilitation and faculty modelling are pivotal to successful IPE didactic instruction, especially during the exposure phase. New learners may struggle with the relevance of IPE; many already consider themselves proficient communicators and team players. Teaching methods must actively engage students in activities that

EXHIBIT 8.3 Resources for Developing Interprofessional Learning

Resource/ URL	Description
Guide to Effective Interprofessional Education Experiences A National League for Nursing IPE Tool Kit http://www.nln.org/docs/default-source/default-document-library/ipe-toolkit-krk-012716.pdf?sfvrsn=6	A free guide for designing and implementing effective interprofessional education (IPE) and collaborative practice experiences in nursing. Site includes sample lesson plans for didactic, simulation, and clinical education.
National Center for Interprofessional Practice & Education: Resource Center https://nexusipe.org	A national web resource center hosting an extensive digital library that includes IPE assessment tools and instruments.
CompTIME: University of New England Online Modules Addressing IPE Competency Development www.une.edu/wchp/ipec/comptime	A set of five free interactive online modules designed to support students and faculty in learning about IPE competencies and collaborative practice. Content is creatively presented through weaving a clinical patient story throughout the module series.
American Interprofessional Health Collaborative https://aihc-us.org	A forum that showcases national IPE and collaborative practice efforts. Audio presentations and PowerPoint slides of recent webinars are archived for review. In 2017, will launch a strategic webinar series to assist faculty in how to get started with IPE.
Institute for Health Improvement Open School www.ihi.org/education/ihiopenschool/Pages/default.aspx	An online community providing modular education to support the delivery of safe, high-quality patient care. Select modules address IPE competencies, including communication, teamwork, and leadership. Courses are free to all students and faculty with an "edu" email address.

are developmentally meaningful to them, with teachers guiding discussions to assure that IPE learning objectives are met. Facilitation assists in transitioning students from concrete knowledge formation to engagement in reflectivity and critical thinking. Even in the context of disciplinary-specific instruction, faculty play an important role through infusing perspectives of another discipline into discourse or immediately addressing biases and stereotypes that students may voice about other professions.

Utilization of the arts—for example, theater, visual arts, and literature—is a relatively underused method in nursing and health profession education. When integrated effectively, the arts engage affective knowing, emotional intelligence, and critical thinking—all essential capabilities for nursing practice. Stories impart ethical dilemmas, calling forth issues of human dignity, empathy, value-based care, and the exigencies of poor communication in ways that traditional lecture cannot. Readers Theater is a particularly salient deployment of the arts in health profession education, especially when the key players represent different professional groups dramatically narrating the story of vulnerable patients and situations. As with all aspects of IPE instruction, opportunities for participants to engage in nonjudgmental reflection and guided debrief amplify learning.

In 2014, the Josiah Macy Jr. Foundation panel (2014) called upon health profession educators to integrate patients and families as contributory partners in developing and teaching health profession education. Stories of patients *from* patients are perhaps the most transformative of learning experiences for students. Patient stories told in non-clinical, real-life terms remind students that any one of us could at any given time be a person facing a life-altering health situation. Inviting patients and their care providers to the classroom to share their care experience narratives has the added benefit of expli-cating how collaboration works or fails to work. Exhibit 8.4 offers sample teaching and learning strategies appropriate for IPE didactic instruction.

EXHIBIT 8.4 Sample Active Learning Strategies for Didactic Interprofessional Education

IPEC Competency Domain	Sample Active Learning Strategy
Values/Ethics for Interprofessional Practice	View an online video presenting the story of Sue Sheridan (Agency for Healthcare Research and Quality website www.ahrq.gov/teamstepps/instructor/videos/ts_Sue_Sheridan/Sue_Sheridan-400-300.html) or Josie King (YouTube www.youtube.com/watch?v=JMs-gNFPgm8). Assemble students into small groups to work together in identifying and analyzing issues related to patient safety and quality care. Prompt students to propose interprofessional (IP) practices and processes to address these issues.
Roles and Responsibilities for Collaborative Practice	Assemble students into small IP groups with access to the Internet. Assign students to complete a Web Quest in researching similarities and differences in roles and responsibilities of various health disciplines (e.g., roles of physical therapy, occupational therapy, speech therapy, leisure/recreation therapy). Have students create a graphic or visual to capture their findings.
Interprofessional Communication	Assemble students into small IP groups and provide TeamSTEPPS® communication resources (materials are free at Agency for Healthcare Research and Quality website www.ahrq.gov/teamstepps/index.html). Instruct students to examine together as a team two assigned communication tools (e.g., SBAR, Teach-back, CUS). Have students prepare a 5-minute tutorial, including a sample role-play, to illustrate the select communication technique. Teams then present their assigned communication tool to one another and discuss clinical uses and implications.

(continued)

IPEC Competency Domain	Sample Active Learning Strategy
Interprofessional Teamwork and Team-Based Practice	Assemble students into small IP groups. Assign students to work together in completing a teamwork activity found on the web (e.g., paper chain challenge, Lego® tower challenge, marshmallow challenge). Debrief by analyzing the process:

How did you work as a unit?

What was the process like?

Did a leader emerge? If so, how?

Who assumed what role in completing the activity?

What did the team do when different ideas were expressed?

Any observations regarding communication?

Who negotiated? How were problems solved?

What would you do differently next time?

Questions for the winning team:

What was your process like?

How does this compare to the other teams? |

CUS, concerned, uncomfortable, safety; IPEC, Interprofessional Education Collaborative; SBAR, situation, background, assessment, recommendation.

SIMULATION LEARNING

The simulation laboratory provides an unparalleled environment for cultivating and assessing IP capabilities. Consistent with prior definitions, interprofessional simulation (IPE-SIM) occurs when faculty, facilitators, and students from two or more disciplines participate together in a shared simulation experience to realize mutually identified goals or learning outcomes (Decker et al., 2015, p. 294). As simulation is a behavioral, performance-based strategy, this reflects an immersion level of IPE (Charles et al., 2010). The focus of IPE-SIM centers on the skills of teamwork, communication, collaboration, and problem solving, thereby providing opportunities to enact behaviors characteristic of collaborative health profession practice (Boet, Bould, Layat Burn, & Reeves, 2014). This attention to the process of care and working together as a team differs from discipline-specific simulation, thus requiring joint faculty collaboration and new scenario development to achieve IP learning outcomes.

A team-based approach to simulation development, in which involved faculty stakeholders use their own clinical experiences as a guide, renders scenario development that is both authentic and relevant for the disciplines involved. Scenarios should provide learners an opportunity to elicit knowledge, behaviors, and attitudes reflective of the IPEC competencies, and these desired outcomes should be jointly identified by the faculty planning team from the onset. A solid IPE scenario does not have to be complex to be effective, but it does have to be true to real-life patient and provider experiences.

One common pitfall in IPE-SIM occurs when too many disciplines are involved at the same time, or different professions are linked in a manner that does not reflect the realities of patient care delivery. In such situations, students quickly disengage, as provider relationships are forced, unnatural, and artificial. The IPE-SIM development team needs to consider authentic clinical situations and associated opportunities for disciplinary collaboration, as well as the points in the care delivery continuum where these collaborations occur.

For example, an IPE-SIM was created by an IP faculty workgroup addressing the collaborative practice care of a young woman with life-altering injuries from a motor vehicle accident. This unfolding case was designed so that student IP teams could assess and plan care for the simulated patient and her husband across the continuum from acute hospitalization to rehabilitation to home. Chronic pain, loss of mobility, self-care deficits, relational role strain, financial pressures, and questions about childbearing options characterize the issues set forth in this multi-session IPE-SIM. Students from nursing, medicine, physician assistant, dental hygiene, dental medicine, social work, pharmacy, and occupational and physical therapy all provided meaningful contributions at various points in time to this simulated patient and her husband. The IP exchange and multi-session sequence allowed students to get to know one another and their varied expertise. This served to enhance student understanding as to what collaborative patient-centered team skills look like in action. Additionally, students described greater confidence in their own professional identity from this IPE-SIM and enhanced ability to communicate and work effectively on a team.

The organization of IPE-SIM reflects the same best practice process found in any discipline-specific simulation experience, including a prebrief, simulation, and debrief. Chapter 7 provided an excellent overview and helpful guidance for the design and implementation of simulation. Interprofessional debriefing can be challenging for even the most experienced simulation facilitators. While there are numerous valid methods for debriefing, key to a successful IP debrief is faculty determination of a consistent model or set of questions during the scenario development phase. The temptation to digress into discipline-specific clinical content is bypassed when clear IPE objectives guide the debriefing. Providing each student opportunity and active encouragement to reflect and express his or her point of view uncovers learner progress, with areas of confusion addressed through additional faculty guidance and facilitation. One indicator of success is when students articulate how IPE-SIM will change or influence their future practice as a result of the experience and opportunity for reflection. Exhibit 8.5 provides tips for conducting a successful IP debriefing.

There are numerous challenges that commonly arise in the design and delivery of IPE-SIM, and anticipating obstacles is an important step in the planning process. Logistical factors include aligning multiple professional programs with differing calendars and curricular sequences, thereby making a common time for IPE-SIM difficult. Administration may be reticent to provide sufficient faculty release time for shared IPE-SIM development, or similarly dedicate adequate faculty coverage during the execution of IPE-SIM (Boet et al., 2014). Financial support may be problematic in determining how and which program resources will be used to fund IPE-SIM (Boet et al., 2014). Additionally, faculty may express discomfort in working with learners of differing education levels, clinical experience, and perceived inequalities in professional authority (Boet et al., 2014).

Addressing these challenges requires flexibility, creativity, and "out of the box" thinking. Early collaboration with administration can clarify the importance of IPE-SIM, which may contribute to protected time and financial investments from an institutional level. Providing administration with an overview as to how simulation activities simultaneously meet learning outcomes for different disciplines highlights the advantage of common infrastructure and financial investment. IPE-SIM represents a new

EXHIBIT 8.5 Tips for Interprofessional Education-Simulation Debriefing

- Was the process of care in interprofessional education-simulation (IPE-SIM) comfortable or difficult? What contributed to the process experience?
- Were roles and responsibilities well understood?
- How were problems or concerns handled? Who assumed leadership? Why?
- Directly inquire as to the care processes addressing participant communication, teamwork, collaboration, and use of disciplinary roles and responsibilities.
- Reflect aloud on facilitator observations related to verbal and nonverbal communication, evidence of teamwork, professional roles, and collaborative leadership.
- Inquire as to any change in assumptions and perceptions from inception to conclusion of IPE-SIM.
- Discuss influences that contributed to the identified changes.
- What process aspects should be reinforced on future IPE-SIM experiences? What approaches should be changed?
- Provide a clear summation of the content that was discussed during the IPE-SIM debrief.

frontier, with opportunities for extramural grant funding and faculty research, potentiating fiscal growth and faculty scholarship.

Asynchronous IP communication and collaboration activities are effective tools for addressing disciplinary scheduling challenges. Learners do not necessarily need to be in the same physical space during simulation, and can successfully share information and plan care through e-mail, texts, phone calls, or live Internet communications like Skype or Zoom. As an example, while participating in on-campus simulation, baccalaureate nursing students were provided cell phone contacts of pharmacy students who were off campus on a clinical rotation. Students collaborated in real time in the care of simulated patients while maintaining different program-specific curriculum schedules. Through careful IP faculty planning, this strategy successfully addressed the logistical challenges of scheduling simulations and provided students with authentic, real-world clinical collaborative practice learning experiences.

CLINICAL LEARNING

Interprofessional clinical learning is experiential in nature, providing a pedagogical bridge between what students learn in the classroom and what occurs in the practice workplace. This represents an immersion level of learning (Charles et al., 2010), as students use foundational concepts gleaned through didactics to inform processes and practices for high-quality care provision. The opportunity to work with other health disciplines in the actual care of patients, families, or communities further extends and deepens nursing students' practical know-how for IP practice. These experiences, however, will be variable, as not every student will have the same opportunity or engagement with clinical IPE. The culture of select settings and care foci reflect an inherent disposition toward teamwork and collaboration. Rich IP clinical learning opportunities are common for nursing students engaged in geriatric, rehabilitation, hospice, substance abuse, diabetes, ambulatory care, and rural health rotations.

Interprofessional clinical learning may be realized thorough numerous approaches. Job shadowing is one potential activity, allowing students to observe other professions in action. How does the practice of the observed discipline compare with nursing practice? What roles overlap with those of nursing? Observing in vivo demonstration of others' skills encourages students to reflect on how and when working together serves to achieve best practice. Such experiences also illustrate referral processes, explicating how and why nursing recommends the engagement of another discipline. Faculty prompts further guide student reflection and critical observation. Students might orally present their job shadowing findings related to communication, roles, and teamwork as part of a clinical postconference. Alternatively, students may journal on their shadowing experience, providing time for reflection on disciplinary approaches, dialogue observed, and application for future practice.

Patient rounding presents another experience for IP clinical learning. This setting-dependent practice provides students with an opportunity to engage and problem-solve with patients and other health disciplines involved in care delivery. The student experience may assume numerous forms: observational in noting team participant interactions or direct if providing care to the patient in question. Rounding also provides opportunities for nursing students to observe leadership skills and identify differences in approaches or styles in leading care teams. These observations constitute useful topics for clinical postconference, allowing students to analyze the impact of leadership on clinical care delivery and patient outcomes.

Some clinical settings (for example, hospice and long-term care) commonly conduct case conferences to assess how care is being provided and to establish future clinical goals. Ideally, case conferences are patient-centered, thereby including perspectives not only from providers but also from the patient and family. Participation in or observation of case conferences affords nursing students additional experience in examining how communication, teamwork, and collaboration impact the process and outcomes of clinical care.

Through coordination with IP colleagues, faculty may discover other professional disciplines on clinical rotation at the same time as a given nursing rotation. This presents possibility for shared pre- or post-conferences, as well as opportunity for collaborative care planning assignments. If the rotation involves community health, it might be possible to arrange joint home visiting experiences for IP students. Faculty collaboration and creativity are essential in discovering and advancing IP clinical learning for nursing students.

EVALUATION OF IPE

Evaluation of IPE outcomes begins with a clear identification of the desired knowledge, skills, and abilities engendered through IP learning. Early IPE endeavors involve exposure or introduction of foundational concepts; thus, the determination of student learning can be achieved through direct assessment techniques such as examinations, student writing/reflections, or focus groups. Faculty colleagues collaborating on exposure IPE experiences should determine from the onset what artifacts will be used as evidence of student learning. Foundational outcomes commonly address participant knowledge about communication, roles and responsibilities, and the process of collaboration, as well as determination of any changes in attitudes or perceptions about working together on teams. Although there is value in validating that students have cognitively grasped collaborative practice principles, what matters more is whether students demonstrate IP capabilities in the actual provision of patient care. As a result, an IPE evaluation plan generally assumes a longitudinal, multi-step design.

Immersion learning supports student performance of collaborative behaviors, and is accomplished through simulation or observation in the clinical practice setting. It is important to clearly identify the action or behavior to be evaluated, with IP competency statements subsequently integrated as part of simulation performance rubrics or as items on clinical evaluation tools. This process invites students and supervising faculty to narratively describe situations and associated actions or behaviors performed that evidence collaborative practice capabilities. Additionally, valid and reliable IP tools are available at the National Center for Interprofessional Practice and Education web site (https://nexusipe.org). Each instrument in the resource center is accompanied by a description as to use, target audience, intended outcome/competency, and authorship. The National Center provides an invaluable resource for nurse educators in the IPE evaluation process.

Finally, questions addressing IP learning may be incorporated into departmental/college alumni satisfaction surveys. Students may not realize the value of collaborative practice lessons until well engaged postlicensure in day-to-day clinical practice. Determining graduate perceptions of IPE learning serves to inform curricular efficacy, and supports future refinements and improvements.

SUMMARY

This chapter provides pedagogical guidance in the design, implementation, and evaluation of IPE in nursing education. Opportunities for broad curricular integration, including didactic, simulation, and clinical learning, are explored. Numerous exemplars and resources are provided to support faculty newly embarking on IP teaching and learning.

It is essential for nursing education to adopt and integrate IPE, thereby cultivating nursing graduates who are knowledgeable about disciplinary roles and responsibilities and are competent in communication, teamwork, and collaborative leadership. Learning together for future practice together supports national calls for health profession education reform and produces practice-ready nurses prepared for today's collaborative, team-based workforce.

REFERENCES

Barr, H. (2013). Toward a theoretical framework for interprofessional education. *Journal of Interprofessional Care, 27*, 4–9. doi:10.3109/13561820.2012.698328

Begley, C. M. (2009). Developing inter-professional learning: Tactics, teamwork and talk. *Nurse Education Today, 29*, 276–283. doi:10.1016/j.nedt.2008.09.006

Bertrand, Y. (2003). *Contemporary theories in education and practice.* Madison, WI: Atwood Publishing.

Berwick, D., Nolan, T., & Whittington, J. (2008). The triple aim: Care, health, and cost. *Health Affairs, 27,* 759–769. doi:10.1377/hlthaff.27.3.759

Boet, S., Bould, M. D., Layat Burn, C., & Reeves, S. (2014). Twelve tips for a successful interprofessional team-based high-fidelity simulation education session. *Medical Teacher, 36*, 853–857. doi:10.3109/0142159X.2014.923558

Buring, S., Bhushan, A., Broeseker, A., Conway, S., Duncan-Hewitt, W., Hansen, L., & Westberg, S. (2009). Interprofessional education: Definitions, student competencies, and guidelines for implementation. *American Journal of Pharmaceutical Education, 73*(4), 59.

Canadian Interprofessional Health Collaborative. (2010). *A national interprofessional competency framework: Quick reference guide.* Retrieved from http://www.cihc.ca/files/CIHC_IPCompetenciesShort_Feb1210.pdf

Centre for the Advancement of Interprofessional Education. (2016). *Home.* Retrieved from http://www .caipe.org

Charles, G., Bainbridge, L., & Gilbert, J. (2010). The University of British Columbia model of interprofessional education. *Journal of Interprofessional Care, 24*(1), 9–18. doi:10.3109/13561820903294549

Committee on the Robert Wood Johnson Foundation Initiative on the Future of Nursing at the Institute of Medicine. (2011). *The future of nursing: Leading change, advancing health.* Retrieved from http:// www.nap.edu/catalog.php?record_id=12956

Decker, S. I., Anderson, M., Boese, T., Epps, C., McCarthy, J., Motola, I., . . . Scolaro, K. (2015). Standards of best practice: Simulation standard VIII: Simulation-enhanced interprofessional education (Sim-IPE). *Clinical Simulation in Nursing, 11,* 293–297. doi:10.1016/j.ecns.2015.03.010

Greiner, A. C., & Knebel, E (2003). *Health professions education: A bridge to quality.* Washington, DC: National Academies Press.

Hean, S., & Dickinson, C. (2005). The contact hypothesis: An exploration of its further potential in interprofessional education. *Journal of Interprofessional Care, 19,* 480–491. doi:10.1080/13561820500215202

Hewstone, M., & Brown, R. (1986). Contact is not enough: An intergroup perspective on the "contact hypothesis." In M. Hewstone & R. Brown (Eds.), *Contact and conflict in intergroup encounters* (pp. 1–44). Oxford, UK: Blackwell.

Institute of Medicine. (1972). *Educating for the health care team.* Washington, DC: National Academy of Sciences.

Institute of Medicine Committee on Quality of Health Care in America. (2000). *To err is human: Building a safer health system* (L. T. Kohn, J. M. Corrigan, & M. S. Donaldson, Eds.). Washington, DC: National Academies Press.

Institute of Medicine Committee on Quality of Health Care in America. (2001). *Crossing the quality chasm.* Washington, DC: National Academies Press.

Interprofessional Education Collaborative. (2016). *Core competencies for interprofessional collaborative practice: 2016 update.* Washington, DC: Author.

Interprofessional Education Collaborative Expert Panel. (2011). *Core competencies for interprofessional collaborative practice: Report of an expert panel.* Washington, DC: Interprofessional Education Collaborative.

Josiah Macy Jr. Foundation. (2014). *Partnering with patients, families, and communities: An urgent imperative for health care.* Conference Recommendations. Retrieved from http://macyfoundation.org/ docs/macy_pubs/JMF_ExecSummary_Final_Reference_web.pdf

Kolb, D. (1984). *Experiential learning: Experiences as the source of learning and development.* Englewood Cliffs, NJ: Prentice Hall.

LatDict. (2016). *Collaborare.* Retrieved from http://latin-dictionary.net

Mezirow, J. (1998). On critical reflection. *Adult Education Quarterly, 48*(3), 185–191.

Oandasan, I., & Reeves, S. (2005). Key elements for interprofessional education: Part 1: The learner, the educator and the learning context. *Journal of Interprofessional Care, 19*(Suppl. 1), 21–38. doi:10.1080/13561820500083550

Pardue, K. T. (2013). Not left to chance: Introducing an undergraduate interprofessional education curriculum. *Journal of Interprofessional Care, 27*(1), 98–100. doi:10.3109/13561820.2012.721815

Pardue, K. T. (2015). A framework for the design, implementation, and evaluation of interprofessional education. *Nurse Educator, 40,* 10–15. doi:10.1097/NNE.0000000000000093

Pettigrew, T. (1998). Intergroup contact theory. *Annual Review of Psychology, 49,* 65–85.

Reeves, S., Goldman, J., & Oandasan, I. (2007). Key factors in planning and implementing interprofessional education in health care settings. *Journal of Allied Health, 36,* 231–235.

Speakman, E. (Ed.) (2017). *Interprofessional education and collaborative practice: Creating a blueprint for nurse educators.* Washington, DC: National League for Nursing.

Thibault, G. E. (2011). Interprofessional education: An essential strategy to accomplish the future of nursing goals. *Journal of Nursing Education, 50,* 313–317. doi:10.3928/01484834-20110519-03

Wenger-Trayner, E., & Wenger-Trayner, B. (2015). Introduction to communities of practice. Retrieved from http://wenger-trayner.com/introduction-to-communities-of-practice

World Health Organization. (2010). *A framework for action on interprofessional education & collaborative practice.* Geneva, Switzerland: Author. Retrieved from http://www.who.int/hrh/resources/ framework_action/en

Teaching in a Learning Laboratory
and Clinical Setting

Learning Laboratories as a Foundation for Nursing Excellence

CAROL F. DURHAM AND DARLENE E. BAKER

OBJECTIVES

- Describe the process of skill development and implications for teaching in learning laboratories
- Analyze the role of the learning laboratory in nursing programs
- Describe the effective setup and operations of learning laboratory
- Describe best practices for teaching in a learning laboratory

Skills acquisition is an important component of nursing education, beginning early in the curriculum and continuing throughout the nursing program. Learning laboratories provide a safe environment for initial psychomotor skills acquisition while offering opportunities to socialize students into the professional role of a nurse. The phrase *learning laboratory* used in this chapter refers to what may frequently be termed a resource center, learning center, or skills laboratory. The phrase is used to allow for a broader understanding of the function and purpose of this environment, which may encompass a wide range of learning activities, processes, supplies, and equipment to enhance clinical reasoning and provide for deliberate practice prior to applying knowledge, skills, and attitudes in patient care. While simulation is discussed in a different chapter, the pedagogy in this chapter is applicable.

The learning laboratory is designed to simulate the clinical setting and to be a nonthreatening space for the development of knowledge, skills, and attitudes that are foundational to clinical practice. Students enter learning laboratories excited about becoming nurses, and they often envision the psychomotor skills taught there as being *what* nurses do. The challenge for nurse educators in the laboratory is to assist students in understanding that acquisition of psychomotor skills is foundational to nursing practice but is only one component of being a nurse. Educators in laboratory settings are charged with encouraging the development of a strong foundation of learning so students can advance in their understanding of the depth and breadth of the art of nursing.

This chapter provides practical strategies embedded in educational pedagogy of skills acquisition. Students' ability to perform skills is essential to safe and high-quality patient care. Acceptable competence of clinical skills is a prerequisite to developing competency at the expert level. Professional performance of psychomotor skills is not simply automated; it requires sound judgment, careful planning, critical thinking, and decision making to ensure safe and effective patient care. This knowledge is integral to the successful implementation of psychomotor skills, and it represents a critical cognitive component of skill mastery. It is critical that learners not only *understand* and are able to *perform* the skill, but also comprehend the *rationale* for the skill. Educators and learners have to understand that knowing and doing are two different things. As an example, memorizing the skills checklist for evaluation may demonstrate knowledge of the steps, but does not prepare a learner to perform the skill in a safe and competent manner in the dynamic context of patient care. Patients expect nothing less, as they rate nursing as the most trusted profession for the 15th consecutive year (Norman, 2016). The privilege and responsibility for our profession to fulfill that trust is incumbent on all components of nursing education and begins in the laboratory.

SKILL DEVELOPMENT: ESSENTIAL CONCEPTS

A solid understanding of the skill and ability to perform it enables learners to develop their competence and confidence as practitioners, allowing them to consider the clinical situation in a broader context. Diers (1990) provides a succinct description of the complexity of skills acquisition that can be shared with students as they begin learning in the laboratory and embarking on their nursing career:

> Skills are thought to be the rudiments of more complicated things, and therefore rote, unchanging, mechanical. But the acquisition of skill is neither easy nor automatic. Once learned, however, a skill is absorbed into the banks of memory and the fibers of the nervous system so it can be called up and counted upon with instant reliability. Carefully learned skills free the mind for analysis, for decision-making, for innovation and choice. Skill implies mastery, but skill mastery does not define excellence in practice. It is only one of the spring boards from which a leap to excellence becomes possible. (p. 66)

The automation of basic skills mentioned by Diers allows the learner to examine what is going on with the patient at a higher level. However, reflecting on Ericsson's (2004) deliberate practice, discussed later in the chapter, it is important to not move too quickly to automation of nursing skills.

In the learning laboratory, educators should understand that they are working with novice learners, defined by Benner (1984) as "beginners [who] have had no experience of the situations in which they are expected to perform" (p. 20). Because "novices have no experience of the situation they face, they must be given rules to guide their performance" (p. 21). Students' experiences in the learning laboratory have an important role in developing their understanding of skills in a contextual framework. Students are embarking on a career with its own culture, language, and application of skills that are unique in the health care field. Often educators expect learners to be expert in skill performance prior to beginning clinical rotations. However, only basic performance of skills should be expected, because skills have just been introduced. Clinical and laboratory educators have to create opportunities for students to continue developing their skills through application with frequent feedback and opportunity for refinement. For example, when designing laboratory experiences, nurse educators can teach some skills early, such as donning sterile gloves and universal precautions. As students progress through subsequent laboratories, learning more complex skills, they should continue to be held accountable for the earlier skills such as sterile gloving and universal precautions as they are expected to do in clinical practice.

This scaffolding of learning is essential for moving learners toward expert skill development. Benner (1984) suggested that an expert "no longer relies on an analytic principle (rule, guideline, maxim) to connect her or his understanding of the situation to an appropriate action" (p. 31) because the expert nurse has "an enormous background of experience" (p. 32). Only through practice and experience can students advance in their skills development. This enormous amount of experience takes time. Some suggest that it may take approximately 4 hours of practice per day for 10 years to achieve a level of mastery for more complex knowledge and professional skills (Colvin, 2008; Ericsson, 2008; Levitin, 2006). Therefore, it is important for educators to establish an expectation of acceptable performance early on, with the understanding that skills development continues throughout a professional career.

The importance of solid skills development cannot be underestimated for the patient, nurse, or employer. Patients equate excellence in care with the ability of their nurse to perform the skills necessary for their care. The confidence of nurses is intertwined with their ability to competently perform those same skills. The employer relies on nurses to deliver excellent care, which requires high levels of knowledge and psychomotor skills development. Competent performance of skills is expected through a nurse's last day of clinical practice. If this important foundation is not established properly early in the curriculum, then the students will continue to struggle with skills and will adopt poor practices that can have a negative impact on the quality and safety of nursing practice. These poor practices not only become ingrained in that nurse's clinical performance, but can also become a poor standard of care for a given clinical setting as that nurse precepts new nurses and students.

PHASES OF SKILL DEVELOPMENT

Fitts and Posner (1967) described three phases of skills development: cognitive, associative, and autonomous. The *cognitive phase* requires a lot of attention and is focused on understanding the skill, how best to implement the skill, and the evaluation of the skill. The *associative phase* is devoted to refining the skill so the performance is more consistent with less variability. The *autonomous phase* is more habitual and automatic, requiring less attention and freeing the learner for higher level thinking. Students in learning laboratories are in the cognitive phase and may begin to move to the associative phase near the end of their laboratory experience, depending on the amount of practice and instructor feedback they obtain. It is more likely that the associative and autonomous phases will occur in professional practice, where certain skills such as washing hands, introducing self, and surveilling the environment will become second nature. These automatic abilities require initial skill learning followed by practice and then repeated performance in a variety of patient care scenarios, both simulated and real. For example, it is important that learners be able to automate select skills, such as assessing blood pressures of a rapidly deteriorating patient, without having to think about the sequence of steps needed to assess the blood pressure.

DELIBERATE PRACTICE

Automation of all skills, however, is not the end goal for *expert* performance. To facilitate the journey to expert performance, it is helpful to consider deliberate practice. Ericsson (2004) defined deliberate practice as "engaging in practice activities with the primary goal of improving some aspect of performance" (p. S73). He delineated the steps as first identifying an area for improvement for a well-defined task, then receiving immediate feedback, and finally problem-solving for improved performance through repetition of the task (Ericsson, 2004). Ericsson (2008) cautioned, however, that those who are trying to achieve expert performance must work to counteract automaticity by striving for continual improvement. For example, students arrive at the school of nursing with hand washing automated from years of washing their hands. However, in health care, we need them to be more deliberate in not only the technique of hand washing but also in the frequency and timing of hand washing. Educators are not trying to automate the *task* but are trying to automate the *expectation* that hand washing will be done on entering the patient's room and prior to patient care.

For high-risk patient safety skills such as medication administration, it is important that they are not automated. There is a risk of disengaged thinking while performing repetitive psychomotor motions during a skill such as medication administration. It is essential that learners recognize that these skills require concentration and careful attention to detail for accuracy and safety in the presence of repetition. Ericsson (2008) suggested that with careful evaluation of the procedure as it occurs and with concurrent problem solving for potential areas of improvement, skill development can be enhanced. Many agencies and nurses are reflecting on the practice of medication administration, considering methods to improve the skill of medication administration, and implementing "do not disturb zones" for the medication administration nurse to minimize distractions and associated errors. Faculty members should instill in their learners an expectation that they should personally, as well as within the profession, continually reexamine how skills are performed and explore ways to improve patient care using deliberate practice instead of settling for acceptable performance.

DEVELOPMENT OF PROFESSIONAL CONFIDENCE

The learning laboratory is also essential for establishing the professional confidence that graduates need to begin their nursing career. It can be the milieu where students begin to develop the *therapeutic use of self* (Kardong-Edgren, 2012) and to provide patient-centered care. The Quality and Safety Education for Nurses (QSEN) competencies define *patient-centered care* as "[recognizing] the patient or designee as the source of control and full partner in providing compassionate and coordinated care based on respect for [the] patient's preferences, values, and needs" (Cronenwett et al., 2007, p. 123). Assisting students in learning how to approach patients with respect and dignity, being responsive to their individual needs, being sensitive to cultural differences, and collaborating with the patient and with other members of the health care team in the delivery of safe and quality care are a few of the overarching goals of socialization into the nursing profession. As educators design experiences for students, it is important not to overlook these core values of good nursing care. Learners need the opportunity to practice cognitive as well as motor skills. Educators can embed skills in patient care scenarios to teach these concepts.

ROLE OF FACULTY, STAFF, TEACHING ASSISTANTS, AND PEER MENTORS

The type of nurse educator chosen to teach in a learning laboratory varies based on the objectives and academic considerations. Laboratory educators should be nurses and can include faculty members, staff, or graduate nursing teaching assistants based on staffing needs. Undergraduate peers also may be used with qualified nursing oversight. All educators, regardless of position or experience, require training on the content of each laboratory to promote consistent teaching and demonstration of skills, to enable educators to effectively communicate rationales and evidence-based practice (when available), and to permit them to adequately and consistently assess student performance during evaluation. Training sessions should be held at the start of the academic term and regularly through the semester or quarter. These sessions should be structured to allow review of previously taught material as needed, discussion of upcoming skills to be learned, and demonstration of skills. Educators may practice the skills and receive coaching on skills demonstration as needed. At the end of the term, a wrap-up session should occur to discuss opportunities to refine the teaching plan and improve educational practices.

Faculty members provide supervisory oversight of all activities, including learning module development, laboratory scheduling, and coordination of laboratories with clinical courses, and represent the laboratory on nursing school curriculum and other committees. In addition, faculty members should be capable of teaching skills in an interactive and engaging manner and of facilitating simulation experiences. It is important to know that a great nurse or lecturer does not translate to a competent skill faculty; additional training is required.

Full- or part-time staff members who engage in direct teaching of nursing skills should be nurses. The educational background required to work in a learning laboratory is based on standards and policies established by the state board of nursing. Staff members might be nurses who work at local health care facilities or might be employed solely by the school of nursing. Apart from teaching in the laboratory or simulation settings, staff members might be responsible for laboratory operations such as ordering and maintaining supplies and equipment, supervising the setup and breakdown, and tracking student progress through learning modules and simulation experiences. Staff members might also complete administrative work such as copying, entering grades, scheduling student evaluations and practice sessions, and rescheduling any missed laboratories or evaluations. Some of these administrative duties can be assigned to non-nursing personnel.

Part-time teaching assistants may be graduate nursing students or practicing nurses. If graduate students are available, they provide a great resource for staffing laboratories because they typically bring current clinical expertise to their teaching and benefit from being mentored into the educator role. Many teaching assistants seek the position because they desire to become nurse educators. Because it is likely that teaching assistants can earn more working per diem in a health care agency, recruitment for the position requires an appealing package that includes financial compensation, tuition reimbursement, and health insurance coverage. In addition, work schedules must coordinate with academic schedules. To provide teaching assistants with a more holistic understanding of the laboratory environment beyond teaching content and skills, they also should be trained to assist with the laboratory setup and breakdown and routine cleaning tasks, and to input data to monitor student attendance. This broader perspective of the complexity of the lab allows them to appreciate all the components that contribute to a quality teaching environment.

If a peer-mentored environment is desired, students in upper levels of the nursing program can be recruited to provide additional practice for beginning students. Peer mentoring allows additional time not only for deliberate practice of psychomotor skills, but also for informal mentoring of students. The peer-mentored system should have established guidelines and expectations of the mentors and identified benefits for the students who participate in it.

EXPECTATIONS FOR LEARNERS IN LABORATORY

To encourage development of the professional nurse role, students should be given a written overview of guidelines and rules for laboratory attendance and preparation that parallels behaviors they will be expected to demonstrate in their role as professional nurses in the clinical setting. This information should be given with or before their first exposure to the learning laboratory. Students should learn about behavioral expectations, which emphasize the importance of personal accountability, patient and nurse safety, and compliance with the Health Insurance Portability and Accountability Act (HIPAA) and Family Educational Rights and Privacy Act (FERPA) standards. In addition to written guidelines, educators should role-model the expected clinical behaviors during laboratory sessions. Students should learn to clean up the bedside work area after patient care and ensure proper disposal of all supplies and equipment according to Occupational Safety and Health Administration (OSHA) and agency guidelines, which parallel the expectations of their behavior in a patient care environment.

Students should be required to dress in a professional manner while performing patient skills in the laboratory, following established guidelines regarding necklines, hemlines, and footwear, which would be appropriate to working in a patient care environment. Some schools of nursing ask students to dress for laboratory experiences, including simulation sessions, in their clinical uniforms. This approach is supported by the work of Adam and Galinsky (2012), who described the basic principle of "[enclothed cognition as having a] co-occurrence of two independent factors—the symbolic meaning of the clothes and the physical experience of wearing them" (p. 922). Their research suggests that donning a laboratory coat as a physician increases the person's attentiveness and carefulness. This can be transferrable to nursing students wearing their uniforms in laboratory settings, affecting their psychological perception of being and acting like a nurse. What they wear in laboratory might have an influence on how they begin to build confidence in their role as a nurse. Consequences of violating expectations of dress and appearance should be clearly outlined in the laboratory guidelines.

INTEGRATION OF LABORATORIES INTO CURRICULA

A successful learning laboratory is one that is integrated throughout the curriculum, allowing students regular, repetitive opportunities for deliberate practice. It is important for skills acquisition to provide a psychologically safe environment in which the learner "is able to behave or perform without fear of negative consequences to self-image, social standing, or career trajectory" (Ganley & Linnard-Palmer, 2012, p. e50). This "safe environment" does not diminish teaching and holding learners accountable for the standard of care, but rather creates space for the learner to focus on learning versus shutting down from fear of consequences. The climate of the learning laboratory is that of collaboration. Achievement of acceptable psychomotor skills demonstration (a designated level of performance, determined by nurse educators using evidence-based practice and best standards of practice) and attainment of related knowledge is the joint responsibility of the students and educator. Students are responsible for participating in designated learning activities to attain knowledge and promote acceptable skills acquisition. Although students may be able to perform a skill at the time of assessment, skills can be retained only with practice (Oermann, Muckler, & Morgan, 2016). Educators are responsible for providing opportunities for practice, feedback, and repeated practice at regular intervals, not only in the laboratory but also in the clinical setting.

Many learning laboratories include not only psychomotor skills acquisition but also simulation experiences, using computerized manikins, task trainers, standardized patients, and virtual reality with case-based scenarios. These provide an opportunity for students to apply what they are learning in the laboratory to patient care scenarios that simulate clinical practice. Simulation can be integrated throughout the curriculum beyond content for adult health, pediatrics, and obstetrics courses to include leadership, community health, mental health, and interprofessional experiences. Chapter 7 discusses the pedagogy of simulation in the learning laboratory.

TYPES OF LEARNING LABORATORIES

A variety of laboratories associated with both clinical and nonclinical courses may be offered throughout the prelicensure program and in graduate nursing programs. Schools of nursing vary in the sequencing of skills across the curriculum, usually beginning with basic foundational skills and advancing to more complex skills. There is no consensus on what constitutes a complex skill; however, hand washing is a basic skill, whereas central line care is a complex skill. Grouping of skills should be a deliberate decision by faculty to meet the learning needs of their students as they move from laboratories to practice settings. The established flow of clinical experiences in a nursing program will also influence how skills are grouped. Beyond beginning with foundational skills and building to complex skills, there is no consensus on what sequence skills should be taught (Table 9.1). In the graduate curriculum, laboratories can be offered for advanced health assessment, diagnostic reasoning, development of skills, and various content-specific learning experiences.

Table 9.1 provides an example of typical laboratories offered in a nursing program, listed by course and purpose, examples of skills taught for each course, and necessary preparation by students and laboratory personnel. The table includes prelicensure laboratories and also more advanced laboratories that may be offered, such as a laboratory in a diagnostic reasoning course for graduate students in nurse practitioner programs and an interprofessional education laboratory to provide essential immersive environments for interprofessional learners to develop essential skills in communication, collaboration, and teamwork.

SAMPLE LEARNING MODULE

Teaching materials and instruction guides pertaining to each specific laboratory taught should be standardized across content to promote consistency in teaching between individual educators. The materials included in Appendix A can serve as sample templates in the development and revision of learning laboratory documents in the reader's own institution. Appendix A provides the reader with seven documents for the laboratory: (a) teaching environment setup: equipment, supply use, and reset guide; (b) lesson plan; (c) teaching box supply list; (d) standardized learning module overview; (e) example provider's order; (f) example medication administration record; and (g) example skill competency evaluation checklist (Appendices A.1–A.7).

TABLE 9.1 Types of Learning Laboratories

Learner Groups

- Scheduled laboratory groups (can be based on clinical assignments, arbitrarily assigned, or self-selected)
- Small group for deliberate practice (students self-select attendance days and times)
- One-to-one skills review and/or deliberate practice (completed at the request of students or faculty/staff)
- Small simulation sessions (tabletop exercises such as problem-based learning and patient care scenario-based case studies)

Course and Purpose	Sample Skills Focus Areas	Preparation
Fundamentals Skills Laboratory/Basic Medical Surgical Skills Laboratories (can bridge across several clinically oriented courses or be contained in one fundamentals nursing course) Learn, practice, and refine: • Communication skills • Bedside psychomotor nursing skills • Increase students' confidence in the clinical setting	Basic to advanced patient care skills based on course requirements. Generally encompass aspects of: • Microbial safety and vital signs • Personal care • Immobility interventions • Safe patient handling and movement • Medication administration techniques for various nonparenteral routes • Injections • Intravenous therapy • Wound care • Elimination • Respiratory interventions • Gastrointestinal (GI) intubation • End-of-life care • Central venous access devices • Venipuncture	Provide learning modules in advance for student review prior to the laboratory session. Set up supplies, equipment, and charts specific to the skills to be taught in each laboratory.
Health/Physical Assessment Laboratories Learn, practice, and refine: • Communication and interviewing skills • Body system assessment skills • Documentation skills	Conduct body system assessment specific to each session's content. Provide regular practice, integrating the systems learned each week into a cohesive patient assessment.	Provide learning modules in advance for student review prior to the laboratory session. Online format: No room or laboratory resources needed Classroom format: Laboratory setup

(continued)

TABLE 9.1 Types of Learning Laboratories (*continued*)

Course and Purpose	Sample Skills Focus Areas	Preparation
		Provide a private space with appropriate diagnostic equipment for the body systems reviewed in each session.
		Set up additional learning resources such as simulators and anatomical models.
Advanced Medical Surgical/Capstone Laboratories Refresh previously learned communication and psychomotor skills. Increase students' confidence with psychomotor skills.	Basic to advanced patient care skills based on course requirements. Generally encompasses aspects of: • Medication administration: oral, injectable, intravenous, gastrostomy, central line flushes • Sterile dressing changes • Tracheostomy care • Catheterization • Health/physical assessment • Venipuncture • Equipment review	Provide learning modules in advance for student review prior to the laboratory session. Set up supplies and equipment for: • Applicable medication administration routes • Selected bedside clinical skills • Health/physical assessment review
Pharmacology Competency Laboratories Synthesize content from multiple courses (health/physical assessment, fundamentals, pharmacology). Integrate pharmacologic knowledge with medication administration procedures.	Interpretation of laboratory values Use of pharmacologic references Medication administration includes: • Recognizing and/or averting medication errors • Medication administration skills: oral, topical, eye, ear, injectable, intravenous Health/physical assessment skills pertinent to each scenario Effective communication with health care team	Provide learning modules in advance for student review prior to the laboratory session. Instruct students to perform a focused review of content: • Applicable medication administration procedures from fundamental skills training • Selected drug classifications and categories, including but not limited to the medications found in the scenarios • General health assessment skills Set up supplies, equipment, and charts for each patient care scenario.

(continued)

TABLE 9.1 Types of Learning Laboratories (*continued*)

Course and Purpose	Sample Skills Focus Areas	Preparation
Pediatric and Family Health Laboratories Review previously learned skills in a pediatric and family-oriented context. Practice patient-specific skills and interventions for the pediatric population.	Generally includes practice in: • Medication administration: oral, injectable, intravenous • Use of infusion devices • Infant bathing, feeding, and diapering	Provide learning modules in advance for student review prior to the laboratory session. Instruct students to review required modules prior to laboratory.
Review equipment.	GI intubation: insertion, feedings, medications, removal • Urinary catheterization and specimen collection • Ostomy care as applicable to area • Tracheostomy care as applicable to clinical setting	Set up supplies, equipment, and charts for: • Medication administration • Infant care skills • Bedside procedures
Maternal and Newborn Health Laboratories Review previously learned skills in the context of a labor patient, a newborn, and a postpartum patient. Practice patient-specific skills and interventions for the maternal/newborn population. Review equipment.	Generally includes practice in: • Labor support techniques and interventions for the patient and family • Fetal heart monitoring • Postpartum assessment checklist • Newborn assessment and medication administration • Practice counting newborn heart rate and respiratory rate	Provide learning modules in advance for student review prior to the laboratory session. Set up supplies, equipment, and charts specific to the skills to be reviewed.
Public/Community Health Laboratories Review previously learned skills in the context of a community setting. Develop and practice patient education and intervention skills in a community-oriented context.	Generally includes review of: • Vital signs: use of manual and/or nonelectronic equipment • Glucometer use • Basic wound care Use of patient education materials: posters, supplies, equipment, models	Provide learning modules in advance for student review prior to the laboratory session. Set up supplies, equipment, and charts specific to the skills to be reviewed.
Diagnostic Reasoning Laboratories	• Body system assessment specific to each session's content	Provide learning modules, case studies, and integrated clinical scenarios as required.

(continued)

TABLE 9.1 Types of Learning Laboratories (*continued*)

Course and Purpose	Sample Skills Focus Areas	Preparation
(Graduate student nurse practitioner laboratories for various specialty areas) Practice and refine body system assessment skills. Refine communication and interviewing skills with a provider-oriented focus.	• Regular practice integrating systems learned each week into a cohesive assessment	Provide a private space with appropriate diagnostic equipment for the body systems reviewed in each session. Set up additional learning resources such as simulators and anatomical models. Set up audio or video equipment as required based on scenario needs and objectives.
Interprofessional Education Laboratories Learn, practice, and refine: • Interprofessional communication skills • Principles of teamwork and collaboration Practice skills and procedures within interprofessional teams.	• Basic to advanced patient care skills and assessment techniques based on patient care scenarios • Practice integration of teamwork, collaboration, and communication skills	Provide learning modules in advance for student review prior to the laboratory session. Set up supplies, equipment, and charts specific to the skills to be reviewed.
External Clients Nursing skills refresher for skills development laboratories: • Practice specific skills and procedures • Improve communication skills Videotaping education offerings.	• Basic to advanced patient care skills and assessment techniques based on course requirements	Provide learning modules in advance for student review prior to the laboratory session. Set up supplies, equipment, and charts specific to the skills to be reviewed.

Source: Copyright Education-Innovation-Simulation Learning Environment, School of Nursing, The University of North Carolina at Chapel Hill, 2017. Reprinted with permission.

LABORATORY ORGANIZATION

INSTRUCTOR-TO-STUDENT RATIO

The instructor-to-student ratio in laboratory is determined based on several criteria and can vary based on the intent of each laboratory. Several laboratory groupings are suggested at the top of Table 9.1. Room size, number of staff available to teach, availability and amount of equipment and supplies, student level in the program, and technical difficulty of skills in a particular laboratory all influence the instructor-to-student ratio. The evolving learning styles of students also should be considered. Ratios may range from 1:8 or 1:10 to mimic the clinical setting or can be 1:12 or higher with a large group focus. Because skills acquisition requires more than theoretical knowledge, students need the opportunity to practice with timely feedback, which may be difficult to offer in laboratories with a high student-to-faculty ratio.

STUDENT ASSIGNMENT

Students can select their laboratory section through a registration process, which allows for individual preferences, or might be placed in laboratories based on predetermined criteria such as clinical group assignments. Educators can be assigned to specific laboratory groups for the term or to laboratory sections on a rotational basis. Assigning educators to a specific laboratory section across the term provides them an opportunity to become familiar with the students in that section and to better understand the students' learning styles. It also can establish an atmosphere of trust and collegiality. However, rotating educators between laboratory groups can provide learners with an opportunity to experience diverse teaching styles and to learn strategies for working within contingency teams, an arrangement that parallels staffing patterns in clinical practice.

STAGING AREA

Organization of the laboratory is essential to the success of the laboratory and nursing program. The need for organization cannot be overestimated: when done well, organization makes the laboratory environment seem to run effortlessly. The learning laboratory requires a lot of consumable supplies, durable equipment, staff, and logistical systems to manage both staff and the flow of large numbers of students. Because supply and equipment management is essential to a well-run laboratory, the laboratory requires a staging area. The staging area is more than a storage room. In fact, if called *storage*, facility management committees may be tempted to move the laboratory storage area to an inconvenient location, making it challenging to access. If the focus of the space is on *staging*, the space is recognized as being an integral component of the laboratory operations. The staging area is the center of infrastructure activity of the learning laboratory.

Functionality of the staging area is dependent on appropriate building structure and a high level of organization and tidiness to allow for accessibility of equipment and supplies when needed. It should to be equipped with at least one sink for cleaning and resetting equipment such as intravenous (IV) fluids and suction canisters. A sink is also essential to prepare supplies for laboratories that require simulated liquids such as IV fluids, parenteral nutrition (PN), blood, urine, gastrointestinal fluids, and fake stool samples. The staging area also requires adequate shelving and power sources to store supplies and equipment, flat work areas for assembling and packing, and appropriate carts for item transport. A variety of cleaning supplies should be readily available to assist in harvesting used supplies. It is helpful to have various adhesive removers to use for removing adhesive residue from tubing, manikins, and other surfaces. Basic office supplies, from scissors, tape, and markers to printers and label-making equipment, should be accessible, but it is preferred that they be made available in the staging area workspace.

LABORATORY ACTION PLAN

Standardization of room setup across simultaneously occurring laboratories promotes consistent educational experiences among separate laboratories. To promote standardization, it is helpful to create a room setup guide outlining how to prepare the space and/or manikins for student learning and practice. Appendix A.1 provides the Teaching Environment Setup: equipment, supply use, and reset guide. It provides guidelines to follow before, during, and after each teaching session. The guide should be reviewed by each educator prior to beginning the session to ensure familiarity with the setup equipment, supplies, and procedures.

In addition to the room and laboratory setup guidelines, there should be a lesson plan that both outlines the content to be covered and indicates the amount of time to be spent on each topic. Recommendations for possible teaching strategies, such as observation, participation during the educator's demonstration (round table practice, discussed further later in the chapter), and practice after observation should be included on the lesson plan to guide the educational experience allowing consistency among educators. Appendix A.2 provides an example of a lesson plan.

To enhance efficiency and consistency in each laboratory and between rooms, a teaching box can be created for each module (Figure 9.1). A teaching box is prepared and restocked after each teaching session. If there are concurrent sessions, the educator can create a teaching box for laboratory room and store the restocked teaching boxes in the staging area, ready for the next session (Figure 9.2). Module-specific equipment and supplies

FIGURE 9.1 Examples of teaching boxes used for laboratory setup.

FIGURE 9.2 Teaching boxes stored in laboratory staging area.

Source: Copyright Education-Innovation-Simulation Learning Environment, School of Nursing, The University of North Carolina at Chapel Hill, 2017. Reprinted with permission.

are placed in the teaching box, along with a list of contents. Items that are necessary for the laboratory but do not fit into the teaching box can also be listed, along with the storage location of those items. The content list should indicate where to obtain replacement supplies if needed. Appendix A.3 provides a template for creating a teaching box supply list.

LEARNING MODULES

Students should enter each laboratory experience with a basic understanding of the content to be covered in that laboratory. Each learning module should start with a standardized overview of expectations for student preparation, required supplies, laboratory objectives, required and recommended readings, and a list of the skills to be covered in the laboratory. Specialized module content should include the key theoretical concepts and outline the procedures for the skills to be covered, giving students a standardized baseline from which to start skills acquisition. A standardized learning module overview is found in Appendix A.4.

Providing students with the key concepts underlying individual skills is a component of teaching any skill. Learning the theoretical underpinnings and patient care application of skills assists the learner to understand how the knowledge can be used in practical clinical situations. Making the connections between acquiring and using knowledge is what Benner, Sutphen, Leonard, and Day (2010) refer to as *teaching for a sense of salience* (p. 94). This sense-making assists students to understand the nuances of skills, their application to patient care, and how skills acquisition affects their professional development as a nurse.

Learning modules can vary from locally prepared documents to ones obtained from commercial publishers and nursing organizations. They should be available to learners for either printing or downloading to meet different reading and learning styles. Faculty members should ensure that content found in the course textbook and learning resources matches the laboratory modules. These documents need to be revised each year to stay current with practice, national guidelines, articles, textbooks, and other resources used in the course. If learning module content differs from these resources, that fact should be noted in the module, with a rationale for the difference to assist the learner to understand how evidence-based practice may evolve quicker than the supporting textbook.

Some programs of study provide didactic content prior to lab where the skills are covered in lecture with a subsequent lab. Other programs provide conceptual themes, such as immobility, without didactic content related to the skills related to immobility. An additional teaching/learning aid is to provide an audio file to deliver standardized key theoretical or procedural content, eliminating the possibility of inconsistent coverage of material in individual laboratories. Additionally, the podcast allows students who are auditory learners an alternative method for acquiring the content. Students read the module and have the option of listening to a podcast of the content prior to attending the laboratory session.

LEARNING LABORATORY SESSIONS

It is important for students to review the content before attending the laboratory session, to avoid spending a significant amount of time during the laboratory discussing key concepts and to allow for more time for practicing skills. To encourage student review and a basic level of preparation, a quiz might be administered online or in person before the laboratory session or as the first component of the session before teaching begins. The frequency of these quizzes may vary from preceding each laboratory session to being given randomly throughout the course. The aim of these quizzes is to assess preparation for the laboratory and understanding of key concepts, not to assess skill application.

Ideally, all students will have an opportunity for supervised practice of all skills (either by the educator or by a fellow student observing using the procedure guide). Another option is to have students view video recordings that demonstrate the skills and include evidence-based practice. Students can then use laboratory time to apply what they have learned in case-based scenarios. A third approach, referred to previously as *round table practice*, is used when students move through the steps of a skill together. As an example, students can arrange the overbed tables in a half circle as the educator demonstrates and walks the students through a skill (such as donning sterile gloves) in a step-wise manner. Students continue to practice while the educator walks around the room to critique technique and offer feedback. The best approach depends on the learners, content, space and time constraints, and expertise of the educator. During the laboratory sessions, students should have practice time, with feedback after skills are demonstrated to allow them the opportunity for deliberate practice to improve performance. Some skills can be practiced outside the laboratory setting, but others require specialty laboratory equipment and supplies (for example, tracheostomy suctioning); adequate time in the laboratory environment is an important consideration. Regardless of where skills are practiced, it is important to provide specific criteria to facilitate accurate practice.

REALISM

Realism in the learning laboratory enhances preparation of students for actual patient care. Realism should be enhanced as much as possible within the constraints of the learning laboratory to encourage students to immerse themselves in the patient care scenario. There are many ways to promote a realistic environment, from setting up simulated hospital rooms with patient records and manikins in the beds to obtaining the actual equipment and supplies available at local facilities.

Cost is always a consideration when determining how realistic a laboratory can be. The school of nursing must make a decision whether to purchase or create a facsimile of the necessary items for teaching, such as call bells and medication labels. For example, call bells can be made from pictures downloaded from the Internet, which are then laminated or affixed to a surface and attached to a cord. The cord can be a purchased electrical cord or a cloth or cable that is made to represent a hospital call bell cord. Simple computer software found free on the Internet can be used to simulate medication labels, or labeling systems can be purchased from a vendor. Learning laboratory personnel constantly have to balance educational needs and funding constraints.

Another way to create realism is to provide paperwork that mimics affiliate agencies' paperwork that the student will need when performing the skill and will use for documenting when completed. For medication administration in a laboratory, a provider's order sheet, medication administration record, and other pertinent documentation forms should be available for the specific laboratory content. The forms can be hard copies or in an electronic charting format. In the interest of patient safety and to clearly differentiate simulated documents from actual patient care documents, it is important to label these forms and documents "For Educational Use Only—Not for Actual Patient Care." Appendix A.5 provides an example of a provider's order sheet. Appendix A.6 is an example of a medication administration record (MAR).

SUPPLY BAGS

Skill acquisition requires manipulation of materials and lots of practice. To enable hands-on practice, supply bags can be assembled, providing the student with a select list of supplies for skill development. Bags can be purchased for a specific nursing course or periodically throughout the program to meet specialized clinical requirements. The contents of each bag will reflect the skills that the faculty consider most important for students to gain competence in performing. Supply bags can be funded with a separate fee that students pay in addition to other course costs, or they can be provided as part of the required lab fees. Supply bags can promote student responsibility while providing all students with the same level of supplies, either new or used. Students are responsible for bringing and maintaining their supplies for labs across the semester. Providing supplies up front to students can decrease the amount needed in laboratories, which has implications for space utilization, storage, and funding. Decisions should be made about the specific contents to offer in the supply bag, such as whether to supply needles and syringes for practice and appropriate disposal or recycling of used supplies at the end of training.

PRACTICE LABORATORIES

Practice laboratories allow deliberate practice of skills taught in laboratories and can enhance student performance. Practice laboratories can be regularly scheduled or can occur on an as-needed basis, depending on the requirements of the specific course and nursing program. Practice laboratories can be open to general practice of any skill requiring refreshment or refinement, or they can be geared toward preparation for an upcoming performance evaluation with a focus on the set of skills to be evaluated. Practice laboratories for evaluation should not be considered a time to reteach laboratory content, but rather a time for skill refinement using deliberate practice. These laboratories do not have to be tied to a specific clinical course; instead, they can be offered to any student who needs to refresh skills or who requires remediation.

Staffing decisions for practice laboratories depend on the availability of resources, both personnel and physical. Ideally, all practice laboratories should be staffed with a qualified educator, and the ratio of educators to students should be low to allow for more direct supervision of and feedback to students as they practice skills. If the decision is made to offer practice laboratories without an educator present, space access and accountability issues have to be addressed. Practice laboratories should occur with the same room setup as the one in which skills were taught, which can result in competition for space and faculty. Decisions also have to be made about when to offer practice laboratories and what equipment and supplies will be made available to students during them. General practice laboratory policies and procedures should be in place and available for students, including cleaning and resetting the laboratory space for later students, timeliness and attendance requirements, and penalties for nonattendance. When students do not attend scheduled practice labs, they prevent other students from having the benefit of that laboratory practice time.

INDIVIDUAL DELIBERATE PRACTICE

Individual deliberate practice sessions, which are also known as 1:1 teaching time, can benefit students who are struggling to grasp a specific skill or concept in the laboratory or group practice sessions or who want to improve their competence through practice. Individual practice sessions should not be used in place of initial teaching or group practice, but should be used as an adjunct to maximize resource utilization. Clear guidelines for the use of deliberate practice time have to be established to ensure the most equitable availability for all students who seek assistance. Consideration should be given to the frequency of deliberate practice time, the best qualified educator to guide learning in the session, and policies for determining the frequency of individual student access because of limited resources.

COMPETENCY EVALUATIONS

Demonstration of skills through competency evaluation provides visible evidence of the student's psychomotor skill learning. Competency in skill performance should be assessed in periodic performance evaluations throughout the term, but it can also be assessed only at the end of the term. Designated levels of performance expected in clinical practice and determined by faculty are the traditional ways to constitute skills competence. Skills evaluation can be formative or summative. Formative evaluation judges students' progress in developing skills and is focused on diagnostic feedback without assigning a grade to the evaluation experience. Summative evaluation, in contrast, is end-of-instruction evaluation to determine what the student has learned. Summative evaluation provides a basis for grading and other high-stakes decisions (Oermann & Gaberson, 2017).

Formative skills competency evaluation occurs through an informal assessment of selected skills, such as when an evaluator observes a student performing a dressing change and provides real-time feedback about the student's technique and ability to perform the skill at a safe and competent level. A summative skills competency evaluation of the same dressing change skill is a formal assessment of the student's ability to perform the skill according to predetermined criteria on a checklist. Proceeding without feedback from the evaluator, the student attempts to perform the skill at a safe and competent level. At the end of the summative evaluation, the student receives feedback that counts toward a weighted evaluation of the skill demonstrated. Both types of evaluation are essential components in learning laboratories (Table 9.2). More in-depth discussion about formative and summative evaluation can be found in Chapter 12.

TABLE 9.2 Types of Competency Evaluations

Formative Evaluation	Summative Evaluation
• Skills to be evaluated can be randomly selected or preassigned • Informal assessment of selected skills • Uses skill procedure checklists • Immediate feedback provided throughout procedure	• Skills to be evaluated can be randomly selected or preassigned • Formal assessment of selected skills • Performance evaluation based on predetermined criteria (pass–fail or graded) • Feedback provided at end of evaluation • Can be partial or complete (e.g., demonstrate either a complete head-to-toe examination or a selected body system)

Decisions concerning the amount and type of feedback to be offered during skills performance have to be made, reviewed, and agreed on by all evaluators to promote standardized evaluation criteria. At the beginning of the term, provide an evaluation study guide for student reference. Students should refer to the guide when they are introduced to the skill in laboratory, while refining their technique in practice laboratory, and when preparing for the competency evaluation. Knowledge of the underlying cognitive components relative to skills is essential to skills acquisition and is evaluated through laboratory quizzes, course examinations, and competency evaluations.

Consistency in teaching skills is evident at the point of evaluation; inconsistency places the learner at a disadvantage for the performance evaluation. Students need to be assured that they have been taught what is necessary to be successful, not only on the competency exam, but also for practice. Standardized evaluation checklists are important to enhance consistency among evaluators and can be developed based on the course material, based on a skills guide, or generated locally. Evaluations can be awarded a grade or a successful result can be considered a pass–fail requirement for a course. The importance of skills evaluation as a component for successful completion of the course must be outlined in the course syllabus. The selection of skills for evaluation can vary based on local agency and nursing program requirements.

Skills to be evaluated might be a predetermined set that all students complete, or they might be randomly assigned from the skills to be demonstrated. Evaluations can be documented on paper or in an electronic format. Electronic formats are easy to send to students for review after each evaluation is complete, and the educator can upload the performance evaluation checklists into a secure student file. With an electronic format, the laboratory educator can access the checklist at the time of the evaluation and then save it into the student file after the evaluation (Figure 9.3). Verbal feedback given at the end of the evaluation can be followed up with an e-mail attachment of the actual checklist documentation. This provides students the opportunity to review what was missed as they prepare for return demonstration of the skill at a later time. As with all testing instruments, information security concerning evaluation forms must be in compliance with established academic standards.

When the instructor creates student evaluation checklists, it is helpful for both students and evaluators to know which critical steps are mandatory for successful completion of the skills. If there are critical patient or nurse safety elements that, when omitted, would require students to repeat the evaluation, both evaluator and student should be aware of those elements. However, students should not expect to pass skills

FIGURE 9.3 Faculty using an electronic form to record student performance evaluation.

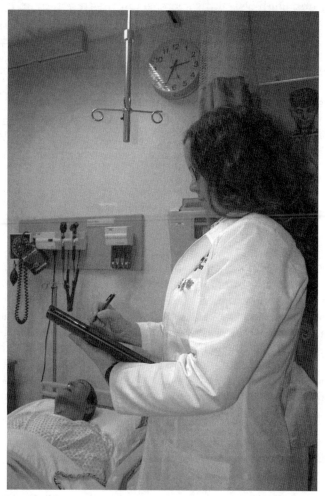

Source: Copyright Education-Innovation-Simulation Learning Environment, School of Nursing, The University of North Carolina at Chapel Hill, 2017. Reprinted with permission.

if only the critical steps are completed, but other less critical but important steps are not demonstrated.

A star system is an example of a transparent evaluation system that triages the steps of skills into different levels. A star system, assigning one, two, or three stars to each step of the skill, encourages students to understand the critical steps in a skill, promotes patient and nurse safety, and reinforces the understanding that all steps have a rationale and degree of importance. If students omit or do not perform correctly a one-star step, they can be required to be reassessed for that skill, regardless of how well they perform the rest of the steps. If students omit or do not perform correctly two of the two-star steps, they need to be evaluated again, and so forth. Appendix A.7 provides an example skill competency evaluation checklist.

Students should be able to review the evaluation results, especially if they will be required to be reassessed on those skills at a later date. When students do not perform a skill satisfactorily, they are usually evaluated again on the same skill.

Students can, however, be required to perform a different skill in subsequent evaluations, based on local policy and depending on the importance of the skill or underlying concept. High-risk skills such as administration of an IV push medication would benefit from a second attempt at the same skill, possibly with a different medication.

Performance evaluation can contribute points to a course grade or be pass–fail. If evaluations are pass–fail, students might not attend to the important work of skills acquisition due to competing priorities. If points (even minimal points) are attached to skills performance, students may give higher priority to the laboratory content. The number of allowable reassessments should be incorporated into the course syllabus to avoid a situation in which students continually fail performance evaluations but still pass the course. The consequences of not obtaining a satisfactory pass after the established numbers of allowable attempts must be determined and communicated to students at the beginning of the course.

LOGISTICS

SCHEDULING

Scheduling is a key consideration when running a learning laboratory. The need for multiple student interactions requires close scheduling to avoid conflict and meet staffing requirements. Regularly scheduled teaching laboratories, practice laboratories, evaluations, opportunities to be reassessed on the performance of skills, and remediation sessions have to be coordinated around the students' class and clinical schedules. Laboratories and simulation experiences for students in different terms of the nursing program have to be interwoven because of competition for space and staffing. The schedule should be developed and maintained centrally in the learning laboratory to minimize conflicts and accidental overbooking.

SIGN-UP TOOLS

Scheduling students for practice laboratories, evaluations, and individual practice time can be accomplished in different ways. Students can be allowed to sign up independently, or they can be scheduled for activities by laboratory personnel. If students are allowed to sign up on their own, the method chosen must be accessible to all students. They should be notified in advance when the sign-up will be available, thereby providing equal opportunity for selecting preferred timeslots. Guidelines should be in place for determining how many times students can sign up for recurring activities, when sign-up will open and close, how students notify learning laboratory personnel if they cannot attend a scheduled laboratory, and any penalties for nonattendance.

INVENTORY TRACKING

An inventory system for tracking equipment needs to be in place in the learning laboratory. Personnel should be able to track equipment purchases; schedule and complete maintenance; and check out equipment to students, staff, and faculty members. The inventory tracking system can be hardcopy or electronic, but must include a labeling system to track each individual piece of equipment. Regular inventory checks should be accomplished to ensure that all equipment is available and tested for usability. Equipment needing an upgrade can be noted in the inventory for future purchasing opportunities.

BUDGET AND PURCHASING

The budget for learning laboratories varies across schools of nursing and can range from minimal to substantial. It can come from different sources, both internal and external. The budget for the learning laboratory should include recurring supply purchases, plans for one-time equipment purchases, and personnel salaries, if applicable. A purchasing and budget tracking system should be in place, using both hardcopy forms and electronic tracking processes. Information concerning warranties, recall notices, and items purchased via outside sources for the laboratory should be kept with purchasing and budget documents to facilitate continuity in equipment maintenance, planning, and utilization of funds.

The fiscal costs of running a laboratory include obtaining sustainable equipment and consumable supplies. Sometimes laboratories acquire used beds, overbed tables, bedside tables, and other equipment when area hospitals purchase new items. Additionally, purchasing from companies that have refurbished equipment can lower costs, but it is recommended to complete a reference check to ensure that the equipment has been adequately refurbished. Laboratories make large financial investments in computerized simulation manikins, static manikins, and task trainers. As good stewards, learning laboratories need to care for these teaching aids to maximize their longevity. Even with excellent care, equipment will eventually have to be replaced. Replacement considerations should be included in annual fiscal planning for the laboratory.

Consumable supplies are a large expense for laboratories. If schools have the option to affiliate with a medical facility purchasing department to order supplies, it can be cost effective because of bulk ordering. Additional fees such as stocking fees charged by the medical facility must be calculated into the budget. Outside vendors also are a viable resource for laboratory supplies. Often it is beneficial to have accounts with multiple supply vendors to allow for access to various products, competitive cost comparisons, and flexible shipping timelines.

EXTERNAL CLIENTS

Given the rich resources of a learning laboratory, there are often external clients that request utilization of the laboratory to equip their learners. External clients may include health care continuing education programs, local hospitals, emergency services, and researchers, among others. External clients benefit from having a laboratory located nearby to provide an easily accessible space for learner practice. Researchers can use a laboratory to properly train employees in such tasks as blood collection, taking vital signs, and medication administration. Depending on legal requirements and local needs, a business contract outlining the details of staffing, funding, reimbursement, and purchasing should be established.

SUMMARY

Learning laboratories exist both to create meaningful learning experiences during skills acquisition and to nurture the development of professional nurses who can provide safe and quality care. For learning laboratories to function effectively, they should be integrated into the curriculum to provide students the opportunity to review skills and engage in deliberate practice, while applying skills across the patient care continuum. Although educators who work in the learning laboratory might come from a variety of backgrounds or hold varied positions, they should all agree on the importance of the learning laboratory in the greater context of nursing education. Teaching in learning laboratories can be a rewarding role because students enter the laboratory excited about learning psychomotor skills, and the educator has the opportunity to encourage depth and breadth of professional competency.

When planning learning laboratory content, educators must consider staffing needs, training requirements for laboratory educators, expectations of and by students, the educator-to-student ratio, and the depth and breadth of student assignments and evaluations to be completed. Storage and staging of equipment and supplies, the action plan for laboratory setup and breakdown, the type and quantity of supplies available to students, and efforts to promote realism in the laboratory setting must also be considered within budgetary constraints. Laboratory content should be structured and presented in a timely manner, preferably at the same time as or close to the time that applicable course content is taught. Careful development of learning experiences that provide consistent opportunities for all learners is an important consideration when determining the flow of laboratory content. The availability and frequency of psychomotor skills practice, including the amount of deliberate practice that can be provided, has to be balanced with the need to present new content, evaluate skills acquisition, and provide simulation experiences. All of these factors, while challenging, contribute to making the learning laboratory an environment that is both rewarding and renewing with each new influx of students.

Learning laboratories should be vibrant, educational hubs for engaging learners to be immersed in deliberate practice to provide quality and safe patient care. Faculty members are responsible for providing creative learning experiences that move the learner from knowing about to implementing those skills, while considering how to provide optimal care in each unique patient situation. Laboratory educators are privileged to be a guide for learners during this portion of their journey from novice to expert practitioner.

REFERENCES

Adam, H., & Galinsky, A. D. (2012). Enclothed cognition. *Journal of Experimental Social Psychology, 48*(4), 918–925. doi:10.1016/j.jesp.2012.02.008

Benner, P. (1984). *From novice to expert: Excellence and power in clinical nursing practice.* Menlo Park, CA: Addison-Wesley.

Benner, P., Sutphen, M., Leonard, V., & Day, L. (2010). *Educating nurses: A call for radical transformation.* Standford, CA: The Carnegie Foundation for the Advancement of Teaching.

Colvin, G. (2008). *Talent is overrated: What really separates world-class performers from everybody else.* New York, NY: Penguin.

Cronenwett, L., Sherwood, G., Barnsteiner, J., Disch, J., Johnson, J., Mitchell, P., . . . Warren, J. (2007). Quality and safety education for nurses. *Nursing Outlook, 55*(3), 122–131. doi:10.1016/j.outlook.2007.02.006

Diers, D. (1990). Learning the art and craft of nursing. *American Journal of Nursing, 90*(1), 64–66.

Ericsson, K. A. (2004). Deliberate practice and the acquisition and maintenance of expert performance in medicine and related domains. *Academic Medicine, 79*(Suppl. 10), S70–S81.

Ericsson, K. A. (2008). Deliberate practice and acquisition of expert performance: A general overview. *Academic Emergency Medicine, 15*(11), 988–994. doi:10.1111/j1553-2712.2008.00227.x

Fitts, P. M., & Posner, M. I. (1967). *Human performance.* Belmont, CA: Brooks/Cole.

Ganley, B. J., & Linnard-Palmer, L. (2012). Academic safety during nursing simulation: Perceptions of nursing students and faculty. *Clinical Simulation in Nursing, 8*(2), e49–e57. doi:10.1016/j.ecns.2010.06.004

Kardong-Edgren, S. (2012). Non-technical skills vs therapeutic use of self: An observation. *Clinical Simulation in Nursing, 8*(2), e35. doi:10.1016/j.ecns.2011.12.003

Levitin, D. J. (2006). *This is your brain on music: The science of a human obsession.* New York, NY: Dutton.

Norman, J. (2016). Americans rate healthcare providers high on honesty, ethics. *Gallup 2016.* Retrieved from http://www.gallup.com/poll/200057/americans-rate-healthcare-providers-high-honesty -ethics.aspx

Oermann, M. H., & Gaberson, K. B. (2017). *Evaluation and testing in nursing education* (5th ed.). New York, NY: Springer Publishing.

Oermann, M. H., Muckler, V. C., & Morgan, B. (2016). Framework for teaching psychomotor and procedural skills in nursing. *Journal of Continuing Education in Nursing, 47,* 278–282. doi:10.3928/00220124 -20160518-10

10

Clinical Teaching in Nursing

LISA K. WOODLEY

OBJECTIVES

- Describe the importance of effective clinical teaching in nursing
- Summarize research related to clinical teaching in nursing
- Differentiate between the various components of the process of clinical teaching, including learning outcomes, student learning needs, clinical learning activities, student guidance in the clinical setting, and evaluation of student performance

The clinical teacher plays a pivotal role in shaping the learning for nursing students in the clinical setting. Because of this, it is essential that clinical teachers exhibit effective teaching behaviors and best practices in teaching nursing, and that they inspire students. This chapter explains why effective clinical teaching is so critical, the process of clinical teaching, and how the clinical teacher should best address learning outcomes for students. Specific teaching strategies are discussed, such as how to create a learning climate that is inviting and supportive to students, how to foster effective relationships in the clinical setting, how to design an effective and inspirational clinical orientation, and how to choose best patient assignments for students. This chapter also describes other best clinical teaching practices, such as structuring and organizing the clinical day, creating clinical conferences and other learning activities that enhance student learning, and giving guidance and feedback to students in the clinical setting. The concepts and teaching strategies described in the chapter are applicable across clinical settings and other sites in which students have practice experiences. Models of clinical teaching, such as dedicated education units and other types of partnerships, are described in Chapter 13, and clinical evaluation is discussed separately in Chapter 14.

THE IMPORTANCE OF EFFECTIVE CLINICAL TEACHING

The clinical experience has long been recognized as a significant and essential component of nursing education. Because of the importance of clinical learning experiences, and because resources are limited, clinical teachers need to optimize clinical practice opportunities. Clinical teachers have a responsibility not only to their students, but also to patients, families, and the nursing profession to identify and exhibit highly effective clinical behaviors.

Many clinical teachers, however, have had little formal preparation for this complex teaching role. New clinical teachers might have clinical competence and have completed a graduate program related to advanced practice nursing, but might have little to no experience or formal education in how to effectively teach students. While novice teachers are often excited at the opportunity to contribute to the education of nursing students, they may encounter reality shock as they try to meet the many responsibilities inherent in the role of clinical faculty (Jetha, Boschma, & Clauson, 2016). Additionally, complex practice areas, increasing patient complexity, and acuity in patient conditions add to the challenges faced by clinical faculty (Hewitt & Lewallen, 2010; Spurr, Bally, & Ferguson, 2010). Highly specialized interventions, new and ever-changing technology, and a focus on nursing excellence and patient safety despite high patient turnover also contribute to the challenges faced by today's clinical teachers and highlight the importance of using effective and innovative teaching strategies (Phillips & Vinten, 2010). Shortages of faculty can make it challenging to hire and retain effective clinical faculty members with current expertise in the clinical area (Maguire, Zambroski, & Cadena, 2012).

Clinical teachers represent a pivotal component of the clinical experience for students. Consider a unit that has wonderful learning opportunities for students, rich patient experiences, and a helpful staff. If the clinical teacher working on that unit with students lacks teaching skills, students might have a negative learning experience. Conversely, students might be placed in a clinical setting with less optimal learning experiences, but when the teacher is highly effective and inspirational, students will likely have a positive learning experience. In essence, the clinical teacher can promote learning regardless of experiences available in the clinical setting, and can hamper learning despite valuable experiences being available (Oermann, Shellenbarger, & Gaberson, 2018). Additionally, clinical teachers are instrumental in teaching nursing students core professional values, such as care, compassion, and empathy (Richardson, Percy, & Hughes, 2015). These values are essential in the development and socialization of the student into the profession of nursing.

The clinical experience offers nursing students the opportunity to apply theory from the classroom setting into the practice setting, solve complex clinical problems, reflect on care observed or provided, think creatively to meet patient and family needs, and carry out nursing skills within the context of the health care system (Ironside, McNelis, & Ebright, 2014). However, simply placing a student in the clinical area does not guarantee that this learning will occur. Without an effective clinical teacher, students might develop poor habits and disillusionment because they might view the classroom and clinical environments as two completely separate worlds. It is up to the clinical teacher to help students navigate the clinical setting and to assist students in merging these two environments. For instance, students might say that the dressing change materials in the hospital setting are "completely different" from the ones they practiced with in the laboratory setting of the school of nursing. It would be easy for the student in such a scenario to become frustrated. However, by pointing out the principles that govern this skill and helping the student see how to safely adapt the materials to comply with those skill-related principles, the clinical teacher can guide the student in merging the two worlds of clinical and classroom learning.

RESEARCH RELATED TO CLINICAL TEACHING

The literature suggests that for clinical teachers to be effective, they need to possess a variety of teaching behaviors. These behaviors fall into several categories, including knowledge and clinical judgment, teaching skills, interpersonal skills, personal characteristics, and evaluation skills (Knox & Mogan, 1985). Knowledge and clinical judgment refer not only to having extensive, up-to-date knowledge, but also to the ability to clearly communicate that knowledge to students and facilitate their development of clinical judgment. Teaching skills include such activities as helping students organize their thoughts about patient problems and being well prepared and organized. Interpersonal skills are reflected in a clinical teacher's ability to display mutual respect; listen to students; and be supportive, and encouraging, yet challenging. Personal characteristics include being approachable and enthusiastic, being a strong role model for students, admitting mistakes, and having a sense of humor. Evaluation skills include the ability to provide feedback and evaluate students fairly, constructively, and in a manner that will facilitate learning (Knox & Mogan, 1985). Beginning and senior-level students emphasize the importance of similar clinical teacher behaviors, and note that clinical teachers need to possess behaviors in all five categories to be deemed effective.

Other research shows that students' view of the effectiveness of clinical faculty directly relates to their motivation for learning (Valiee, Moridi, Khaledi, & Garibi, 2016). In fact, student confidence flourishes when the clinical teacher practices a holistic approach to education, demonstrated by supporting students and promoting their independence (Valiee et al., 2016). Clinical teachers should have a passion for collaboration with students and should genuinely care about individual students, including building a comfortable and supportive relationship with students. They should also demonstrate a passion for seeing students succeed and reach excellence, for the profession of nursing, and for the teacher–student relationship (Edgecombe & Bowden, 2009; Richardson et al., 2015; Spurr et al., 2010).

Research on clinical teaching in nursing reflects that students experience a variety of stressors in the clinical practice area. One very real stressor is the fear of making mistakes in the clinical setting, including medication errors, potentially impacting not only the patient safety but also the student's confidence and self-worth (Koharchik & Flavin, 2017; Zieber & Williams, 2015). Other student stressors include being unfamiliar with the clinical setting and clinical practices; experiencing different types and acuity of patient conditions; interacting with patients, staff members, and other health care providers; and interacting with and being observed by clinical faculty members. Some settings, such as pediatrics, may create more stress for students because of the vulnerability of pediatric patients and the frequent but potentially intimidating involvement of families in patients' care. Additionally, clinical faculty are essential in helping students successfully navigate the clinical environment. For instance, if nursing students experience incivility from staff nurses, clinical faculty, or other health professionals, they are more likely to develop emotional exhaustion and burnout (Babenko-Mould & Laschinger, 2014). Clinical educators are instrumental in ensuring that this does not happen, and if it does, to help the student work through the experience. It is essential for clinical teachers to be aware of how stressful the clinical experience can be for students, and to reassure students that the role of the clinical teacher is not just to evaluate, but rather to teach, mentor, and help students learn. Keeping clinical feedback instructional and not overly personal or critical can also reduce students' stress and increase student motivation to learn (Oermann et al., 2018).

It is important to note that the stress experienced by nursing students does not diminish as they advance through the program. Senior students who are about to graduate might be anxious about passing their licensing examination, fear whether they know enough to practice competently, and experience the anxiety of job hunting while they are completing their studies. The need for clinical teachers to role-model excellence in nursing and to support and guide senior students remains just as paramount as when working with beginning nursing students.

Stressors exist for clinical teachers as well. Clinical teachers report stress related to multiple demands and role expectations, balancing heavy teaching workloads with other activities, receiving less-than-desirable compensation, and feeling physically and emotionally drained at the end of the clinical day (Whalen, 2009). Working with students who are ill-prepared for the clinical experience, and working with borderline or failing students in the clinical setting, are situations that are also stressful for faculty (Whalen, 2009). At times, working with borderline and failing students can create power struggles and feelings of blame experienced by both faculty and students; this in turn also increases faculty stress (Poorman & Mastorovich, 2014). Developing teaching strategies for dealing with these issues can help the clinical teacher remain positive and cope effectively. Enjoying the personal satisfaction that develops as the result of being professionally competent can also counterbalance this stress for clinical faculty.

Additionally, multiple authors describe the increasing diversity of nursing students, including those who come from ethnically and linguistically diverse backgrounds, as a challenge for clinical faculty (Abu-Arab & Parry, 2015; Debrew, Lewallen, & Chun, 2014; Koch, Everett, Phillips, & Davidson, 2015; Starkey, 2015). These are challenges that must be met effectively by clinical faculty for nursing to retain these students and increase the diversity of its membership.

RELATIONSHIPS WITH STUDENTS AND STAFF

The clinical learning environment has a much more complex context than the more controlled classroom environment, and is essential in socializing students into the profession of nursing, through positive role modeling, encouragement, support, and quality feedback (Edgecombe & Bowden, 2009). It is important for clinical teachers and students alike to remember that the clinical learning environment is an established health care or community setting, and that students and clinical teachers are guests in that site. The clinical teacher's role, in addition to mentoring, guiding, planning for, and teaching students, is also to act as a culture broker or boundary spanner in this clinical setting (Oermann et al., 2018).

As much as possible, clinical teachers should have input into clinical site selection and should advocate for stability in their clinical site placements, so that relationships with staff and administrators can be forged and maintained. When staff get to know and can build a trusting, collaborative relationship with clinical faculty, a positive experience ensues for all involved. Staff nurses will often watch for additional opportunities for students to learn when a known and respected clinical teacher is present on the unit, and the teacher can feel confident in having students team up with staff for additional learning experiences, or tap into additional learning resources within the clinical area.

As a gatekeeper in the clinical setting, it is critical that the clinical faculty member keep lines of communication open between students and staff (Oermann et al., 2018).

Keeping staff informed and up-to-date about the specific activities in which students will be engaging from week to week helps avoid confusion and frustration on the part of both students and staff. Patient safety is also maintained as a result of clear communication among faculty, students, and staff. Further discussion pertaining to the relationship between clinical teachers and students is woven throughout this chapter.

PROCESS OF CLINICAL TEACHING

Clinical teaching includes identifying the outcomes for learning, assessing student learning needs, planning clinical learning activities, guiding students, and evaluating their learning and performance (Oermann et al., 2018). This chapter addresses outcomes for learning, assessing learner needs, planning clinical learning activities, and guiding students. Clinical evaluation is discussed in Chapter 14.

LEARNING OUTCOMES

Learning outcomes of the clinical experience can be intended as well as unintended. Intended learning outcomes for students relate to three domains of learning. Each of these domains of student learning can be fostered through effective clinical teaching behaviors and strategies, which promote learning and student confidence.

Cognitive learning reflects students' growing knowledge level, an ability to engage in clinical reasoning and problem solving, and the development of students' higher-level thinking skills (Oermann et al., 2018). Faculty can promote the achievement of cognitive learning outcomes by engaging students as participants in patient-centered discussions, encouraging students to examine patient situations from multiple points of view, and engaging students in rigorous yet supportive questioning, thereby teaching students how to *think* rather than to memorize.

A second domain of learning, psychomotor learning, reflects students' skill acquisition, including the ability to perform skills in a safe, effective, accurate, and fluid manner over time (Oermann et al., 2018). Faculty can encourage psychomotor learning outcomes through careful patient selection, and by providing guidance, support, and encouragement for students during skills and procedures. These learning outcomes can also be fostered by positive role modeling on the part of the clinical teacher and by encouraging students to use clinical resources effectively. Within this domain, students also need to learn organization, priority setting, and time management skills to function effectively in complex health care environments. Clinical nurse educators can teach students these skills using tools, group discussions, and role modeling.

Within the third domain of learning, the affective domain, students develop professional attitudes, beliefs, and values that form an essential part of nursing practice (Oermann et al., 2018). Faculty can provide clear expectations and directions, role-model professional behaviors, and use other teaching strategies to develop and challenge students within the affective domain of learning.

In addition to the intended learning outcomes previously noted, students might also experience unintended learning outcomes as a result of the clinical experience. These unintended learning outcomes can be positive, such as the student considering the specialty area as a potential career choice and developing a passion for that area of nursing. Unintended outcomes, however, can be negative and long lasting, such as students losing self-confidence, becoming disengaged, being "turned off" to the clinical area, or even questioning their own ability to become nurses. All of these unintended learning outcomes hinge directly on the clinical teacher and the teacher's interactions with students in the clinical setting.

ASSESSING LEARNER NEEDS

Today's clinical teachers have the added challenge of working with multiple groups of students, each with the unique learning needs and diversity that these student groups bring. Faculty working in all types of nursing programs often teach a diverse student population, with differences in race, gender, age, work experiences, and life experience. Faculty working with undergraduate students might be working with an added layer of diversity: traditional baccalaureate students as well as accelerated second degree nursing students (those with at least a bachelor's degree in another field). The research on relationships between faculty and second degree students remains primarily descriptive and anecdotal, but it is apparent that accelerated second degree nursing students may present challenges and have a unique set of needs (D'Antonio et al., 2010). Second degree students appear to anticipate intellectual challenges in nursing programs, but also experience emotional challenges related to their tremendous workload (D'Antonio et al., 2010). In turn, some faculty members express unease when teaching those students, finding them driven and potentially intimidating, whereas others enjoy the challenges and rewards that come with working with accelerated students. Similarly, faculty members teaching in advanced practice nursing programs may have an equally diverse student population, with differences in prior work and life experiences. It is essential that discussions occur among *all* students and faculty members on a regular and ongoing basis about how individual students learn best, and how faculty and preceptors can foster that learning, so that congruent expectations can be achieved (D'Antonio et al., 2010).

Creating an effective learning experience with students in the clinical setting also begins with assessing individual learner characteristics and learning needs (Edgecombe & Bowden, 2009). Even before the clinical experience starts, faculty members can get to know students through learner assessments. Additionally, a carefully planned and orchestrated clinical orientation can help teachers assess students' learning needs, as well as establish a climate for nursing. Further discussion of learner needs is found in the section concerning clinical orientation in this chapter.

PLANNING CLINICAL ACTIVITIES

CREATING AN EFFECTIVE LEARNING ENVIRONMENT

Planning clinical activities for students starts with shaping the clinical environment so that it will be a safe and enjoyable place in which to learn. Creating an effective learning environment for nursing students begins with the clinical teacher establishing a partnership with the clinical site even before the course begins. By orienting to the clinical agency, the faculty member gains familiarity with the clinical environment and patient population. This familiarity is essential in guiding students (Oermann et al., 2018). The clinical teacher might shadow a seasoned staff nurse, or work alongside staff for several shifts, home visits, or other experiences, before teaching begins in that site. During this time, the faculty member can also communicate clear expectations to staff and managers in the setting about the roles that the clinical teacher, students, and staff will take during the upcoming clinical course and establish collaborative relationships with staff. It is important to remember that in traditional clinical courses, teachers and students are typically guests within a larger, more stable health care setting and that interactions with staff reflect this. In partnerships, these roles vary, as discussed in the next chapter.

ESTABLISHING THE CLIMATE FOR LEARNING: CLINICAL ORIENTATION

A well-thought-out student orientation is a key aspect of the clinical experience. It is essential that the clinical teacher take every opportunity during this critical time to establish a positive climate for learning. Consider, for example, the clinical faculty member who arrives late to orientation, does not have his or her materials ready, talks about the upcoming experience without eliciting students' input or responses, and makes little effort to learn about the students themselves. Students will likely be given the impression that the clinical teacher is disorganized, is intimidating, and does not care about them as individuals or partners in learning. In turn, these students are likely to become concerned about having to guess what the teacher wants, might "hide" when the faculty member is present, or might be afraid to ask questions. Because clinical time is so limited and valuable to student learning, it is important that faculty maximize every learning opportunity for students, and those opportunities begin with orientation.

The teacher should consider developing a folder for each student, to be distributed electronically to students or as hard copies within the first few minutes of clinical orientation. These folders can contain such documents as a clinical schedule; an outline of a typical day on the unit, in the clinic, in the home, and so on; descriptions of clinical assignments; documentation examples; and key resources that are site and specialty dependent. A folder (paper or electronic) made individually for each student provides a personal touch. It also provides concrete evidence that the faculty member cares enough about individual students to provide them with key materials to get them started in the course. This is a simple but effective way to begin building the student–faculty relationship. Students can be encouraged to add to these folders as they progress through the course, with relevant articles, policies and procedures, clinical assignments, and so forth. Through these actions, students learn the importance of building their own professional portfolio and developing a vehicle for evidence-based practice, professional growth, and lifelong learning.

Clinical orientation provides an opportunity to get to know students individually, as well as an opportunity to establish the climate of the clinical group. By emphasizing that the clinical group will act as a team that will learn together and support each other in the clinical setting, the faculty member sets the expectation that students will assist each other and not compete with one another for faculty time or for learning experiences. This is another important concept to establish at the outset, to prevent clinical groups from becoming competitive or polarized.

Clinical orientation can be an excellent time to introduce the use of analogies to inspire students. A sample analogy useful to share during clinical orientation related to professional growth, group teamwork, and the development of nursing competence in the clinical setting is found in Appendix B.1.

Additional key questions to ask students during orientation, to achieve the goals of establishing the climate for learning, might include the following:

- *What are students excited about as they begin this clinical course? What are they nervous about?* These types of questions encourage students to begin sharing and establish that the clinical group and setting is a safe environment in which to learn where students will be supported and stimulated. This kind of initial dialogue is also important for student engagement and underscores the importance of transparency in the clinical teacher–student relationship.

- *What are the students' expectations of the clinical teacher?* Students might be surprised to hear this question, as faculty typically spend a great deal of time discussing expectations of students. That question, too, should be discussed, but if students are *first* asked expectations of faculty, they can be put more at ease, and the *partnership* of learning can be established. By articulating what they expect from the clinical teacher, students invariably will reflect on what *they* also bring to the learning situation, including past learning experiences that have been positive or negative and why. This question also allows for a frank and open discussion about which student expectations might be easily met (for instance, that the faculty member is approachable) versus expectations that might be unrealistic (for instance, that they would prefer to observe care interventions prior to carrying them out themselves). Having an honest discussion of this nature is an excellent way to enhance group cohesiveness, clear up misconceptions before they have a chance to surface and, again, establish the learning climate as a partnership where both students and teachers share responsibility. This dialogue informs faculty about individual students' previous experiences as learners in the clinical setting, and makes it easier for faculty to avoid assumptions about the types of experiences that students might or might not have had. It also sets the stage for another, slightly different discussion: faculty expectations of students.

- *What are the clinical teacher's expectations of students in the clinical setting?* Once student expectations of faculty have been discussed, students are more receptive to hearing, understanding, and caring about faculty expectations of them. If students feel respected as adults and as individuals and understand that their clinical teacher is committed to the partnership of teaching and learning in the clinical setting, student motivation increases and so does students' commitment to learning. The open discussion of faculty expectations of students during clinical orientation provides students with clear guidelines. Students, as a result, do not have to spend valuable time during the clinical course itself guessing what the faculty member wants. Issues such as clinical preparation, when and under what circumstances teacher supervision is required, types of learning activities that will take place during the clinical experience, what student activities are appropriate during "down time," specific skills that students cannot engage in, and the progression of activities that will occur over the course are important topics to address within the context of faculty expectations of students.

   Students cannot be expected to remember all the verbal details shared with them during orientation, as they are likely experiencing some degree of anxiety at the time, and there is often a great deal of information shared in orientation. Because of this, it is helpful for students to be given a written copy of key faculty expectations as a part of the orientation packet. This copy should be shared and reviewed with orientation, and they should be encouraged to keep this information with them during the clinical experience. These faculty expectations can be labeled "Clinical Guidelines" or a similar title. These clinical guidelines can include such information as where, when, and under what circumstances to contact the clinical teacher outside of the clinical setting, contact information, expected student behaviors, guidelines for submitting written work, directions for clinical preparation, and so forth. Additional information about the clinical site, the types of common patient and family problems, common interventions, and other information can also be shared in these clinical guidelines (Exhibit 10.1).

EXHIBIT 10.1 Sample Clinical Guidelines to Share With Students in Orientation

- Clinical teacher contact information (preferred method of contact, don't call after X pm, etc.)
- Clinical site contact numbers
- Clinical site information (short description of the clinical setting where students are practicing, including phone number, typical patient population, types of common patient and family problems, common interventions, typical staffing, etc.)
- What students should do if absent or late
- Preparing for clinical practice (process, student and teacher roles, clinical worksheets, preconferences, etc.)
- Expected student behaviors (important actions if unsure about care or have questions; need for communication and sharing pertinent information about patient with nurse, teacher, and others; school dress code and why important; new orders and process; documentation; working as a team)
- Typical day in the clinical setting (hospital unit, in the clinic, in a community agency, during a home visit, etc. depending on type of clinical practice)
- Written assignments and submission information

Additional topics to cover during clinical orientation should include the following:

- *What are the ways in which individual students in the clinical setting learn best?* By asking students this during the initial orientation session, teachers communicate that they care about each student individually and that students are respected as unique, adult learners. When students are required to articulate how they learn best, they need to reflect on their own learning styles, consider what has and has not worked well in the past, and take responsibility for themselves as learners. Establishing how individual students learn best sets the stage for the rest of the clinical experience and also allows the opportunity to have frank discussions. For instance, in response to students who indicate that they learn best through demonstration, the clinical teacher has an opportunity to dispel any misconceptions about the clinical experience. It might be worthwhile to point out that although sometimes the opportunity to observe might be present, there might be other times in which unique clinical experiences present themselves. In the latter case, provided that the student has the requisite skills and knowledge, faculty can assert that they will not demonstrate first, but will rather support the students as they engage in the particular activity. By having this open discussion in orientation, expectations can be clarified and student anxiety can be diminished.

- *Are individual students visual, auditory, and/or kinetic learners?* This question can help guide clinical teachers in providing each student with a method of teaching that best matches individual student learning styles. Given that the clinical environment is fraught with anxiety for students, it makes sense for faculty members to minimize that anxiety in whatever way possible, and matching teaching to individual student learning styles is a small but powerful way to achieve this. There is no sense in teaching students in a way that they will not learn.

Consider the following scenario. A nursing student in the clinical setting has attention deficit hyperactivity disorder (ADHD) and cannot take her ADHD medications because she is pregnant. She is a student who articulated during orientation that she is a visual learner, who also benefits from using concrete directions. She is attempting to administer medications with a staff nurse who becomes very frustrated and approaches the clinical teacher, saying that the student is "ill-prepared and doesn't know what she is doing." The clinical teacher seeks out the student to gather more information and finds her crying in the medication room. After learning about the situation and calming the student, the clinical teacher reminds the student of her aptitudes, and issues a vote of encouragement to the student. She then has the student write down an appropriate medication ratio on a paper towel in the medication room, and further reviews key steps of the procedure in a written format. The student relaxes, takes a deep breath, and says "I've got it." She proceeds to carry out the skill without further difficulty. She later reflects on the experience, and realizes that her current situation makes her more emotional and also makes auditory learning particularly difficult for her. She reflects that when placed in the situation with a staff nurse who was trying to verbally explain the procedure, she blanked out and then panicked. The use of alternate methods of teaching and learning (e.g., visual learning through the use of the written math ratio; the use of concrete, step-by-step directions as a guide to follow; and giving encouragement to the student), allowed the student to relax, process the information, learn, gain confidence, and successfully engage in reflective practice. Because the clinical teacher asked key questions during orientation and remembered these details about the individual student, the faculty was able to effectively teach the student not just about the skill, but about herself as well.

- *What is at least one personal goal that each student has in terms of this clinical experience?* Involving the students in guiding their own learning within the clinical experience is critical for their personal and professional growth, and this should be done at the outset of the course, in orientation. Questions such as their personal goals of what they want to achieve in the course help students become personally invested in each clinical course. Students can be encouraged to use the acronym "SMARTER" when formulating their goals, whereby the goals are specific, measurable, attainable, relevant, and timely, and can be evaluated and reevaluated (Baird, 2008). Articulating these goals and putting them in writing can make students invest more personally in the clinical experience.

- *What are some good and bad experiences from previous clinical courses?* Asking students to share these with clinical faculty in private or through a writing exercise provides transparency for students and faculty alike, and it allows all to have a similar starting point. It might be difficult for some students to share openly, particularly if they have had a previously negative clinical experience. However, if trust is established with the teacher beginning with the first clinical day, and the message is sent that the teacher is asking this information to help students learn, then students can feel empowered.

Another topic that should be included in orientation to the clinical setting is the system used by the clinical agency for electronic medical records and documentation. In acute and long-term care settings, a treasure hunt can be planned for this learning, and an example is provided in Appendix B.2. Additional topics are professional dress, including what students should wear when they visit the clinical agency, home, or other setting, and what constitutes appropriate student identification; typical timeline of a clinical day; timeline of the course, including when assignments are due; demonstrations of patient care-related equipment; and when and where to find agency policies and why doing so is important. The use of an analogy, as shown in Exhibit 10.2, emphasizes student accountability and responsibility for their own learning, clarifies expectations of both student and clinical teacher, and underscores the importance of a team approach where faculty and other students' time is considered.

EXHIBIT 10.2 Example Analogy for Communication of Student Expectations

A simple analogy of a baseball game can be helpful in discussing student responsibilities with respect to new nursing procedures and interventions, which require teacher or preceptor guidance, in the clinical setting. This analogy assumes that students have obtained the requisite knowledge in the learning laboratory, have been shown where appropriate documentation can be located in the clinical setting, where supplies and equipment are kept, and where they can find appropriate nursing policies.

Starting a baseball game requires communication among team members. Students need to communicate to their clinical teacher, the patient, and the preceptor/clinician with whom they are working that they are planning on carrying out a specific procedure. They also need to consider other members of their team (their peers and the need for students to have access to the clinical teacher or preceptor). Use of this baseball analogy allows for a more streamlined student–teacher interaction and allows the clinical teacher or preceptor to be available for other students.

- Getting to first base. Students can be expected to locate and verify the care provider's order for the skill. If the student has taken the time to verify the order, then he or she can effectively show it to the clinical teacher or preceptor and save valuable time searching through the medical records.

- Getting to second base. Students can also be expected to find and review the relevant nursing policy. The teacher or preceptor can then review key points of the procedure with the student and increase efficiency, rather than taking the additional time to *locate* the policy with the student.

- Getting to third base. Students should gather the equipment and supplies for the procedure.

- Getting to home plate. Students can now locate their clinical teacher or preceptor and begin a brief focused discussion of the steps of the procedure. Students gain in self-confidence and independence by doing this additional preparatory work prior to spending one-to-one time with the teacher or preceptor. Because the student has gone around the bases, he or she should be able to quickly identify the provider order to verify, show the teacher or preceptor the equipment and supplies gathered, be prepared to discuss why those items were chosen (building problem-solving and organizational skills), and review key points of any relevant nursing policies. Use of this analogy also underscores the importance of nursing students using and thinking about agency policies, an important aspect of safe, professional nursing care.

CHOOSING CLINICAL ASSIGNMENTS

It is essential for faculty to keep the clinical objectives, or competencies, in mind when choosing patient assignments and other clinical activities. Specific patient assignments should be made purposefully, with the idea that, by caring for the patient or engaging in other types of activities, the students will work toward meeting the clinical objectives for the course. Specific goals for each week should be transparent to students and faculty alike, and learning activities should provide opportunities for students to meet those goals. Although students might take a more simplified approach to patient selection, such as desiring the opportunity to engage in a particular psychomotor skill or interact with a parent in the clinic, clinical teachers should keep goals in mind and consider all types of learning opportunities for students. The potential to engage in a particular kind of communication with a patient or family member, chance to explore patient advocacy issues or ethical concepts with patients, and opportunity to be exposed to diversity all represent examples of valuable learning experiences for the students.

Keeping track of student experiences can assist the clinical teacher in ensuring that each student obtains a variety of learning opportunities during the course. Creating a simple table, reflective of essential learning activities, and tracking each student's activity over the course is an easy way to stay organized and ensure that students are exposed to a diverse set of learning experiences.

It is also helpful to obtain student input regarding patient selection and other learning experiences. By doing so, clinical teachers again convey that they care about the student as an adult learner and value student input in creating each student's own learning opportunities. For example, in pediatrics, students might be asked which patient ages they are most or least comfortable with. Faculty can then solicit student input as to whether they would rather be eased into new experiences, depending on their comfort level, or just "jump in" with teacher, preceptor, or clinician support. Each student will respond individually, and by honoring those responses whenever possible, the teacher–student relationship deepens through collaboration and trust.

Patient assignments do not always need to take the traditional form, where one student is assigned to one patient. Clinical teachers should be encouraged to think creatively about patient assignments and various configurations for these assignments. For instance, two beginning students can be assigned to one more-complex patient, or students may work collaboratively with staff nurses, among other models. Students can also be offered learning activities in the clinical setting that enhance professional behaviors. For instance, students can learn leadership skills by buddying with a team leader for an experience or learn management skills by working for a short time with a case manager or first-level or middle manager (Oermann et al., 2018).

In some clinical settings, teachers might use a form to record students' assignments for use by students and staff; these forms should be clear, specific, and individualized each week. Clarity on the assignment form can help avoid misunderstandings about who is responsible for what patient care when the students are in the setting. The form should include the teacher's contact information if staff need to contact the faculty member outside of the clinical hours. It should be specific about the starting and finishing times for the students and the activities in which each student will be engaged. In addition, it is important to be clear that the staff nurse remains the primary patient caregiver, so miscommunication is avoided.

Faculty must be intentional about how much information to give to students about their patients in writing. Patient privacy and confidentiality laws prohibit faculty from posting patient assignment forms in areas that might be visible to visitors and others, and assignment forms should not include identifying information about patients, such as full names or medical record numbers. Some clinical teachers post the same assignment form in several places on the unit; other teachers share the assignments electronically or orally with students. It is helpful if staff have access to a copy of the assignment form to avoid duplication of care and ensure that all members of the health care team are working together. A sample patient assignment form that can be used when teaching in a hospital or long-term care setting is found in Exhibit 10.3. This would be modified for learning activities in the community, home, and other settings.

In some states, the State Board of Nursing outlines specific skills that students may not perform under any circumstances. Clinical teachers in each state should be aware of this information so as not to put the student, patient, family, staff member, or themselves at risk.

Learning objectives should become more complex as students progress through a given clinical course and as they progress through the nursing program.

EXHIBIT 10.3 Sample Nursing Student Assignment Sheet

- School of Nursing
- Course Number and Name
- Clinical Teacher, Credentials
- E-mail Address and Contact Phone Number
- Dates of Care: _____
- Clinical Activities: Nursing students are responsible for the following activities: Basic care of the assigned patient including hygiene, assisting with patient nutrition, vital signs, and so forth. The assigned staff nurse remains the primary caregiver for the patient.
- Clinical Hours: x to x

Student Name	Patient Initials	Room Number

Patient assignments and other clinical learning activities should reflect this increasing complexity of learning objectives. The clinical teacher needs to decide whether students will engage in certain activities during a given day. This can depend on the comfort and confidence level of teacher and students, the acuity and needs of the patients, and other experiences that might be happening in the clinical area that day. This information should be communicated clearly to students and staff.

It is helpful to periodically ask students to identify their goals for learning. These goals can reflect course or clinical objectives or their personal goals and needs. The teacher can then use these to inform patient assignments and other clinical activities for the student. Students can be encouraged to use the SMARTER (specific, measurable, attainable, relevant, timely, evaluated, and reevaluated) acronym for their goals, as this process teaches students about professional growth.

GUIDING STUDENTS: KEY TEACHING STRATEGIES

There are a multitude of teaching methods that can be used to enhance student learning in the clinical setting. Some of these teaching methods are described here.

ORGANIZATION FOR FACULTY AND STUDENTS

Being organized is paramount to having the clinical experience run smoothly. Clinical teachers have a great deal of responsibility: to students, patients, families, and staff nurses and other clinicians. Teaching in the clinical environment can be exhausting and stressful. Organization is a key strategy to not just survive, but to flourish as a faculty member.

Organizational strategies for faculty include being well prepared for the clinical experience, carefully selecting patients and other learning activities for students so that specific learning outcomes are achieved, and learning about the patients to guide the questions asked of students. Clear directions are essential for students and staff as to what students will be doing and not doing and the times that the students will be in the setting. It is also helpful to provide structure for students regarding what activities they might engage in during "down time," for example, in an acute care setting when their patient is sleeping or in the clinic between appointments. Guidance for students in terms of how to access the faculty member and staff if they are not immediately visible on the unit is also helpful to discuss. The use of a pager system and texting the faculty member are strategies that can help with this and make the teacher's presence on the unit more apparent.

Specific learning objectives should also be shared with staff and students. By having clear directions provided to them, all parties are aware of the goals, and the students can function as an organized, cohesive unit. For example, faculty teaching beginning students might want to strategize whether all students will perform certain skills in a given clinical day or whether a controlled approach is more appropriate, such as a few students giving medications early in the day, and other students giving medications in the latter part of the day.

As simplistic as it sounds, the better organized and more prepared clinical teachers are for the clinical course, the more effective they will be as nurse educators. Faculty need to take the necessary time to review patient histories and problems, so as to be able to ask students specific questions about them and to be familiar with each patient's *unique* health experience. It does not do the student any good for the faculty member to ask "blind" questions.

STRUCTURE WITHIN THE CLINICAL DAY

The clinical teacher and preceptor, or other clinician with whom the student is working, are key in helping students organize their patient care. It is essential that students learn to practice patient- and family-centered care in the clinical setting, and not focus only on tasks (Forbes, 2010). This can be challenging in the face of the unpredictability of the clinical setting, and the fact that a patient's status often changes during the course of the clinical day, with new nursing actions as a result. Similarly, clinics, homes, and other settings in which students have clinical experience can be equally unpredictable. Teachers should collaborate with students to help them organize their day using patient-focused strategies (Forbes, 2010). For example, a student performing a task such as a dressing change might often focus only on the dressing change itself and have tunnel vision. As the teacher accompanies the student to the bedside and guides performance, the teacher can engage the patient in an individualized way. During the dressing change, the faculty member might talk with the patient about what is important, discuss patient-centered goals, or simply just get to know the patient better. In this way, the faculty member demonstrates the importance of considering the whole person while performing a skill and role models this for the student. At the same time, it is important for the clinical teacher to realize that considering the whole person while simultaneously performing a psychomotor skill is a developmental process for many students, and that the student will improve with time and practice and gain confidence. This same principle is applicable to guiding performance in other types of practice settings.

Teachers can provide students with tools to help them organize their patient care. Some clinical teachers provide students with course-specific tools for use in preparing for clinical practice, giving direction to the student as to what information they need to know about their patients prior to engaging in their care. In addition, other tools can be used, such as a time sequence plan, to give students structure with which to organize their day. Even though the clinical environment and the patient's status might change, having some beginning structure to the experience lessens student anxiety and gives students a framework from which to begin their care. As students become more comfortable in the clinical setting, they can be encouraged to develop their own tools for organizing nursing care. Examples of organizational tools are found in Appendices B.3 and B.4.

CLINICAL CONFERENCES

Clinical conferences are essential to the learning and support of nursing students. They can provide an environment that facilitates learning, offer opportunities for brainstorming and problem solving, and allow the clinical teacher to gain knowledge about the students' understanding of the patient or patients for whom they will be caring. When structured carefully and intentionally, clinical conferences can underscore that the clinical environment is a safe place in which to learn, and promote active learning among all student members of the group. Clinical conferences can also help students derive meaning from their clinical day, and afford faculty opportunities to use active learning strategies to enhance student learning (Megel, Nelson, Black, Vogel, & Uphoff, 2013).

From the outset, during orientation, clinical teachers should establish the notion of the group working together as a team and that team members will support and learn from each other. The clinical group should form an environment where students are free to ask questions, challenge each other, and not always have to have the right answer. They should be free to debate a topic without becoming threatened, and learn to respect others' points of view. If the clinical faculty member emphasizes that questions can be asked freely, that debates and differences of opinions are celebrated, and that faculty are approachable, then students can relax and focus on learning, instead of feeling intimidated.

The literature suggests that clinical teachers spend much of their time in the clinical setting asking lower level questions, and should try to use higher level questioning (Hsu, 2007). Group conference time is an ideal time to introduce higher level questioning. Done in a safe, nonthreatening, and supportive manner, higher level questioning can stimulate not only individual students, but the clinical group as a whole, where the group is challenged as a team to respond to faculty questions.

If students are struggling in response to higher level questions, it is helpful for the clinical teacher to rephrase questions and sequentially ask a lower level question. When students are able to successfully answer a lower level question, they gain confidence in their own knowledge base and skill level. This, in turn, increases their confidence at responding to higher level questions. Words of encouragement such as "you can do this" or "I know you know this" also remind students that faculty have faith in their abilities. This in turn boosts their self-confidence, making many students want to learn more.

McAllister, Tower, and Walker (2007) suggest that students need to "practice engaging in critical reflection, dialoguing, being sensitive to difference, being compassionate in caring, and using creative thinking" (p. 306). Clinical conference is one such arena in which faculty can employ strategies not only to get students to learn about patients and nursing care, but also to engage them in transformative learning. Teachers want students to pause for a moment and think critically beyond the tasks.

CLINICAL PRECONFERENCE

One type of clinical conference is the preconference, which typically takes place prior to the students engaging in patient care, depending on the course and type of agency. Clinical preconferences can have several purposes. One important purpose is to provide an opportunity for the teacher to assess students' knowledge and understanding about their patients. During preconference, the teacher assesses whether students have the knowledge required to care for patients and in areas in which they need further information and guidance.

Another purpose of a clinical preconference is to encourage students to think critically and creatively about their patients. To do this effectively, faculty members should feel comfortable and confident with information about the patient and clinical context to ask challenging and stimulating questions. The preconference, therefore, can provide the venue for teachers to ask a variety of lower and higher level questions to develop students' thinking. For clinical courses in which the teacher has a group of students, a preconference also affords an opportunity for students to ask questions in a group setting, where the environment is safe, group members are supportive, and students learn from each other.

It can be helpful for teachers to ask pointed questions of the group, such as a question about a particular approach students might have to a challenging psychosocial situation. Questions such as "Tell me about your nursing priorities for the day," "What do you anticipate as expected outcomes for your patient today?," "What might be the worst case scenario for your patient, how would you recognize it, and what would you do about it?," and so forth allow students the opportunity to develop their thinking skills and apply theory to practice. Additionally, a focused discussion of students' patients and families allows students to compare individuals and situations, encourages them to learn about patients' experiences in differing stages of an illness, and helps them compare different interventions or treatments modalities. Students are able to compare the impact of family and culture on a patient's health trajectory and on how patients at different life stages cope. In this way, students learn about important nursing concepts across patients and situations.

Clinical preconferences can also serve to build relationships among students. For instance, assigning students buddies during preconference sets up a partnership among students for the rest of the day. A buddy system allows students to get to know more than one patient, affords students a fall-back person who can help them with care, and can also expose students to multiple approaches without having the additional responsibility of actually caring for that patient. Students can also gain additional learning experiences as they watch out for and interact with each other's patients.

During clinical preconferences, clinical teachers can provide students with an opportunity to briefly present their patient(s) to the rest of the group. This gives them practice at being concise and developing the skills needed later for handoff. In addition, the preconference offers a venue for faculty to discuss certain practical issues, such as any special learning activities planned for that day, reminders of what students can and cannot do, and other information.

CLINICAL POSTCONFERENCE

A second type of clinical conference, the postconference, provides different opportunities for student learning. It is important to note that postconferences do not have to take place at the end of the clinical day, although in many cases that can be the most opportune and convenient time for students and faculty to convene. Clinical teachers, however, should consider the best time for students to engage in postconference without being distracted by patient care and other activities.

An important component of clinical postconferences is the opportunity for students to debrief (Hsu, 2007; Megel et al., 2013; Oermann et al., 2018). Some students might have had a particularly trying experience with a patient, family member, or staff member. Strategies such as role-playing, active listening, having other students offer suggestions, and group discussion can make individual students feel supported and can stimulate further learning. Questions from clinical teachers such as, "If you could do anything different, what would it be and why?" or "What was particularly useful that you learned today that might influence your clinical practice next week?" can be useful in helping students learn reflection and reflective professional practice. Megel et al. (2013) suggest that of all the activities that can take place in the clinical setting, the support that the clinical faculty display for students to understand and find meaning in their clinical day is the most valued by students and faculty alike.

A clinical postconference can also augment student learning in other ways. Students can share perspectives of clinical situations, teach each other, gain self-confidence and appreciation for each other's contributions, and enhance the sense of teamwork among students. Postconferences can be used in other ways. Students can be given an assignment in which they need to present a patient to each other and compare the care they gave based on evidence. Students need preparation time to be successful at this activity. Student peers can be invited to ask higher level thinking questions of each other, thus allowing student presenters to hone their problem-solving skills as well as their confidence in oral skills. Nurses often present and discuss patients with other members of the health care team, so being able to articulate themselves successfully and confidently is an essential skill for students to learn.

Clinical teachers should be free to use whatever creative strategies they can develop to enhance student learning in postconferences. "Pass the problem" is one such strategy to get other clinical group members involved. In this strategy, one student presents a clinical situation or problem that he or she encountered that day. The next student offers an analysis of that situation, and a third student then critiques this analysis. When done in a supportive and open manner, this is an excellent strategy to foster critical thinking, and it underscores the importance of having more than one solution to a clinical problem.

During postconference, students can also be asked to write a 1-minute care plan in which they draw an algorithm pertaining to their patient, the nursing priorities they focused on, and where those priorities were at the end of the day (Oermann et al., 2018). Students can be creative and then share their ideas with their peers. Some faculty members use postconferences as an opportunity to enlist guest speakers, who can have their own topic area that they present. Though potentially effective, this type of conference should not be done frequently, as students' time might be better used in active engagement with each other, rather than listening to a minilecture.

CASE STUDIES

Case studies can be helpful in assisting nursing students to develop advocacy and delegation skills in a safe and nurturing environment (Powell, 2011). Students can be given opening case scenarios, and then given additional patient information as they respond to the scenario. These cases can be an excellent platform for developing skills, enhancing group teamwork, and augmenting self-confidence of students. Case studies can also take the form of problem-based learning in the clinical setting, which can promote student-directed solutions, group work and dynamics, and cooperative learning (Oja, 2011).

CONCEPT-BASED LEARNING ACTIVITIES

Concept-based learning activities, such as having students focus on a particular concept in a given day, can enhance critical thinking. Students can then be asked to compare this concept across the various patients that the group cared for during that clinical day (Lasater & Nielsen, 2009). For instance, in a pediatric setting, students might be asked to collectively analyze how the concept of fluid and electrolytes compared in some of the patients the group cared for that day, such as an infant with short bowel syndrome, an adolescent with Crohn's disease, and a toddler with leukemia.

NURSING ROUNDS

Conducting nursing rounds during the clinical day is another teaching strategy that can enhance nursing students' critical thinking skills and problem-solving abilities, as well as their confidence in communicating with other health care team members. During nursing rounds, one or two students per week present their patient and the care they have been engaged in to the clinical group, clinical teacher, staff nurses, and other available health care team members. This provides a valuable opportunity for students to learn to present their patients to other team members in a confident and concise manner, advocate for patients, ask questions of and collaborate with the health care team, consider multiple approaches to care, and so forth.

STUDENT PRESENTATIONS

Providing students with an opportunity to conduct a short presentation within their peer group is an additional teaching strategy that clinical teachers can employ to enhance student learning. Students might be asked to share a few key points about their patient from a previous week, focusing on one aspect of nursing care that intrigued them. They can then be asked to retrieve a nursing article related to evidence-based practice about that aspect of nursing care and compare the care they observed or engaged in with the article. Other students in the group can be asked to pose critical thinking questions to the presenter or, alternatively, the presenter can ask questions of the group. Opportunities such as these can boost students' thinking skills and self-confidence in communication.

LAB BLITZES

In addition to one-to-one discussions with individual students about their patients, in clinical courses in hospitals, or in outpatient or community settings, it can be helpful to use an occasional clinical conference for group discussions of key patient data, such as laboratory results that are often poorly understood by students. Teachers should use as many creative strategies as possible when conducting laboratory blitzes. For instance, sample laboratory results from one of the patients can be printed, with all patient identifying information removed. Students can then be asked to analyze these results, determine possible diagnoses for the patient, and identify nursing priorities based on these laboratory results.

Alternatively, students can be given pointers, such as Ten Key Questions to Ask Yourself about Your Patient, and laboratory values can be incorporated into these questions. As an example, students might be directed to look up the patient's potassium level for any patient receiving diuretics. This can, in turn, stimulate a rich discussion about the effects of some diuretics versus others, how these medications relate to their patient's unique health status, what other laboratory results in addition to potassium level might be affected by diuretics and why, and so forth. Laboratory blitzes are most effective if they are kept short, focused, and fun.

SHORT WRITTEN CLINICAL ASSIGNMENTS

Different types of written clinical assignments can be used, depending on the learning to be achieved in clinical practice. For an affective learning outcome, students might be asked to provide in a journal a short reflection about what went well and what did not go well in their experience with their patient, what they would change for next time, and events that had an impact on them during the experience. This activity can enhance students' critical thinking, and it also helps teachers understand challenges that the student faced that day that they might not have otherwise verbalized (Chan, 2013).

Cognitive learning can also be enhanced through short written clinical assignments (Oermann et al., 2018). Ideally, students are given guided questions within the assignment, specific to the clinical objectives. Examples of guided questions might include the following: How were the safety needs of your patient met? What were the developmental needs of your patient based on concepts of growth and development, and how did these developmental needs compare to those of the actual patient today? Did your perceptions about the patient and home environment change between this home visit and the prior one? In addition to encouraging the student to explore a select clinical situation, written assignments can enhance writing skills and the ability to convey ideas in a clear, succinct manner.

USE OF GUIDANCE AND FEEDBACK IN THE CLINICAL SETTING

Because the student–teacher relationship is critical to the learning and development of the student, feedback from the teacher needs to be consistent, specific, transparent, honest, and encouraging. Students respond well to the *feedback sandwich*, in which constructive feedback is placed between two pieces of "bread" (i.e., positive feedback). Rather than saying, "You were disorganized during that nursing procedure," the teacher can explain, "I liked how you were able to find the policy for that nursing procedure in the clinic. It seemed as though your organization needed improvement, because you forgot a few supplies, but you did an excellent job of engaging the patient during the procedure itself." It is important to remember that teacher observation is a major source of stress for many nursing students, so keeping feedback instructional versus punitive is key.

Also, teachers should be sensitive to how, where, and when feedback is delivered in the clinical setting. Feedback in front of the patient, peers, staff, or in a public area has potential for the student to feel criticized and should be avoided.

Guidance in the clinical setting can take many forms. When carrying out care, it is most helpful to students if the teacher provides guidance before student interaction with the patient. Students can be independent with the behind-the-scenes activities (for example, verifying a provider order and reviewing the agency policy and procedure). However, it is essential that the teacher review what students will do before they interact with patients, anticipate patient responses and challenges, prepare students for those, and elicit a brief self-evaluation by the student concerning what went well and what changes might be made for next time. This provides an opportunity for giving feedback to the student.

Formative written feedback should also be provided to students on a regular basis during the clinical course. Koh (2008) suggested that high-quality formative feedback enhances learning and student achievement. A running log of brief written faculty comments, shared electronically with students on a weekly basis, as well as the student contributions to a written clinical portfolio about the nursing care they provided, ensures open communication between faculty and student—and that evaluation is a collaborative process. The provision of prompt, specific, and regular feedback, both verbal and written, is critical to the learning process, allowing the students opportunities to correct mistakes before they become patterns and to feel supported and mentored during the clinical experience. With this feedback, summative evaluations are fair, do not pose surprises for the student, and are less anxiety-producing. Examples of weekly feedback are found in Exhibit 10.4.

EXHIBIT 10.4 Sample Weekly Student Feedback

Student Name:

Clinical Teacher:

Dates of Clinical Practice:

Week 1	Clinical orientation, introduction to the clinical area.
	You were self-directed in terms of your learning needs, asked thoughtful questions, and demonstrated therapeutic communication with your patient. You submitted a well-thought-out beginning clinical worksheet, which was complete and was supported by the evidence you summarized. A good start to this clinical course—keep up that energy and enthusiasm!
Week 2	You came well prepared for the clinical experience as evidenced by your clinical worksheet and participation in our preconference. You provided thorough basic care for your patient and were aware of her needs. You appear to be more comfortable with the electronic charting system, and your documentation was clear and specific about your patient's change in condition. Remember that a full assessment needs to be documented in the patient record by 0900; I would like to see you work on this more next week. Keep up the good work!
Week 3	You were astute in your care of your patient this week, identifying key changes in the patient's respiratory status, including changes to breath sounds, and communicating those to the staff nurse. Glad to see you following through on a thorough morning assessment—the fact that you did this allowed you to discover the patient's respiratory changes. Your organization needed some work this week with wound care—you reviewed the appropriate policy and understood the rationale but were missing several supplies. Make sure you gather all your supplies before you begin next time and review them with me. I'm impressed with your energy and passion for nursing.
Week 4	You demonstrated critical thinking and clinical judgment this week in your analysis of the relationships among your patient's pathophysiology, lab work, medications, and nursing interventions. This was evidenced by your participation in preconference and nursing rounds as we discussed the patient and discharge needs. You showed confidence and competence in caring for a patient with complex medical and psychiatric problems, and you demonstrated patient-advocacy skills.

SUMMARY

The clinical experience for nursing students is often brief, expensive to operationalize, and dependent on limited resources, and yet it is the environment in which students learn to apply theory to practice and become socialized into the profession. The effectiveness of the clinical teacher is pivotal to student learning. It is essential that clinical teachers in nursing be effective, inspirational, and motivational, and that they engage in best teaching practices.

Many clinical teachers in nursing have had little formal education on how to effectively teach students and on best teaching practices in the clinical setting. Other challenges also face clinical teachers, such as advanced technology in the clinical setting, patient acuity, and balancing multiple demands and a heavy workload in the clinical teaching role, among others. These factors can be sources of stress for clinical teachers. For clinical teachers to be effective, they need to have knowledge and clinical judgment, teaching skills, interpersonal skills, personal characteristics, and evaluation skills. Passion for nursing and teaching is paramount as well.

The process of clinical teaching includes identifying learning outcomes, assessing learner needs, planning clinical learning activities, guiding students, and evaluating students' learning and performance. Learning outcomes can be intended or unintended. Intended outcomes reflect cognitive, psychomotor, and affective domains; the clinical teacher can employ a variety of teaching strategies to facilitate learning in each of these areas. Unintended learning outcomes can range from being positive to negative, and they are closely tied to the effectiveness of the clinical teacher.

When assessing learner needs, clinical teachers need to recognize and honor the diversity of the student population with whom they are working and use best teaching practices accordingly. They also need to assess individual learner characteristics and learning needs.

Planning clinical activities begins with creating an effective learning environment. The clinical teacher can influence the learning environment before the students begin their clinical course, through establishment of a collaborative teacher–staff relationship; becoming comfortable with the clinical practices in that setting; and clarifying teacher, student, and staff expectations and roles. A carefully planned and orchestrated clinical orientation for students also helps to establish a climate conducive to learning. Planning clinical activities involves the careful selection of learning activities that will enhance learning and students' confidence levels. Patient assignments and selection of other clinical activities should be made thoughtfully and intentionally, and they should provide opportunities for students to achieve learning objectives as well as personal goals.

To effectively guide students in the clinical setting, the clinical teacher should use teaching methods that reflect best practices. Some of these methods include organizing the clinical experience, providing structure and clearly stated expectations for students, and conducting clinical conferences that are meaningful for students. Other teaching strategies that are helpful in guiding students include nursing rounds, student presentations, and short writing exercises. Guidance and feedback in the clinical setting also involve sharing feedback with students in a consistent, specific, and encouraging manner; balancing positive and constructive feedback; and providing formative written feedback regularly.

REFERENCES

Abu-Arab, A., & Parry, A. (2015). Supervising culturally and linguistically diverse (CALD) nursing students: A challenge for clinical educators. *Nurse Education in Practice, 15*, e1–e9. doi:10.1016/j.nepr.2015.02.006

Babenko-Mould, Y., & Laschinger, H. (2014). Effects of incivility in clinical practice settings on nursing student burnout. *International Journal of Nursing Education Scholarship, 11*(1), 145–154. doi:10.1515/ijnes-2014-0023

Baird, K. (2008). *Raising the bar on service excellence: The healthcare leader's guide to putting passion into practice.* Fort Atkinson, WI: Golden Lamp Press.

Chan, Z. C. Y. (2013). A systematic review of critical thinking in nursing education. *Nurse Education Today, 33,* 236–240. doi:10.1016/j.nedt.2013.01.007

D'Antonio, P., Beal, M., Underwood, P., Ward, F., McKelvey, M., Guthrie, B., & Lindell, D. (2010). Great expectations: Points of congruencies and discrepancies between incoming accelerated second-degree nursing students and faculty. *Journal of Nursing Education, 49,* 713–717. doi:10.3928/01484834-20100831-08

Debrew, J., Lewallen, L., & Chun, E. (2014). Outsiders in nursing education: Cultural sensitivity in clinical education. *Journal of Professional Nursing, 30,* 149–154. doi:10.1016/j.profnurs.2014.08.005

Edgecombe, K., & Bowden, M. (2009). The ongoing search for best practice in clinical teaching and learning: A model of nursing students' evolution to proficient novice registered nurses. *Nursing Education in Practice, 9*(2), 91–101. doi:10.1016/j.nepr.2008.10.006

Forbes, H. (2010). Issues in Nurse Education: Clinical teachers' approaches to nursing. *Journal of Clinical Nursing, 19,* 785–793. doi:10.1111/j.1365-2702.2009.03078.x

Hewitt, P., & Lewallen, L. (2010). Ready, Set, Teach! How to transform the clinical nurse expert into the part-time clinical nurse instructor. *The Journal of Continuing Education in Nursing, 41,* 403–407. doi:10.3928/00220124-20100503-10

Hsu, L-L. (2007). Conducting clinical post-conference in clinical teaching: A qualitative study. *Journal of Clinical Nursing, 16,* 1525–1533. doi:10.1111/j.1365-2702.2006.01751.x

Ironside, P., McNelis, A., & Ebright, P. (2014). Clinical education in nursing: Rethinking learning in practice settings. *Nursing Outlook, 62,* 185–191. doi:10.1016/j.outlook.2013.12.004

Jetha, F., Boschma, G., & Clauson, M. (2016). Professional development needs of novice nursing clinical teachers: A rapid evidence assessment. *International Journal of Nursing Education Scholarship, 13*(1), 1–10. doi:10.1515/ijnes-2015-0031

Knox, J., & Mogan, J. (1985). Important clinical teacher behaviours as perceived by university nursing faculty, students, and graduates. *Journal of Advanced Nursing, 10*(1), 25–30.

Koch, J., Everett, B., Phillips, J., & Davidson, P. (2015). Is there a relationship between the diversity characteristics of nursing students and their clinical placement experiences? A literature review. *Collegian, 22,* 307–318. doi:10.1016/j.colegn.2014.03.007

Koh, L. C. (2008). Refocusing formative feedback to enhance learning in pre-registration nurse education. *Nurse Education in Practice, 8,* 223–230. doi:10.1016/j.nepr.2007.08.002

Koharchik, L., & Flavin, P. (2017). Teaching students to administer medications safely. *American Journal of Nursing, 117*(1), 62–66.

Lasater, K., & Nielsen, A. (2009). The influence of concept-based learning activities on students' clinical judgment development. *Journal of Nursing Education, 48,* 441–446. doi:10.3928/01484834-20090518-04

Maguire, D., Zambroski, C., & Cadena, S. V. (2012). Using a clinical collaborative model for nursing education: Application for clinical teaching. *Nurse Educator, 37,* 80–85. 10.1097/NNE.0b013e3182461bb6

McAllister, M., Tower, M., & Walker, R. (2007). Gentle interruptions: Transformative approaches to clinical teaching. *Journal of Nursing Education, 46,* 304–312.

Megel, M., Nelson, A., Black, J., Vogel, J., & Uphoff, M. (2013). A comparison of student and faculty perceptions of clinical post-conference learning environment. *Nurse Education Today, 33,* 525–529. doi:10.1016/j.nedt.2011.11.021

Oermann, M., Shellenbarger, T. & Gaberson, K.(2018). *Clinical teaching strategies in nursing* (5th ed.). New York, NY: Springer Publishing.

Oja, K. (2011). Using problem-based learning in the clinical setting to improve nursing students' critical thinking: An evidence review. *Journal of Nursing Education, 50,* 145–151. doi:10.3928/01484834-20101230-10

Phillips, J., & Vinten, S. (2010). Why clinical nurse educators adopt innovative teaching strategies: A pilot study. *Nursing Education Perspectives, 31,* 226–229.

Poorman, S., & Mastorovich, M. (2014). Teacher stories of blame when assigning a failing grade. *International Journal of Nursing Education Scholarship, 11*(1), 1–10. doi:10.1515/ijnes-2013-0081

Powell, R. (2011). Improving students' delegation skills. *Nurse Educator, 36*(1), 9–10. doi:10.1097/NNE.0b013e3182001e2e

Richardson, C., Percy, M., & Hughes, J. (2015). Nursing therapeutics: Teaching student nurses care, compassion and empathy. *Nurse Education Today, 35,* e1–e5. doi:10.1016/j.nedt.2015.01.016

Spurr, S., Bally, J., Ferguson, L. (2010). A framework for clinical teaching: A passion-centered philosophy. *Nursing Education in Practice, 10,* 349–354. doi:10.1016/j.nepr.2010.05.002

Starkey, T. (2015). The critical factors that influence faculty attitudes and perceptions of teaching English as Second Language nursing students: A grounded theory research study. *Nurse Education Today, 35,* 718–725. doi:10.1016/j.nedt.2015.01.017

Valiee, S., Moridi, G., Khaledi, S., & Garibi, F. (2016). Nursing students' perspectives on clinical instructors' effective teaching strategies: A descriptive study. *Nurse Education in Practice, 16,* 258–262. doi:10.1016/j.nepr.2015.09.009

Whalen, K. (2009). Work-related stressors experienced by part-time clinical affiliate nursing faculty in baccalaureate education. *International Journal of Nursing Education Scholarship, 6*(1), 1–18. doi:10.2202/1548-923X.1813

Zieber, M., & Williams, B. (2015). The experience of nursing students who make mistakes in clinical. *International Journal of Nursing Education Scholarship, 12*(1), 1–9. doi:10.1515/ijnes-2014-0070

Partnerships With Clinical Settings: Roles and Responsibilities of Nurse Educators

KAREN L. GORTON AND KATHERINE FOSS

OBJECTIVES

- Describe historical and current trends in academic–practice partnerships
- Describe the steps required to establish a sustainable academic–practice partnership using one framework

Nursing is a practice discipline. The core of nursing education is the clinical education of nursing students. Academic–practice partnerships exist at several levels for the purpose of preparing the nursing workforce to meet nursing practice realities and contemporary health care challenges. Partnerships developed by nurse leaders in a nursing program and a clinical setting are defined as intentional relationships, based on mutual goals, respect, and shared knowledge (American Organization of Nurse Executives [AONE]-American Association of Colleges of Nursing [AACN] Academic–Practice Partnership Steering Committee, 2015).

This chapter provides guidelines for establishing meaningful partnerships. Nurse educator roles and responsibilities are explored relevant to school of nursing collaboration with clinical settings. Specific examples are provided to illustrate concepts and strategies to improve the educational preparation of nurses and ultimately the quality and safety of patient care.

The purpose of this chapter is to present ideas about establishing and sustaining meaningful partnerships between education and practice to stimulate collaborative, contemporary models of clinical nursing education. The nature of education–practice partnerships is explored within the context of quality and safe patient care and excellence in clinical education. The chapter includes a discussion of the value and significance of academic–practice partnerships, characteristics of meaningful partnerships, role and responsibilities of the nurse educator in establishing and sustaining effective partnerships, and relevant research and evidence for concepts underlying exemplar clinical education partnerships.

VALUE AND SIGNIFICANCE

EVOLUTION OF ACADEMIC–PRACTICE PARTNERSHIPS

Historically, academic–practice partnerships were established for a wide range of purposes relevant to advancing religious missions, delivery of patient care with physicians, government programs, and hospital initiatives. Hospitals and universities began forming alliances later to address the need for nursing care delivery and to prepare the future nursing workforce. The Institute of Medicine (Greiner & Knebel, 2003) established an overarching expectation that health care professionals are responsible to ensure collaborative practice and education. Emphasis is placed on opportunities for students to provide patient-centered care as members of a collaborative interprofessional team within a context of evidence-based practice, quality improvement, and informatics.

The looming nursing shortage, access to health care, and the need for continuous quality care and improved patient safety outcomes illuminate shared interests among academic and health care service organizations. Community and regional workforce development initiatives and health care consumers are joining together to address the issues of preparing the future nurse. As a result, academic programs, service agencies, and regulatory or policy-making bodies also need to align and leverage resources to meet the challenges of educating the health care workforce and building safer delivery systems (AACN, 2016; Joynt & Kimball, 2008).

CURRENT STATUS OF ACADEMIC–PRACTICE PARTNERSHIPS

The AACN *Essentials of Baccalaureate Education for Professional Nursing* (2008) recognizes ongoing collaborative academic–practice partnerships as a quality indicator for promoting student learning. Schools of nursing and clinical agencies are challenged to determine capacity for optimizing clinical learning during times of expanding nursing programs and increasing enrollments. The AACN (2016) and others (Broome, 2009; Ridenour, 2009) highlight the value and significance of partnerships in improving the quality and effectiveness of nursing education and have called for support and collaboration among stakeholders. Collaboration is necessary to maximize use of limited resources and build capacity to educate more nurses. An additional impetus is the IOM report, *The Future of Nursing: Leading Change, Advancing Health* (Committee on the Robert Wood Johnson Foundation Initiative on the Future of Nursing at the Institute of Medicine, 2011), which recommends increasing the proportion of baccalaureate-prepared nurses to 80% by 2020.

In 2012, the AONE and AACN provided evidence of support for the development of academic–practice partnerships. Nurse leaders participated in a task force to explore the nature of partnerships, including components and strategies that were deemed to be characteristic of good partnerships and effective in achieving desired outcomes. The purpose of formal academic–practice relationships is to advance nursing practice and to improve the health of the public (AONE–AACN Task Force on Academic–Practice Partnerships, 2012). In 2015, AONE and AACN reviewed and modified the guidelines to address the positively changing environment of academic–practice partnerships (AACN, 2015)

The *Summary of Literature Related to Academic–Service Partnerships*, compiled by the AACN–AONE Task Force on Academic–Practice Partnerships (2010), suggests an abundance of examples of formal academic–practice partnerships and provides evidence of a proliferation of partnerships. Partnerships are evolving in significance, purpose, structure, and expected outcomes. Examples of academic–practice partnerships focus on educating nurses, sharing resources, and undertaking projects focused on nursing student clinical education, evidence-based practice initiatives, and professional development or academic progression programs. Additional examples reflect priorities for interprofessional education (IPE), increased use of clinical simulation to develop clinical competency, and the advancement of evidence-based practice initiatives. Efforts and outcomes are perceived to be mutually positive.

However, following the extensive review of the literature over the past decade, the AONE–AACN Task Force concluded that the majority of reports on partnerships were anecdotal, describing examples of specific efforts and providing little databased evidence to support effectiveness or generalizability. In 2013, this anecdotal approach began to change, with the AACN conference highlighting successful academic–practice partnerships. Conference participants were able to gain understanding on steps required to build successful academic–practice partnerships. Since that conference, the number of resources available to assist programs in forming successful partnerships has grown. It has been demonstrated that different types of partnerships can provide examples of best practices that may be beneficial in developing a mutually beneficial relationship or shared goal. For example, a chief nurse officer and dean may identify key components or strategies relevant to achieve a specific shared goal. Faculty may hold joint appointments in both the academic and practice setting. The academic partner may provide additional resources for preceptor training or even contribute to the curriculum for new graduate residency programs or nursing orientation. The academic partner also may support clinical agency evidence-based practice initiatives, development, or research conferences. The practice partner may assist with clinical education within the academic arena via teaching students in the learning laboratory of the academic partner. All of these activities may be mutually valued and can serve to further strengthen the partnership by bridging real or perceived gaps between academic nursing and practice.

In 2016, AACN issued the Manatt Report on health care transformation and the opportunities for academic nursing (AACN, 2016). While this report focuses on nursing and academic health centers (AHCs), much can be applied to the development of academic–practice partnerships outside of the AHC setting. For academic–practice partnerships, the implications of this report, calling for nursing to be a full partner in the practice setting, engage faculty in practice with the partner and in the development of nurses at all levels, including creating nurse-led care models.

As the academic–practice partnership considers and perhaps embraces the recommendations, both members of the partnership can benefit. Engagement of faculty not only in practice, but as valuable members of the organization, can lead to examination of current trends, issues, and problems from a variety of new perspectives. Not only will the faculty member benefit, but the students will benefit as faculty members translate their current practice experiences into the academic setting. Additionally, nurses from the practice environment have the opportunity to shape and change nursing education to address the increasing complexity of patients in a care setting.

ESTABLISHING MEANINGFUL PARTNERSHIPS

From reported initiatives, the AACN–AONE Task Force identified current evidence of four partnership themes: principles, types, benefits, and barriers. Understanding the concepts and strategies underlying these themes is critical to increasing effectiveness and the potential positive impact of academic–practice partnerships. Eight guiding principles identified and endorsed by AACN and AONE (AACN–AONE Task Force on Academic–Practice Partnerships, 2012) provide a useful framework for nurse leaders in academic and practice settings for understanding the development and sustenance of meaningful relationships (Exhibit 11.1).

EXHIBIT 11.1 AACN–AONE Guiding Principles for Academic–Practice Partnerships

1. Collaborative relationships between academia and practice are established and sustained through:
   - Formal relationships established at the senior leadership level and practiced at multiple levels throughout the organization
   - Shared vision and expectations that are clearly articulated
   - Mutual goals with set evaluation periods
2. Mutual respect and trust are the cornerstones of the practice/academia relationship and include:
   - Shared conflict engagement competencies
   - Joint accountability and recognition for contributions
   - Frequent and meaningful engagement
   - Mutual investment and commitment
   - Transparency
3. Knowledge is shared among partners through mechanisms such as:
   - Commitment to lifelong learning
   - Shared knowledge of current best practices
   - Shared knowledge management systems
   - Joint preparation for national certification, accreditation, and regulatory reviews
   - Interprofessional education
   - Joint research
   - Joint committee appointments
   - Joint development of competencies
4. A commitment is shared by partners to maximize the potential of each registered nurse to reach the highest level within his/her individual scope of practice including:
   - Culture of trust and respect
   - Shared responsibility to prepare and enable nurses to lead change and advance health
   - Shared governance that fosters innovation and advanced problem solving
   - Shared decision making
   - Consideration and evaluation of shared opportunities
   - Participation on regional and national committees to develop policy and strategies for implementation
   - Joint meetings between regional/national constituents of AONE and AACN
5. A commitment is shared by partners to work together to determine an evidence-based transition program for students and new graduates that is both sustainable and cost-effective via:
   - Collaborative development, implementation, and evaluation of residency programs
   - Leveraging competencies from practice to education and vice versa
   - Mutual/shared commitment to lifelong learning for self and others

(continued)

EXHIBIT 11.1 AACN–AONE Guiding Principles for Academic–Practice Partnerships (continued)

6. A commitment is shared by partners to develop, implement, and evaluate organizational processes and structures that support and recognize academic or educational achievements:
   - Lifelong learning for all levels of nursing, certification, and continuing education
   - Seamless academic progression
   - Joint funding and in-kind resources for all nurses to achieve a higher level of learning
   - Joint faculty appointments between academic and clinical institutions
   - Support for increasing diversity in the workforce at the staff and faculty levels
   - Support for achieving an 80% baccalaureate prepared RN workforce and for doubling the number of nurses with doctoral degrees

7. A commitment is shared by partners to support opportunities for nurses to lead and develop collaborative models that redesign practice environments to improve health outcomes, including:
   - Joint interprofessional leadership development programs
   - Joint funding to design, implement, and sustain innovative patient-centered delivery systems
   - Collaborative engagement to examine and mitigate nonvalue added practice complexity
   - Seamless transition from the classroom to the bedside
   - Joint mentoring programs/opportunities

8. A commitment is shared by partners to establish infrastructures to collect and analyze data on the current and future needs of the RN workforce via:
   - Identification of useful workforce data
   - Joint collection and analysis of workforce and education data
   - Joint business case development
   - Assurance of transparency of data

AACN–AONE, American Association of Colleges of Nursing and American Organization of Nurse Executives.

Source: From AACN–AONE Task Force on Academic–Practice Partnerships (2012). Reprinted by permission of American Association of Colleges of Nursing.

The ability to establish and sustain effective partnerships is based on shared mission, values, and trust. Relationships are built through effective, clear communication and commitment to addressing conflicts collaboratively. Opportunities for moving from contractual affiliations to meaningful partnerships exist from carefully planning initial discussions to evaluating outcomes. However, the efforts involved in developing and sustaining strong collaborative relationships are complex and time-consuming, and often are influenced by personal commitments or changes to individual representation within the organization.

An interactive toolkit was developed by AACN–AONE in 2012 and revised in 2015 to guide nursing leaders in the development, growth, and evaluation of academic–practice partnerships. Specific questions, as shown in Exhibit 11.2, identify activities relevant to the development and sustenance of a partnership. Exemplars of strong academic–practice partnerships are provided in the toolkit (AACN–AONE Academic–Practice Partnership Steering Committee, 2015).

EXHIBIT 11.2 Questions for Developing and Sustaining Partnerships

1. Players
   a. Selecting Partners
      - How do you identify your partners?
      - Why is this partner a good fit?
      - How do you identify, approach, and get a meeting with the right person in your potential partner's organization?
   b. Preparing for Your First Meeting
      - Where do you meet?
      - What do you need to know about your potential partner and the organization?
      - What does your partner need to know about you and your organization?
2. Partnership Activities
   a. Initial Meeting
      - What is the right partnership activity?
      - What background information about your organizations might be helpful to bring to the first meeting?
      - What do you have to offer?
      - What is the mutual benefit?
      - What is your vision?
      - Does your potential partner share the same or similar vision?
      - What is the potential initiative/activity and who else needs to be involved in both organizations?
      - Are you talking to the top leadership in the organization? What is the business case for the partnership?
      - What are the next steps? Do you have a timeline established at the end of the first meeting?
      - Follow up with a thank-you note and outline of next steps.
   b. Subsequent Meetings
      - Do you have clarity on goals and vision?
      - What are the details and the timeline for the initiative?
      - What resources are needed?
      - Who is our expert for consultation if need be?
      - Will there be an official MOU?
      - What are the expected outcomes of the partnership?
3. Environment
   a. Time
      - Is this the right time for the partnership?
      - What issues are present that may facilitate or impede the development of the partnership? What is the time commitment for the institutions?
      - Whose time will be required, and how frequently/regularly will we meet?
   b. Space
      - What space and equipment are required for the activity?
      - What money is needed?
      - Where are we meeting?
      - Where will we present outcomes?

(continued)

EXHIBIT 11.2 Questions for Developing and Sustaining Partnerships (*continued*)

c. Regulation
- What are the policies or regulatory issues may impede or facilitate the partnership from both sides?
- How will the partnership be funded?
- What are the constraints of both partners?
- What history is present with the partner institutions?

MOU, memorandum of understanding.

Source: Adapted from American Association of Colleges of Nursing and American Association of Nurse Executives Academic–Practice Partnership Steering Committee (2015). Reprinted with permission from American Association of Colleges of Nursing.

Teel, MacIntyre, Murray, and Rock (2011) identified four themes contributing to successful implementation of an innovative academic–practice partnership to increase educational capacity using the coach/preceptor models. Supportive relationships, goodness of fit, flexibility, and communication are examined in Table 11.1. Although additional programmatic research testing is needed in education innovations, it is helpful for the educator to apply strategies associated with the four themes evidenced in successful partnerships.

In a systematic review of the evidence, Nabavi, Vanaki, and Mohammadi (2012) identified four stages related to the formation and implementation processes of academic and service partnerships. The stages, outlined in Table 11.2, are applicable to a variety of partnerships and create a framework for identifying structures, processes, procedures, and outcomes.

TABLE 11.1 Four Themes Contributing to Successful Implementation

Theme	Application Strategy
Supportive relationships	Students, faculty, and preceptors (clinical staff) form a core triad. Elements of supportive relationships: • Pairing of student and preceptor • Orientation of preceptors by faculty • Faculty role as advocate between student and preceptor • Continuity of clinical rotations in a single clinical agency
Goodness of fit	Planning for and assessing the innovation for an appropriate "fit." This includes: • Presence of an organizational culture that values and supports innovation (academic program and clinical agency) • Recognition of vital roles of faculty and preceptors, including various forms of financial support • Assessment and identification of potential participants (students, preceptors, faculty) and program components for the best "fit"

(continued)

TABLE 11.1 Four Themes Contributing to Successful Implementation (*continued*)

Theme	Application Strategy
Flexibility	The partnership stakeholders recognize: • Organizational culture, structure, rules, and needs will influence adaptation of innovation • Willingness to change • The value of feedback from students, faculty, preceptors to be able to adapt and change as needed
Communication	Multiple modalities of communication are needed to foster effective use of resources and information to meet the needs of students, faculty, and clinical partners and increased flexibility in the partnerships: • Printed literature • Interviews of students, faculty, and preceptors • Web sites or portals • E-mail and telephone communication • Regularly scheduled face-to-face meetings with all stakeholders

Source: Adapted from Teel, MacIntyre, Murray, and Rock (2011).

TABLE 11.2 Four Stages of Formation and Implementation of Academic–Service Partnerships

Four Stages	Examples
Mutual potential benefits Discovery of interests or issues which could be served by resources of a partnership	• Nursing workforce shortage • Insufficient number of clinical placements to support increasing enrollments • Insufficient number of qualified/clinically competent faculty • Development of evidence-based nursing practice, including nursing research and translation of nursing research into practice
Moving from competitor to collaborator Planning and development of cooperative structural framework that includes: 1. Identification and coalition of stakeholders,	Senior leadership from each partner (academic, service, legislative, regulatory agencies) or other stakeholders identify mutual interests and set mission, goals, plans, timelines, and deadlines: • Executive/management committee or advisory council

(continued)

TABLE 11.2 Four Stages of Formation and Implementation of Academic–Service Partnerships (*continued*)

Four Stages	Examples
2. Shared decision or policy making, and 3. Structure that facilitates interaction between partners.	• Task force or working groups formed to promote interaction in a partnership. Focus and activities are to implement mission of partnership and develop methods, including supervision or oversight, identification of roles and responsibilities, framework for decision making, and training needs across organizations in partnership • Development of job descriptions • Affiliation agreement and contract auditing • Regulatory education and compliance monitoring • Preceptor development • Continuing education/staff development programs
Joint practice Process of cooperation between the academic and service organizations to meet mutual goals	New structures and procedures in a partnership bring change to roles and responsibilities for employees in each organization and students: • Joint, adjunct, affiliate faculty appointment • Preceptorship Model • Dedicated education unit • Clinical Scholar Model • Service learning • IPE
Mutually beneficial outcomes Three realms of benefits to an effective academic–service partnership: 1. Service/practice 2. Education 3. Profession	• Career progression path for clinical nurses into education • Clinical nurse job satisfaction • Increase in number of clinical faculty • Increased educational capacity and admissions • Supportive learning environments • Improved employment and recruitment opportunities

IPE, interprofessional education.

Source: Adapted from Nabavi, Vanaki, and Mohammadi (2012).

STRUCTURAL FOUNDATIONS OF ACADEMIC–SERVICE PARTNERSHIPS

CAPACITY MANAGEMENT

In 2009, the National League for Nursing (NLN) commissioned a national survey to examine clinical education in prelicensure registered nursing programs (Ironside & McNelis, 2010). Respondents identified organizational and structural barriers and pedagogical challenges faced in optimizing students' clinical learning (McNelis, Fonacier, McDonald, & Ironside, 2011). The most frequently identified barriers were the lack of quality clinical education sites to accommodate student groups and lack of learning experiences that support learning outcomes. Nursing programs are increasingly under pressure to admit and educate more students quickly, given the demand to ease the nursing shortage and to meet the health care needs of an aging population. Yet, baccalaureate and graduate nursing programs in the United States turned away more than 68,000 qualified applicants in 2014–2015 due to an insufficient number of faculty, clinical sites, classroom space, clinical preceptors, and budget constraints (AACN, 2015). Similarly, 78% of associate degree nursing programs in 2014 turned away qualified applicants (National League for Nursing [NLN], 2014).

Although there are limited fiscal capital and human resources, nursing leaders recognize the expertise across education and practice that is needed to address complex challenges in improving patient safety, quality care, and cost-effective outcomes. When determining capacity relevant to preparing nurses, nursing administrators consider the organization's mission and values, as well as the impact on patient care delivery, patient outcomes, and nursing staff resources. For example, hiring policies related to educational preparation required for nursing positions and accreditation such as Magnet™ have begun to provide the framework for the type of academic degree programs the agency will host. Many decisions to host students in the service agency also consider the time, number of resources needed, including personnel, equipment and space, costs associated with those resources, and the overall number of placement requests from nursing programs. Examples of service agency variables in determining clinical capacity are depicted in Table 11.3.

Service agencies also may examine clinical placement requests in terms of their experience and familiarity with the academic curriculum, model of student supervision used for clinical education, and previous experiences with student performance. Requests for preceptorships are carefully considered by agencies in terms of availability of staff with appropriate credentials and educational background, availability and costs associated with preceptor development courses, and preceptor incentives. The distribution of workload and impact on productivity when clinical staff assume a heavy responsibility for clinical education during a preceptorship is an important factor in determining capacity. Assessment and identification of healthy clinical work environments is another critical consideration.

Nurse educators from both academic and practice settings should consider the systems, framework, and practices that support nurses in developing competence to deliver safe and quality patient care. This is the first step in determining if the clinical unit is appropriate and ready for development of clinical learning experiences and student placements. Nursing programs continue to establish partnerships within nontraditional practice settings (ambulatory care, primary care clinics, outpatient care settings) and community-based sites (refugee centers, day treatment centers, respite care centers) to augment student learning experiences. Best practices, noted in the definition of Clinical Practice Environments for Students, include working and learning together

TABLE 11.3 Examples of Service Agency Variables in Determining Clinical Capacity

Operational Systems	Clinical Services
Determination and monitoring of affiliation agreements/contracts and associated policies that determine role, responsibilities of the partnership	Hours of agency operation
	Types of patient services offered and location of services
Providing The Joint Commission standards required for orientation of nonemployees, which includes students, related to basic life safety and agency operations/resources	Opening or closing and expansion of patient care units or services
	Changing staffing, skill mix, patient acuity and census levels that reflect productivity metrics and patient outcome indicators
Electronic medical record access and medication dispensing systems for student use, which includes training, surveillance of proper use, and troubleshooting resources	Existing and anticipated competency-based education, training, and orientation needs of experienced and newly hired staff

with clinical nurse experts, from a wide variety of settings, who serve as preceptors and role models (AACN, 2008).

Academic and practice partnerships may use centralized computer or web-based programs to standardize student placement processes. Additional purposes and functions of these programs are to monitor student placement numbers at clinical sites and on units, identify sites and units not being used but with the potential for development to support clinical learning and course objectives, and improve information sharing between nursing programs and service agencies for decision making about current and future needs for clinical placements. Burns et al. (2011) described academic partnership strategies to address the faculty shortage through use of a centralized system to provide job postings, create a centralized faculty candidate pool, and clarify nursing faculty requirements and resources. Use of data derived from placement platforms, including efficacy and quality measurement to drive innovations in clinical education, is an opportunity for further research. Financial models for sustainability of centralized clinical placement platforms are also evolving, with costs shared between academic/service partners or covered through student use fees.

CLINICAL AFFILIATION AGREEMENTS

The clinical practice environment for students is defined through written agreements, jointly designed to benefit both academic and practice partners with ongoing evaluation and continuous improvement (AACN, 2008). The clinical affiliation agreement is a tool used by a health care agency and an academic program for provision of clinical learning experiences for students. Table 11.4 provides an example of content outlined in a clinical affiliation agreement.

Clinical affiliation agreements typically have multiple clauses that serve to protect the health care agency and academic program. It is common for the affiliation agreement to be reviewed by legal counsel, risk management, human resources, and agency and nursing program administration to ensure that all interests are represented. The health care agency and academic program both have mandates to provide structure to the affiliation agreement. However, the intent of the partnership is to provide a supportive learning environment and associated clinical experiences for students. The signature authority to establish an affiliation agreement is determined by the leadership structure of each organization. A sample of specific health care agency and nursing program responsibilities are outlined in Table 11.5.

Although the affiliation agreement provides the framework for clinical learning experiences, it is important to recognize that the collaboration between academic program faculty and representatives from the health care agency is critical to the selection of appropriate learning environments and experiences to facilitate achievement of

TABLE 11.4 Content Outline of a Clinical Affiliation Agreement

Agreement Component	Description
Shared purpose of health care agency and nursing program	To promote a planned and supervised program of clinical experience for nursing students
Term period and renewal	Commencement and termination date of affiliation, including reference to early termination terms specified in the agreement
	Termination without cause: language includes termination without cause or penalty by either the health care agency or nursing program by giving the other party a written notice within a timeframe, such as 30 or 60 days to termination
Payment terms	Payment for educational services may be stipulated dependent on the type of service provided, and health care agencies typically exclude payment for wages, worker's compensation, professional liability insurance, health insurance, transportation, meals, room, or uniforms for students
Employment status	Students are not deemed employees of the health care agency for any purpose; they are present in the agency solely as a part of clinical course curriculum experience
Responsibilities of the health care agency	The health care agency retains primary responsibility for patient care and treatment
Responsibilities of the academic program	The academic program affirms that a student is fully matriculated into the program

(continued)

TABLE 11.4 Content Outline of a Clinical Affiliation Agreement (*continued*)

Agreement Component	Description
Insurance provisions	Language includes reference to policies from both the health care agency and the academic program regarding general liability and professional liability insurance as necessary to insure itself, agents, employees, and students against any claim or claims for damages arising either directly or indirectly in connection with the performance of activities under the agreement of providing clinical experiences
	Limitations and state government acts may also be described in this section
Modification and waiver, assignments and compliance with laws and regulations	Affiliation agreements have language reflecting compliance with federal, state, and local laws and regulations

Source: From University of Colorado Hospital, UCHealth, Anschutz Medical Campus, Aurora, Colorado. Adapted with permission.

TABLE 11.5 Sample of Specific Health Care Agency and Nursing Program Responsibilities

Health Care Agency	Nursing Program
Provide appropriate supervision of students	Students adhere to health care agency rules, regulations, policies and procedures, including policies related to patient confidentiality, patient rights, and ethical conduct
Provide students access to rules, regulations, policies, and procedures of the agency	
Provide orientation to the clinical environment that meets regulatory body standards and requirements	Students meet health and immunization status of the health care agency
Provide appropriate emergency care for students incurring sudden-onset illness or injury during the clinical experience, including accidental exposure to patient blood or body fluids	Verification of a criminal background check
	Verification of a negative drug screen
	Student proficiency in written and verbal skills
	Student citizenship or visa status

Source: From University of Colorado Hospital, UCHealth, Anschutz Medical Campus, Aurora, Colorado. Adapted with permission.

specific learning outcomes. The collaborative effort extends to the determination of the type of student supervision required in the clinical environment or model of clinical instruction used.

Affiliation agreements and student placements may also be supported by associated internal policies within the health care agency. Policies describe the circumstances under which students may have clinical experiences as part of an academic program. Accountability of agency personnel and students are identified in these policies, which include the steps in the process for clinical placement of students, orientation of students to the agency, and process for determination and evaluation of clinical placements in the agency. Recordkeeping of placements and audits of compliance with aspects of the affiliation agreement are also components of an agency's policy. Sample policies from the University of Colorado Hospital, Anschutz Medical Campus (AMC) (Aurora, Colorado) are listed in Table 11.6.

TABLE 11.6 Sample Policies

Health Care Agency Internal Policy	Description Relevant to Clinical Placements
Student affiliation experiences	Circumstances for the provision of clinical experiences as part of academic programs
Preceptor policy	Processes by which employees and students are precepted, as well as the process by which preceptors are selected, trained, and evaluated
Background screening policy	Processes and procedures related to reasonable inquiry into the background of employees, vendors, and prospective employees and vendors
Drug- and alcohol-free workplace	Processes and procedures to maintain a drug- and alcohol-free workplace
Urine drug screen multidrug point-of-care testing	Process used for performing CLIA-waived, multidrug screening tests on urine
Employee/volunteer health screens	Procedures for preplacement physicals, fitness-for-duty evaluations, and return-to-work procedures

CLIA, Clinical Laboratory Improvement Amendments.

Source: From University of Colorado Hospital, UCHealth. Anschutz Medical Campus, Aurora, Colorado. Adapted with permission.

ALLIANCE FOR CLINICAL EDUCATION

The Alliance for Clinical Education (ACE) is an example of an academic–practice partnership with representation of more than 70 nursing schools, health care organizations, and professional and regulatory entities in the Denver metropolitan and surrounding region. The purpose of ACE is to promote collaboration between practice and education in preparing a nursing workforce for the future. The ACE group meets quarterly as a forum to share ideas and information and to make recommendations surrounding best practices, community standards, and regulatory compliance, in an effort to provide the optimum clinical student learning experiences (Article I of the Alliance for Clinical Education Bylaws, 2015).

This alliance between education and health care organizations not only addresses clinical nursing education issues as a primary focus, but also serves as a forum to connect and inform members of initiatives and changes affecting nursing workforce development occurring within individual organizations, the State of Colorado Board of Nursing, the Colorado Area Health Education Councils, the Colorado Center for Nursing Excellence, and the Colorado Nurses' Association. The ACE bylaws, scope of work, meeting minutes, and documents are open-source materials and can be found at www.coloradonursingcenter.org/center-special-initiatives/ alliance-for-clinical-education-ace.

EXPLORATION OF MODELS OF CLINICAL EDUCATION

The IOM (Committee on the Robert Wood Johnson Foundation Initiative on the Future of Nursing at the IOM, 2011) calls for nursing faculty to examine the structures and processes associated with clinical education and to determine the extent to which current clinical experiences are preparing students for the future demands of practice. The determination of quality clinical education and associated clinical sites or learning environments is an ongoing dialogue between academic and service leadership (McNelis et al., 2011). Quality clinical experiences are intended to provide students with time and opportunity to synthesize professional values and roles, and cognitive and psychomotor skills, into emerging practice competencies. Support of practice outcome competencies, along the education continuum that includes transition into professional practice, should be a shared priority for academic and service partnerships.

With a changing landscape of health care delivery models and reimbursement, academic and service entities are adding process improvement, research and quality improvement methodologies, and outcomes evaluation into examining the success of their partnerships in preparing the future health care workforce (Beal, 2012). The boundaries of teaching and learning environments in which partnerships function continue to be challenged by paradigm shifts and innovations. As an example, Letcher and Nelson (2014) presented their Culture of Caring Model as "shared ownership of the nursing educational enterprise and excellence in nursing practice" (p. 177). The model weaves together the cultural boundaries associated with nursing education and practice, incorporates evidence-based practice to create a teaching-learning culture that aligns education processes with nursing practice as a shared endeavor, and uses the concept of intervention bundling to promote learning in the practice environment (Letcher & Nelson, 2014).

Traditionally, the Nursing Education Model in the United States consists of an academic faculty in a clinical setting providing direct supervision of a number of students in the application of knowledge and skills acquired in the classroom, laboratory, or simulation setting to assigned patients (Rhodes, Meyers, & Underhill, 2012). The model includes scheduling students into a patient care setting 1 to 3 days per week; scheduling and rotating students into different health care agencies to be exposed to different patient populations (Sullivan, 2010); and requiring students to complete preclinical preparation work and other learning activities such as journaling. As student enrollments increase and faculty pools decrease, nursing programs need to use innovation to determine and provide quality clinical experiences (Rhodes et al., 2012).

Alternatives to traditional models of clinical education are emerging. Five types of academic–practice partnerships reflecting collaboration and innovation are described.

INTERPROFESSIONAL EDUCATION

The need for IPE and core competencies for interprofessional collaborative practice were discussed earlier in Chapter 8. Developing well-functioning teams is a priority because of the complexity of care delivery and need for care coordination among the many providers encountered by a single patient. Interprofessional collaboration focuses on activities that promote integrated models of education and practice among health professions students, including the value of each discipline as a full partner in the delivery and determination of quality and safe patient care. Students learn the professional role and scope of practice of their discipline, and through IPE develop an awareness of other health professional roles and convergence of those roles to achieve the common goal of optimal patient outcomes.

IPE may occur in the classroom, through simulation, activities in the clinical setting, or a combination of these throughout health professions programs. Teaching strategies and learning opportunities to reframe relationships and use collaboration, negotiation, and communication skills are foundational in developing interprofessional partnerships as a standard in professional practice. During the implementation of IPE initiatives or associated activities, the clinical teacher may be in a position to renegotiate traditional roles and responsibilities among staff and establish new ways of working that promote interprofessional competencies.

EXAMPLE OF INTERPROFESSIONAL EDUCATION AT THE UNIVERSITY OF COLORADO, AMC

The AMC of the University of Colorado was intentionally designed to facilitate collaborative IPE among the health science programs of Dental Medicine, Pharmacy and Pharmaceutical Sciences, Nursing, Physical Therapy, Public Health, Anesthesia Assistant, Physician Assistant, and Medicine. The planning of campus design was purposeful in the desire to bring health professions students closer together in classroom, laboratories, and simulation spaces and create common space and facilities to promote student interaction and socialization.

Within the context of IPE, the IPE Council has developed a robust longitudinal curriculum integrating preclinical and clinical training for all of the health profession students. The Interprofessional Practice and Education Development (IPED) curriculum guides learners in developing competencies in teamwork, communication, collaborative interprofessional practice, ethics, values, and quality and safety with an additional focus on vulnerable and underserved populations. The IPE curriculum is shared across all professional health programs and spans a timeframe adapted to the 2 to 4 years' length of health professions programs. Health professions students start the IPED with an orientation to IPE on the first day of class.

Students begin their IPED through 16 weeks of classroom team-based learning experiences. Students are placed into interprofessional teams of 8 to 14 students and complete a series of specific tasks that are designed to explore roles and responsibilities of different professions and to build teamwork and communication skills. Specific skills developed during through the use of scenarios include: teamwork and collaboration, ethics and values, quality care, and safety. The teams meet every week for 8 weeks over the course of two semesters.

Clinical Transformations in Quality and Collaborative Care is the second step in the IPE curriculum. This is a simulation experience for students and takes place in the Center for Advancing Professional Excellence (CAPE), which includes a high-fidelity simulation center. During the simulation experience, students undergo training in the Strategies and Tools to Enhance Performance and Patient Safety (TeamSTEPPS) curriculum for clinical communications developed by the Agency for Healthcare Research and Quality (AHRQ) and the Department of Defense (AHRQ, 2007). The simulation experience mimics real-life scenarios found in health care. The goal of the simulation is to expose students to complex patient situations in which collaborative care is needed to optimize patient outcomes. The focus of the simulation is communication. Students also learn how to react to situations when unsure of actions to take and use reflection to examine individual and team behaviors to promote quality and safety.

The third step in the IPE curriculum, building on previous content and experiences, allows students to achieve the competencies of the program through authentic clinical experiences. The clinical experiences also meet outcomes for each health profession program and comply with accreditation requirements for each program. The experiences are varied and scheduled within students' existing program and are in alignment with students' educational level. Although structured learning activities form the foundation for this step, Clinical Integrations, flexibility as to where and when the activities can be completed has been critical to the success of the IPED.

PEER TEACHING AND LEARNING

Peer-assisted learning is a collaborative and cooperative teaching and learning strategy, whereby students are active and equal partners. Peers facilitate learning by providing emotional support and feedback through discussions and assisting with physical skills and tasks (Secomb, 2008). Typically, peer-assisted learning is done is small groups. Small group size can foster interaction and support for learning among members, including ability to provide instant feedback. Students reported satisfaction and increased self-confidence with peer teaching (Secomb, 2008). In another study, Pålsson, Mårtensson, Swenne, Ädel, and Engström (2017) found that peer learning improved nursing students' self-efficacy in clinical practice.

Peer teaching and learning may also increase student access and involvement in planned learning activities and potentially decrease demand on faculty resources, although faculty supervision is required for peer learning to be effective (Stone, Cooper, & Cant, 2013). Other important considerations include determining the types of content and skills that can be accomplished by peer-assisted learning, level of involvement and collaboration with faculty or staff in health care agencies, and how to address incompatibility of students.

SERVICE LEARNING

The National Service-Learning Clearinghouse (2016) describes service learning as "a teaching and learning strategy that integrates meaningful community service with instruction and reflection to enrich the learning experience, teach civic responsibility and strength communities." Another description of service learning is an "education experience in which students participate in an activity that meets the needs of a specific community and reflect on the service in such a way as to further understand the course content, the broader role of the discipline and their sense of civic responsibility" (Otterness, Gehrke, & Sener, 2007, p. 40). Service learning requires a relationship between the academic and a community-based agency. Both partners establish a need for an identified activity or service that can be provided by students (Reising et al., 2008) and also connected to structured academic coursework.

Use of a reflective process is a component of service learning that differentiates service learning from a volunteer experience (Brown & Schmidt, 2016; Vogt, Chavez, & Schaffner, 2011). Reflective practices include journaling or participation in structured groups for debriefing. Service learning is linked to increases in student knowledge related to social activism and justice, health care equity (Knight, Mooer, & Groh, 2007; Reising et al., 2008), and cultural diversity (Worrell-Carlisle, 2005), as well as to development of leadership behaviors through implementation of a service-learning project (Foli, Braswell, Kirkpatrick, & Lim, 2014).

Application of the Service-Learning Model as a short-term immersion experience for baccalaureate nursing students, Vogt et al. (2011) describe the use of camp nursing as providing opportunities for practice of physical assessment, relationship building, and chronic disease management skills. In response to students' needs to connect Community Health Nursing Theory to practice and address a decrease in clinical sites and resources, Broussard (2011) described the integration of a service-learning framework that identified potential activities that were linked to a community assigned to students. The activities promoted student interaction with community leaders, residents, and public health and social work professionals (pp. 41–42).

Other types of clinical experiences that could be reframed as a Service-Learning Model directed to meeting community needs include health screening programs, flu vaccine clinics, development of wellness programs for underserved populations or the elderly, food delivery programs, friendly visitor programs, attending local legislative sessions pertaining to health policy, and faith-based outreach programs serving specific congregations. In a literature review of service learning in baccalaureate nursing education, B. S. Murray (2013) indicated that service learning, a valuable teaching pedagogy, should include rigorous methods to evaluate course outcomes.

CLINICAL SCHOLAR MODEL

The Clinical Scholar Model (CSM) originated in 1984 as a joint initiative between the University of Colorado, AMC, College of Nursing and University of Colorado Hospital in Aurora, Colorado. The model has expanded in the past three decades to include 12 service agencies and 30 clinical scholars. The service agencies include acute care hospitals, county public health, and mental health and rehabilitation facilities. The financial modeling of the CSM is varied among the service agencies, which correlates with overall student progression and placement needs and the curriculum objectives. Clinical scholars are expert nurses in service agencies who plan and coordinate students' clinical experiences, teach students, and contribute to the evaluation of their clinical competencies. Additionally, these nurses participate in training, offered by their agency, the academic partner, or an external agency, to introduce them to the concepts related to creating successful student learning experiences within the practice arena.

Qualifications and attributes of the clinical scholar include:

1. Expert nurse who exemplifies professionalism and relationship-centered care in practice and conveys a passion for teaching and learning, particularly in the clinical setting
2. An employee of the health care agency, with time dedicated to planning, coordinating, teaching, and evaluating student clinical experiences
3. Master's prepared in nursing
4. Minimum of 5 years' experience in a nursing specialty practice and 2 years of employment within the health care agency

5. Recruited within the health care agency based on experience in practice and as a preceptor
6. Jointly interviewed and selected for hire by the college of nursing and the health care agency.

Clinical scholars are a valued and integral part of clinical education. They coordinate placements and learning experiences, provide consistent instruction and supervision, and contribute to evaluation of students' clinical competencies. Benefits include streamlined communication, liaison to staff for a smoother integration of students into the clinical setting, consistency of involvement, increased relevance of the clinical experience, and curricular modifications (Preheim, 2008; Preheim, Casey, & Krugman, 2006). Exhibit 11.3 summarizes the roles and responsibilities of the clinical scholar.

EXHIBIT 11.3 Roles and Responsibilities of the Clinical Scholar

1. Coordination
   - Confirms scheduled dates, hours, clinical units preclinical
   - Identifies and negotiates precepted assignments with qualified and available staff nurses
   - Arranges computer training and hospital orientation
   - Assures staff and preceptors are prepared for arrival and engagement of students in learning activities appropriate for the level of student and course outcomes
2. Clinical education
   - Role models professional behaviors to facilitate socialization as a member of the health care team and nursing profession
   - Clarifies expectations and roles using effective communication and conflict management skills to guide the learning experience
   - Assesses critical thinking and clinical skills, and determines knowledge and application of the nursing process specific to the patient assignment
   - Interacts with individual student to model, dialogue, and provide feedback on performance
   - Provides oversight education to ensure the clinical course outcomes are met
   - Conducts clinical conferences to provide an opportunity to reflect on care provided and aspects of professional nursing roles and responsibilities
   - Fosters a trusting and caring relationship, key in developing the student's skills, confidence in performance, and socialization into professional nursing roles
3. Evaluation of student performance
   - Assesses readiness for engagement in clinical practice
   - Serves as a liaison to preceptor and faculty to ensure practice opportunities and skill development according to critical elements for competent practice
   - Consistently evaluates students' clinical performance using standardized clinical evaluation tools and procedures
   - Prepares recommendations for further development and/or revisions of the clinical experience and teaching/learning tools.
   - Facilitates development and implementation of joint research and scholarly activities

Source: From Preheim (2008). Reprinted by permission of Springer Publishing.

DEDICATED EDUCATION UNITS

The Dedicated Education Unit (DEU) Model, developed in the late 1990s at Flinders University of South Australia School of Nursing, is another example of an academic–service partnership. The DEU Model is a triad of students, clinical nursing staff, and faculty members. The DEU is designed to provide an optimal learning environment through collaboration of clinical nurses, agency management, and academic faculty (Moscato, Miller, Logsdon, Weinberg, & Chorpenning, 2007). The key features of the DEU Model are:

1. The clinical unit is an optimal teaching/learning environment.
2. The primary goal is student achievement of learning outcomes.
3. The DEU is used solely by one nursing program.
4. The commitment to attain an optimal practice environment for students and staff is shared through collaborative work efforts and communication.
5. Staff nurses, who indicate a desire to teach, are prepared for the clinical teaching role, and nursing faculty members from the academic program support the staff nurse in the instructor role.
6. Students are paired with staff nurse, who is in the role of clinical teacher (Moscato et al. (2007).

Central to the DEU concept is that staff nurses have a key educational role in students' knowledge and skill acquisition (Moscato et al., 2007). The model facilitates relationship building between academic and practice settings, supports professional nursing development, and enhances student engagement in the practice setting (Ranse & Grealish, 2007; Warner & Burton, 2009; Wotton & Gonda, 2004). The DEU Model also facilitates teaching and learning of quality improvement and safety competencies while decreasing student anxiety, and building trust and student confidence (Masters, 2015; Mulready-Shick, Kafel, Banister, & Mylott, 2009). Beyond the traditional acute care medical/surgical unit, the DEU Model is also found in diverse patient care settings such as long-term care (Melillo et al., 2014), maternal-newborn units (Raines, 2016), and intensive care (Koharchik et al., 2017).

Dedicated education units have increased the capacity of clinical agencies, allowing for increased student enrollments and hosting more students in the practice setting compared to the Traditional Preceptor Model (Hill, Foster, & Oermann, 2015; Moscato, Nishioka, & Coe, 2013); studies report high student and staff satisfaction with the clinical teaching and learning experience (Moscato et al., 2007). Rhodes et al. (2012) examined the impact of the DEU Model on the clinical learning environment. The outcomes included high student satisfaction with their clinical experience, building relationships with DEU nurses that resulted in students' feeling part of the team, and the opportunity for students to witness patient-centered care. Additional outcomes of DEUs included increased staff nurse satisfaction associated with acknowledgment of their clinical practice expertise, the fostering of teamwork to create a supportive learning environment for students, and sparking interest in nurses to return to school (Jeffries et al., 2013; Rhodes et al., 2012).

The DEU agency partners, in an experimental study, reported reduced orientation time for new graduate nurses with DEU clinical experiences (Sharpnack, Koppelman, & Fellows, 2014) and "valuing by staff of students they had educated" (Smyer, Gatlin, Tan, Tejada, & Feng, 2015, p. 296). The development of a DEU for new graduate nurse orientation and role socialization led to improvement in new graduate retention rates, increased medication error reporting, and improved fall rates (Pappas, 2007).

T. A. Murray, MacIntyre, and Teel (2011) evaluated a service-academic partnership DEU and reported that the model was as effective as the traditional model of faculty-led supervision of students. Additionally, there is some evidence of no differences on standardized tests, simulation activities, and classroom tests between students who had the faculty-led model of clinical teaching and students in a DEU (Hendricks, DeMeester, Stephenson, & Welch, 2016; Smyer et al., 2015). Mulready-Shick and Flanagan (2014) identified shifting roles, relationship building, mutual respect, and collaboration between partners as key behaviors and actions for sustaining DEUs. At the unit level, their findings further indicated that the key to sustaining unit DEUs depends on the interest and desire of clinical nurses to teach and to provide support for students' learning. DeMeester (2016) suggested that nursing program faculty have key roles in the evaluation and sustainability of DEUs through their support of clinical nurses, students, and the multiple processes associated with DEUs. A shift in faculty role includes nurturing clinical nurses as teachers, promoting evidence-based nursing practice through mutual sharing of knowledge and expertise, and facilitating a deeper student clinical learning experience, all within the context of a DEU with its own culture and identity (DeMeester, 2016; Jeffries et al., 2013).

Academic–service partnerships are also charged with developing an infrastructure, based on a shared mission and vision, to support all partners involved in the functioning of a DEU. This includes having criteria for matching the clinical unit to learning objectives; selecting clinical nurses as clinical instructors on the DEU; scheduling students and clinical nurses and orienting them; having tools to facilitate consistent communication and shared decision making among students, clinical instructor, and academic faculty member; balancing workloads with unit staffing needs; and identifying evaluation metrics and methods (Glynn, McVey, Wendt, & Russell, 2017; Jeffries et al., 2013; Nishioka, Coe, Hanita, & Moscato, 2014).

Other clinical partnerships that are designed to increase capacity and intentional use of the staff nurse in clinical education, on which the DEU Model is based, build on the relationship between staff nurse and student, and include purposeful development of the expert staff nurse in clinical teaching (DeLunas & Rooda, 2009; Kowalski et al., 2007; Kruger, Roush, Olinzock, & Bloom, 2010). The goal in the clinical learning environment is to promote critical thinking in response to actual patient situations during immersion experiences.

TRANSITION INTO PRACTICE

The successful transition of newly graduated, prelicensure nurses into the practice setting has been a focus of interest for nurse educators and employers for decades. Kramer (1974) described the role and values conflict experienced by new nurses as reality shock. Perceived lack of preparation for entry into fast-paced, acute care settings leaves nurses questioning their career choice and impacts safe, quality care delivery. Casey et al. (2011) described the difficulty new graduate nurses have transitioning to acute care settings and the lack of perceived support from the organization. Challenges, including managing multiple patient care assignments, communicating with physicians, and caring for dying patients, were identified by new graduates. Nursing faculty awareness and ability to prepare students for entry into practice through competency development are critical to the transition.

Schools of nursing can increase the relevancy of clinical education by involving clinical partners in curriculum development and collaborating in teaching and assessment of learning across classroom and clinical settings. Employers recognize the need for structured and specialized orientation, as well as preceptored experiences to coach and advocate for the new graduate nurse. However, the potential impact on quality and safe patient care, nursing turnover of the new graduate nurse, and impact on the health care team suggest that routine efforts to support entry into practice are inadequate. The IOM *Future of Nursing* (Committee on the Robert Wood Johnson Foundation Initiative on the Future of Nursing at the IOM, 2011) report called for the implementation of nurse residency programs, specifically charging state boards of nursing, accrediting bodies, the federal government, and health care organizations to support transition to practice programs.

The emergence of transition-to-practice models and accreditation of new graduate nurse residency programs with a focus on a clinical specialty area demonstrate a response to promote quality and safe care and professional identity. A review of the literature reveals a wide range of definitions, purpose, length, content, and structure of transition-to-practice models, nursing orientation, and nurse residency programs. Common barriers to the design and implementation of a transition program are limited resources and lack of evidence of effectiveness. Despite variations of approaches, the significance of the transition-to-practice issue and need for innovative and comprehensive models are evident.

Examples of transition models include the Vizient/AACN Postbaccalaureate Nurse Residency Program, which is a national model in more than 200 sites in 34 states (Vizient, 2016). A variety of national and state models exist to address specific state needs of education and practice reflected by the nursing shortage and imperative for quality, safe, and cost-effective care. On the national level, the Robert Wood Johnson Foundation, in partnership with the Tri-Council for Nursing and AONE, developed the Academic Progression in Nursing program in 2012 to address the need to increase the academic preparation of nurses to 80% having earned a bachelor's degree or higher by 2020. The program developed and funded statewide models in a number of states. There also are programs that address state-specific needs.

ROLES OF PARTICIPANTS

The value of the education mission must be nurtured and demonstrated first and most fundamentally by the chief nurse officer and nursing school dean or director. The challenge is to establish working relationships through awareness of each other's needs and goals, develop trust and effective communication patterns, and engage to ensure that affiliations move to meaningful partnerships. After the partnership is established, the value of the partnership should be continuously embraced and cultivated by nurse leaders, faculty, and staff responsible for the planning, implementation, and evaluation. Nursing faculty and agency staff activities influence the relationship and contribute to meeting needs and achieving goals. Roles and responsibilities at each level are important determinants of the effectiveness of the partnership.

The nurse educator role is multidimensional, with clear expectations and opportunities relevant to academic–practice partnership development and sustenance. Nurse educator competencies include facilitating learning, promoting development and socialization, using assessment and evaluation strategies, participating in curriculum design and evaluation of program outcomes, functioning as a change agent and leader, pursuing continuous quality improvement in the nurse educator role, engaging in scholarship, and functioning within the educational environment (NLN, 2012). These were discussed in Chapter 1. Within each of these competencies, task statements delineate specific responsibilities aligning with coordination, education, and evaluation of student learning in the clinical setting. Nursing faculty and clinical instructors are responsible, in their roles, to facilitate readiness for transition into practice. Nurse educators' understandings of the factors that facilitate or are barriers to effective partnerships are relevant to role development. Similarly, understanding strategies for articulating goals within the formal partnership and developing action plans to attain those goals are key responsibilities of the nurse educator.

A vast range of opportunities for effective partnerships and collaboration await faculty from the academic program and nurses at the staff or unit leader level at the clinical agency. Mutual respect, valuing, and investment are demonstrated through presence, engagement, and effective communication among faculty and unit staff. Nurse educators and clinical faculty impact the quality of the partnership through planning and preparation for the student learning experiences with unit managers and staff. Students who demonstrate readiness and professionalism contribute to the development of a meaningful and valued role for the team and delivery of quality and safe care. The appropriate level of student engagement, including expectations for patient assessment, nursing interventions, documentation, and supervision, should be clarified to the team members. Team member roles and responsibilities should be explained to the student.

Staff nurses who are prepared for the student's presence and learning needs and are recognized for their expertise feel valued for their contributions to clinical education. Viewing students as unwanted guests or placements as a commodity become barriers to realizing benefits of the partnership. The relationship of faculty and clinical teachers with the nursing staff and nurse leaders at the patient care unit or service level is critical to an effective partnership. Additional evidence of the partnership may be in the form of joint appointments, preceptor training, student scholarships, and participation in unit-based or nursing education committees relevant to quality and safety, and competency development.

Cronenwett and Redman (2003) described four types of clinical agency affiliations with nursing schools. The least effective type of affiliation is perceived to be a negative drain on the organization. For example, conflict and concern for safe patient care may occur if students are inadequately prepared for integration into the clinical unit or accompanied by an unqualified clinical instructor. A second type of affiliation is described as meaningless, with no perceived value or negative impact to the clinical agency. Clinical placements may be viewed as a commodity and routinely requested by the nursing program without consideration of needs or potential benefit to the clinical agency. In the third level of affiliation, value to the partnership is identified. For example, the clinical agency may benefit from a potential source of new graduate nurse employees, and the school of nursing may recognize the relevance of appropriately leveled learning experiences. Significant value of an active partnership is realized only at the fourth level. A clear sense of shared mission and trust are evident with interdependence to achieve goals that could not be accomplished without the partnership. Staff nurses engage in teaching, coaching, and precepting students, increasing nurse satisfaction and contributing to retention. Nursing faculty interact with clinical experts who inform modifications in curricular design or clinical evaluation tools to assess student performance.

Nursing deans and administrators weigh the impact, benefits, and challenges associated with collaboration in the education of the nursing workforce. Seifer and Maurana (2000) identified eight principles for developing and sustaining community-based partnerships. Cronenwett and Redman (2003) recommended assessing how each principle was evident in practice, providing an indication of the value of clinical nursing education to the mission and goals of the clinical agency. The eight principles for developing and sustaining community-based partnerships are in Exhibit 11.4.

EXHIBIT 11.4 Principles for Developing and Sustaining Community-Based Partnerships

1. Agree on mission, values, goals, and measurable outcomes
2. Demonstrate mutual trust, respect, and commitment to partnership
3. Build on strengths and assets, address need for improvement
4. Balance power and enable sharing of resources
5. Communicate with clarity, be open and listen
6. Establish roles, norms, and processes with input and agreement
7. Provide multidirectional feedback to continuously improve partnership outcomes
8. Share credit for accomplishments
9. Recognize that partnerships take time

Source: From Reiniger (n.d.) and Seifer and Maurana (2000).

FUTURE OF ACADEMIC–PRACTICE PARTNERHSIPS

More than a decade ago, the NLN issued a position statement indicating the need for collaboration between educators and health care leadership to prepare the future workforce to function in a complex and rapidly changing health care environment (NLN Board of Govenors, 2003). In 2016, AACN issued the Manatt Report that not only supported the need for collaboration between academic and practice partners, but also called for academic nursing to become increasingly engaged with practice partners to advance health and health care delivery. Nursing faculty and academic nurse leaders need to examine the current status of their partnerships and how they have been viewed and created.

Cronenwett (2004) identified the use of academic and service partnerships to enhance patient care and safety in addition to nursing education and research endeavors. To attain the goal of transforming clinical education and addressing the real-world complexities of health care encountered by students, education and practice innovations should be coupled with teamwork and collaboration among health professionals in academic and service organizations. The goal of transforming clinical education is to improve the level of clinical practice in nursing.

SUMMARY

Academic and service partnerships are forging innovations in clinical education and driving changes in roles for students, faculty, and clinical staff. These innovations and changes will require further evaluation by educators and administrators for curriculum development, additional competencies for practice/teaching, value or cost-effectiveness of the model, and readiness for practice of new graduates. Long-term sustainability of academic–service partnerships should also be examined.

REFERENCES

Agency for Healthcare Research and Quality. (2007). *Team STEPPS™: Strategies and tools to enhance performance and patient safety.* Retrieved from http://www.ahrq.gov/teamstepps/index.html

Alliance for Clinical Education. (2015). *By-laws.* Retrieved from http://www.coloradonursingcenter.org/documents/ace/bylaws_042015.pdf

American Association of Colleges of Nursing. (2008). *The essentials of baccalaureate education for professional nursing practice.* Retrieved from http://www.aacn.nche.edu/education-resources/BaccEssentials08.pdf

American Association of Colleges of Nursing. (2015). Nursing faculty shortage. Retrieved from http://www.aacn.nche.edu/media-relations/fact-sheets/nursing-faculty-shortage

American Association of Colleges of Nursing. (2016). *Advancing healthcare transformation: A new era for academic nursing.* Washington, DC: Author.

American Association of Colleges of Nursing and American Organization of Nurse Executives Academic–Practice Partnership Steering Committee. (2015). *Academic practice partnerships toolkit.* Retrieved from http://www.aacn.nche.edu/leading-initiatives/academic-practice-partnerships/tool-kit

American Association of Colleges of Nursing and American Organization of Nurse Executives Task Force on Academic–Practice Partnerships. (2010). *Summary of literature related to academic-service partnerships.* Retrieved from http://www.aacn.nche.edu/leading-initiatives/academic-practice-partnerships/SummaryLiteratureAcademic.pdf

American Association of Colleges of Nursing and American Organization of Nurse Executives Task Force on Academic–Practice Partnerships. (2012). *Guiding principles.* Retrieved from http://www.aacn.nche.edu/leading-initiatives/academic-practice-partnerships/GuidingPrinciples.pdf

Beal, J. A. (2012). Academic-service partnerships in nursing: An integrative review. *Nursing Research and Practice, 2012,* 1–9. doi:10.1144/2012/501564

Broome, M. (2009). Partnerships: A long walk in the wind. *Nursing Outlook, 57,* 119–120. doi:10.1016/j.outlook.2009.03.006

Broussard, B. B. (2011). The bucket list: A service-learning approach to community engagement to enhance community health nursing clinical learning. *Journal of Nursing Education, 50,* 40–43. doi:10.3928/01484834-20

Brown, J. M., & Schmidt, N. A. (2016). Service-learning in undergraduate nursing education: Where is the reflection? *Journal of Professional Nursing, 32*(1), 48–53. doi:10.1016/j.profnurs.2015.05.001

Burns, P., Williams, S. H., Ard, N., Enright, C., Poster, E., & Ransom, S. A. (2011). Academic partnerships to increase nursing education capacity: Centralized faculty resource and clinical placement centers. *Journal of Professional Nursing, 27*(6), e14–e19. doi:10.1016/j.profnurs.2011.07.004

Casey, K., Fink, R., Jaynes, C., Campbell, L., Cook, P., & Wilson, V. (2011). Readiness for practice: The senior practicum experience. *Journal of Nursing Education, 50,* 646–652. doi:10.3928/01484834-20110817-03

Committee on the Robert Wood Johnson Foundation Initiative on the Future of Nursing at the Institute of Medicine. (2011). *The future of nursing: Leading change, advancing health.* Washington, DC: National Academies Press.

Cronenwett, L. R. (2004). A present-day academic perspective on the Caroline nursing experience: Building on the past, shaping the future. *Journal of Professional Nursing, 20,* 300–304. doi:10.1016/j.profnurs.2004.07.005

Cronenwett, L. R., & Redman, R. (2003). Partners in action: Nursing education and nursing practice. *Journal of Nursing Administration, 28,* 153–155.

DeLunas, L. R., & Rooda, L. A. (2009). A new model for the clinical instruction of undergraduate nursing students. *Nursing Education Perspectives, 30,* 377–380.

DeMeester, D. A. (2016). The lived experience of nursing faculty in a dedicated education unit. *Journal of Nursing Education, 55*(12), 669–674. doi:10.3928/01484834-20161114-02

Foli, K. J., Braswell, M., Kirkpatrick, J., & Lim, E. (2014). Development of leadership behaviors in undergraduate nursing students: A service-learning approach. *Nursing Education Perspectives, 35,* 76–82. doi:10.5480/11-578.1

Glynn, D. M., McVey, C., Wendt, J., & Russell, B. (2017). Dedicated educational nursing unit: Clinical instructors' role perceptions and learning needs. *Journal of Professional Nursing, 33,* 108–112. doi:10.1016/j.profnurs.2016.08.005

Greiner, A. C. & Knebel, E. (2003). *Health professions education: A bridge to quality.* Washington, DC: National Academies Press.

Hendricks, S., DeMeester, D., Stephenson, E., & Welch, J. (2016). Stakeholder perceptions, learning opportunities, and student outcomes in three clinical learning models. *Journal of Nursing Education, 55,* 271–277. doi:10.3928/01484834-20160414-06

Hill, R. Y., Foster, B., & Oermann, M. H. (2015). Dedicated education unit model for a transition into practice course. *Journal of Continuing Education in Nursing, 46,* 403–408. doi:10.3928/00220124-20150821-02

Ironside, P. M., & McNelis, A. M. (2010). Clinical education in prelicensure nursing programs: Findings from a national survey. *Nursing Education Perspectives, 31,* 264–265.

Jeffries, P. R., Rose, L., Belcher, A. E., Dang, D., Hochuli, J. F., Fleischmann, D., . . . Walrath, J. M. (2013). A clinical academic practice partnership: A clinical education redesign. *Journal of Professional Nursing, 29,* 128–136. doi:10.1016/j.profnurs.2012.04013

Joynt, J., & Kimball, B. (2008). *Innovative care delivery models: Identifying new models that effectively leverage nurses.* White paper produced by Health Workforce Solutions and Robert Wood Johnson Foundation. Retrieved from http://innovativecaremodels.com

Knight, D., Mooer, S., & Groh, C. (2007). Service learning as a component of physician assistant Education: The development of a compassionate practitioner. *Journal of Physician Assistant Education, 18*(2), 49–52.

Koharchik, L., Jakub, K., Witsberger, C., Brooks, K., Petras, D., Weideman, Y., & Antonich, M. G. (2017). Staff nurse's perception of their role in a dedicated education unit within the intensive care unit. *Teaching and Learning in Nursing, 12,* 17–20. doi:10.1016/j.teln.2016.11.001

Kowalski, K., Horner, M., Carroll. K., Center, D., Foss, K., & Jarrett, S. (2007). Nursing clinical faculty revisited: The benefits of developing staff nurses as clinical scholars. *Journal of Continuing Education in Nursing, 3,* 69–75.

Kramer, M. (1974). *Reality shock: Why nurses leave nursing.* St. Louis, MO: C.V. Mosby.

Kruger, B. J., Roush, C., Olinzock, B. J., & Bloom, K. (2010). Engaging nursing students in long-term relationships with a home base community. *Journal of Nursing Education, 49,* 10–16. doi:10.3928/01484834-20090828-07

Letcher, D. C., & Nelson, M. L. (2014). Creating a culture of caring. A partnership bundle. *The Journal of Nursing Administration, 44,* 175–186. doi:10.1097/NNA.0000000000000047

Masters, K. (2015). Integrating quality and safety education into clinical nursing education through a dedicated education unit. *Nurse Education in Practice, 17,* 153–160. doi:10.1016/j.nepr.2015.12.002

McNelis, A. M., Fonacier, T., McDonald, J., & Ironside, P. M. (2011). Optimizing pre-licensure students' learning in clinical settings. *Nursing Education Perspectives, 32,* 64–65.

Melillo, K. D., Abdallah, L., Dodge, L., Dowling, J. S., Prendergast, N., Rathbone, A., . . . Thorton, C. (2014). Developing a dedicated education unit in long-term care: A pilot project. *Geriatric Nursing, 35*(4), 264–271. doi:10.1016/j.gerinurse.2014.02.022

Moscato, S., Miller, J., Logsdon, K., Weinberg, S., & Chorpenning, L. (2007). Dedicated education unit: An innovative clinical partner education model. *Nursing Outlook, 55,* 31–37. doi:10.1016/j.outlook.2006.11.001

Mulready-Shick, J., & Flanagan, K. (2014). Building the evidence for dedicated education unit sustainability and partnership success. *Nursing Education Perspectives, 35,* 287–293. doi:10.5480/14-1379

Mulready-Shick, J., Kafel, K. W., Banister, G., & Mylott, L. (2009). Enhancing quality and safety competency development at the unit level: An initial evaluation of student learning and clinical teaching on dedicated education units. *Journal of Nursing Education, 48,* 716–719. doi:10.3928/01484834-20091113-11

Murray, B. S. (2013). Service-learning in baccalaureate nursing education: A literature review. *Journal of Nursing Education, 52*(11), 621–626. doi:10.3928/01484834-20131014-08

Murray, T. A., MacIntyre, R. C., & Teel, C. S. (2011). An analysis of partnerships performance: The St. Johns Mercy Medical Center-Saint Louis University School of Nursing Dedicated education unit project. *Journal of Professional Nursing, 27*(6), e58–e63. doi:10.1016/j.profnurs.2011.08.005

Nabavi, F. H., Vanaki, Z., & Mohammadi, E. (2012). Systematic review: Process of forming academic service partnership to reform clinical education. *Western Journal of Nursing Research, 34,* 118–141. doi:10.177/0193945910294380

National League for Nursing Board of Govenors. (2003). Position statement: *Innovation in nursing education: A call to reform.* New York, NY: Author.

National League for Nursing. (2012). *The scope of practice for academic nursing leaders 2012 revision.* Philadelphia, PA: Wolters Kluwer.

National League for Nursing. (2014). *Findings from the 2014 NLN biennial survey of schools of nursing academic year 2013–2014.* Retrieved from http://www.nln.org/docs/default-source/newsroom/nursing-education-statistics/2014-survey-of-schools—executive-summary.pdf?sfvrsn=2

National Service-Learning Clearinghouse. (2016). *What is service-learning?* Retrieved from https://gsn-newdemo2.s3.amazonaws.com/documents/456/original/Definition%20of%20Service%20Learning.pdf?1308690290

Nishioka, V. M., Coe, M. T., Hanita, M., & Moscato, S. R. (2014). Dedicated education unit: Nurse perspectives on their clinical teaching role. *Nursing Education Perspectives, 35,* 294–300. doi:10.5480/14-1381

Otterness, N., Gehrke, P., & Sener, I. (2007). Partnerships between nursing education and faith communities: Benefits and challenges. *Journal of Nursing Education, 46,* 39–44.

Pålsson, Y., Mårtensson, G., Swenne, C. L., Ädel, E., & Engström, M. (2017). A peer learning intervention for nursing students in clinical practice education: A quasi-experimental study. *Nurse Education Today, 51,* 81–87. doi:10.1016/j.nedt.2017.01.011

Pappas, S. (2007). Improving patient safety and nurse engagement with a dedicated education unit. *Nurse Leader, 5*(3), 40–43.

Preheim, G. (2008). The Clinical Scholar Model: Competency development within a caring curriculum. In M. Oermann (Ed.), *Annual review of nursing education: Clinical nursing education* (Vol. 6, pp. 3–23). New York, NY: Springer Publishing.

Preheim, G., Casey, K., & Krugman, M. (2006). Clinical scholar model: Providing excellence in clinical supervision of nursing students. *Journal for Nurses in Staff Development, 22*(1), 15–22.

Raines, D. A. (2016). A dedicated education unit for maternal-newborn nursing clinical education. *Nursing for Women's Health, 20*(1), 21–27. doi:10.1016/j.nwh.2015.12.005

Ranse, K., & Grealish, L. (2007). Nursing students' perceptions of learning in the clinical setting of the dedicated education unit. *Journal of Advanced Nursing, 58,* 171–179.

Reiniger, A. (n.d.). *Building community campus partnerships in underserved communities: An essential step to effective services.* Case study for the principles of partnership. Best beginnings: A child abuse prevention program in New York City. Community Campus Partnerships for Health Fellows Program.

Reising, D. L., Shea, R. A., Allen, P. N., Laux, M. M., Hensel, D., & Watts, P. A. (2008). Using service-learning to develop health promotion and research skills in nursing students. *International Journal of Nursing Education Scholarship, 5*(1), Article 29. doi:10.2202/1548-923X.1590

Rhodes, M. T., Meyers, C. C., & Underhill, M. L. (2012). Evaluation outcomes of a dedicated education unit in a baccalaureate nursing program. *Journal of Professional Nursing, 28,* 223–230. doi:10.1016/j.prof.2011.11.019

Ridenour, N. (2009). Clinical education reform: Re-envisioning the workforce. *Journal of Nursing Education, 48,* 419–420. doi:10.3928/01484834-20090717-01

Secomb, J. (2008). A systematic review of peer teaching and learning in clinical education. *Journal of Clinical Nursing,* 703–716. doi:10.1111/j.1365-2702.2007.01954.x

Seifer, S., & Maurana, C. (2000). Developing and sustaining community-campus partnerships: Putting principles into practice. *Partnership Perspectives, 1*(11), 7–11.

Sharpnack, P. A., Koppelman, C., & Fellows, B. (2014). Using a dedication education unit clinical education model with second-dgree accelerated nursing program students. *Journal of Nursing Education, 53,* 685–691. doi:10.3928/01484834-20141120-01

Smyer, T., Gatlin, T., Tan, R., Tejada, M., & Feng, D. (2015). Academic outcome measure of a dedicated education unit over time. Help or hinder? *Nurse Educator, 40,* 294–297. doi:10.1097/NNE.0000000000000176

Stone, R., Cooper, S., & Cant, R. (2013). The value of peer learning in undergraduate nursing education: A systematic review. *ISRN Nursing, 2013,* 1–10. doi:10.1155/2013/930901

Sullivan, D. T. (2010). Connecting nursing education and practice: A focus on shared goals for quality and safety. *Creative Nursing, 16*(1), 37–43. doi:10.1891/1078-4535.16.1.37

Teel, C. S., MacIntyre, R. C., Murray, T. A., & Rock, Z. (2011). Common themes in clinical education partnerships. *Journal of Nursing Education, 50,* 365–372. doi:10.3928/01484834-2011-429-01

Vizient™. (2016). Nursing residency programs by state. Retrieved from http://www.aacn.nche.edu/education-resources/NRP-Participants-by-State.pdf

Vogt, M. A., Chavez, R., & Schaffner, B. (2011). Baccalaureate nursing student experiences at a camp for children with diabetes: The impact of a service-learning model. *Pediatric Nursing, 37*(2), 69–73.

Warner, J. R., & Burton, D. A. (2009). The policy and politics of emerging academic-service partnerships. *Journal of Professional Nursing, 25,* 329–334. doi:10.1016/j.profnurs.2009.10.006

Worrell-Carlisle, P. (2005). Service-learning: A tool for developing cultural awareness. *Nurse Educator, 30,* 197–202.

Wotton, K., & Gonda, J. (2004). Clinical and student evaluation of a collaborative clinical teaching model. *Nursing Education and Practice, 4,* 120–127.

Assessment and Evaluation

12

Assessment Methods

MARILYN H. OERMANN

OBJECTIVES

- Compare assessment, evaluation, and grading processes
- Describe methods for assessment and examples of their use in nursing education
- Plan assessment methods for varied learning outcomes in a course

Through the process of assessment, the teacher collects information about student learning and performance. With this information the teacher can determine further learning needs, plan learning activities to meet those needs, and confirm the outcomes and competencies met by the students. Students also assess their own learning and performance, and identify areas in which they need more practice and review. Assessment also provides information on the quality of the teaching, courses, practice experiences, curriculum, and other aspects of the educational program.

This chapter explains assessment, evaluation, and grading in nursing education. Methods are described for assessing learning, and examples are provided for many of these methods. Tests are a common assessment method used in nursing education, and various types of test items are described in Chapter 13. There is a separate chapter (14) on clinical evaluation, and methods such as rating scales are presented in that chapter.

ASSESSMENT

Assessment is the collection of information about student learning and performance. Assessment that provides information about the student's progress in the course and further learning needs is diagnostic: this is feedback for the teacher and students to identify gaps in learning and plan relevant instructional strategies. Assessment also is used at designated times in the course such as midterm and final to confirm the outcomes of learning and determine students' grades. The data collected through assessment provide the basis for students' grades.

Assessment also provides information about the quality of teaching in the course. At the end of a course, students typically evaluate the effectiveness of the teacher and quality of the instructional methods, feedback to students, interactions with them, availability, and other areas. Students, graduates, and alumni assess the nursing program as part of program evaluation. Other uses of assessment are to select students for admission to the educational institution and school of nursing, and placement of students in appropriate courses in the nursing program.

There are five principles the teacher should use when assessing student learning:

1. *Identify the outcomes, objectives, or competencies to be assessed.* Another way of thinking about this is: What is being assessed? The goal in assessment is to determine if students are meeting or have met the intended outcomes, objectives, and competencies.
2. *Select appropriate assessment methods.* The methods for assessing learning, for example, a test or written assignment, should provide information about the particular outcome, objective, or competency being assessed.
3. *Meet students' needs.* The assessment should provide feedback to individual students about their progress in meeting the outcomes and further learning needed. The most important role of assessment is identifying where further learning is needed and planning appropriate strategies to help students learn and improve their performance.
4. *Use multiple assessment methods.* Decisions about learning and performance are often high stakes, having serious consequences for students, and should not be based on one test or assignment. Multiple assessment methods are needed to provide data for determining if the outcomes of a course were met.
5. *Recognize the limitations of assessment when making decisions about students.* One teacher-made test, for example, may not be a true measure of the student's learning about that content. The test may have flaws in its design, and other factors may influence the results (Brookhart & Nitko, 2015).

EVALUATION

Evaluation is the process of making judgments about student learning and performance. The teacher analyzes test scores, collects other assessment data, and then makes a value judgment about the *quality* of learning and performance. There are two types of evaluation: formative and summative. Formative evaluation occurs throughout the instructional process and provides feedback to students (Oermann & Gaberson, 2017). In formative evaluation, the teacher assesses learning, gives prompt and specific feedback to students about gaps in learning and performance and how to improve, and plans further instruction to guide their learning. Giving prompt, specific, and instructional feedback is critical to the learning process and a characteristic of quality teaching. Bourgault, Mundy, and Joshua (2013) compared audio and written feedback on clinical assignments, and students reported that audio feedback was more personal, was easier to understand, included more constructive comments, and was more effective in meeting the course outcomes than traditional written feedback. Data collected through formative evaluation should not be graded.

Summative evaluation "summarizes" what students have learned. This is evaluation at the end of a point in time, for example, at midterm and the end of a course, for determining grades.

GRADING

A grade is a symbol (A through F, pass–fail) that represents the student's achievement in a course. Grades are for summative evaluation, indicating how well the student performed in individual assignments, clinical practice, the skills laboratory, simulation, and the course as a whole.

There are different grading systems that can be used. A common grading system is with letters (A, B, C, D, E or A, B, C, D, F), sometimes combined with + and −. Grades also can be represented by percentages (100, 99, 98, . . .), which, in turn, can be used to assign a letter grade, for example, A = 90% to 100%. There are other grading systems such as Honors (exceptional performance in all areas), High Pass (exceptional performance in most areas), Pass (completely satisfactory performance in all areas), and Fail (unsatisfactory performance), and two-dimensional systems such as pass–fail and satisfactory–unsatisfactory, which are used frequently for grading in clinical courses.

The grade is based on the data collected through the various assessment methods in the course. Each of these methods should be weighted in the overall course grade based on the emphasis of the outcomes and content evaluated by them in the course. For example, a unit examination in an adult health nursing course should count more in the course grade than a journal assignment completed once in clinical practice.

NORM- AND CRITERION-REFERENCED INTERPRETATION

There are two main ways of interpreting test scores and other assessment data. When tests are scored and papers and other assignments are graded, the result is a number. The number itself, however, has no meaning. For example, if the teacher tells students their scores on a test are 20 or 22, what does that mean? Scores need to be referenced or compared to some standard or to other students' scores. A score of 22 might be the highest score possible on the test or the highest score among the students who took it. To interpret a score, there needs to be a reference to compare the score against.

Test scores and the scores resulting from other types of assessment can be interpreted using norm- or criterion-referenced standards. In norm-referenced interpretation, each student's score is compared to those of a norm group. The norm group is often other students' test scores: students who perform better than their peers receive higher scores (Brookhart & Nitko, 2015). Grading on a curve is an example of norm-referenced interpretation. Students' scores are rank-ordered from highest to lowest, with grades based on where a student's score falls in the ranking. For example, the top 10% of students might receive an A and the lowest 10% an F.

In clinical practice, a tool on which student performance is rated on a scale of below to above average is norm-referenced: each student's clinical performance is compared to the group of learners. Norm-referenced interpretation does not indicate what a student can and cannot do; it reflects instead if the student's performance is better or worse than other students in the clinical group (Oermann & Gaberson, 2017).

In criterion-referenced interpretation, students' tests and other scores from an assessment are compared to preset criteria, not to how well they performed in relation to other learners. The grades are based on what the student has learned and can do. With criterion-referenced interpretation, the teacher might indicate the percent of items answered correctly on a test, total score received on a term paper, or competencies met (Miller, Linn, & Gronlund, 2013). In clinical evaluation with criterion-referenced tools, students would be evaluated as to whether they could perform the clinical competencies specified on the tool or have met the outcomes of the clinical course. The competencies are used as the standards for evaluation rather than how other students in the group performed in clinical practice (Oermann & Gaberson, 2017).

OUTCOMES FOR ASSESSMENT

Students need to know what they are expected to learn and the clinical competencies they should develop. Oermann and Gaberson (2017) define learning outcomes as the knowledge, skills, and values students are to achieve at the end of the nursing program or another point in time. Competencies are more specific statements that lead to achievement of these broader learner outcomes (Scheckel, 2016). Some teachers refer to the outcomes of their courses as objectives—the specific knowledge, skills, and values students should exhibit at the end. Regardless of the labels used in a particular nursing program, the outcomes should be clearly stated and measurable, guiding students in their learning and the teacher in developing the instruction and planning the assessment. The teacher selects assessment methods to determine if students have achieved these learning outcomes and developed the competencies.

Outcomes, or objectives, may be written in three domains of learning: they can specify knowledge to be gained (cognitive domain), values to be developed (affective domain), and skills to be performed (psychomotor domain). These domains were introduced in Chapter 4. Each of the domains levels its learning outcomes in a taxonomy. The cognitive domain includes knowledge and higher level cognitive skills. The most widely used cognitive taxonomy has six levels of learning, increasing in complexity: remembering, understanding, applying, analyzing, evaluating, and creating (Anderson & Krathwohl, 2001; Bloom, Englehart, Furst, Hill, & Krathwohl, 1956). These are defined in Exhibit 12.1 with an example of an objective written at each level. The taxonomy of the cognitive domain is valuable in planning the assessment because it helps the teacher focus the test item or other assessment method on a particular cognitive level (Oermann & Gaberson, 2017). If the outcome relates to application, the assessment should determine if students can apply what they are learning to a new situation or in a new context. By using the taxonomy, the teacher can avoid assessment methods that focus on recall of facts and memorization when the intended outcomes of learning are at a higher level.

EXHIBIT 12.1 Cognitive Domain Taxonomy

1. *Remembering*: Recall of facts and specific information
   List two symptoms of heart failure.

2. *Understanding*: Comprehension and ability to explain material
   Describe classes of heart failure based on functional capacity.

3. *Applying*: Use of information in a new situation
   Apply clinical practice guidelines to care of patients with heart failure.

4. *Analyzing*: Ability to break down material into its parts and identify the relationships among them
   Compare psychometric properties of instruments for measuring the quality of life of patients with heart failure.

5. *Evaluating*: Ability to make value judgments based on internal and external criteria
   Evaluate the strength of the evidence related to follow-up care of patients with heart failure.

6. *Creating*: Ability to combine elements to develop a new product
   Develop plan for managing patients with acute decompensated heart failure.

The affective domain taxonomy levels values, attitudes, and beliefs from knowing them to internalizing them as a basis for decisions. The psychomotor domain focuses on the development of motor skills. Learners progress through three phases of learning: cognitive (understanding what needs to be done), associative (gradually refining performance until movements are consistent), and autonomous or automatic performance of the skill (Schmidt & Lee, 2005). There are different taxonomies for psychomotor skill learning. Of the three domains, the cognitive taxonomy is used most frequently for planning assessment.

ASSESSMENT METHODS

Tests are a common assessment method for determining students' learning in a course and certifying nurses' knowledge in the clinical setting, for example, competency tests during orientation. While tests are used frequently for assessing students' learning and determining grades, they are not the only assessment method to be used. In a study by Oermann, Saewert, Charasika, and Yarbrough (2009), nurse educators reported using papers, group projects, and case study analyses more frequently than tests for grading in their courses, although the tests counted more in the students' grades. Other assessment methods are: papers and other written assignments (formal papers, reflective journals, short papers, concept maps, writing-to-learn activities, and others); cases; multimedia; electronic portfolios; discussions and conferences; group projects; simulations; standardized patients; Objective Structured Clinical Examination (OSCE); and self-evaluation. Some of these are used predominantly for assessment in the classroom or online environment, such as papers and group projects, and others are designed for assessing learning and performance in simulation or a laboratory setting, such as standardized patients and OSCE.

TESTS

A test is a set of items to which students respond in written or sometimes oral format. Tests are typically scored based on the number of correct answers, are administered in the same way to all students, and are usually timed.

Tests are used for admission to a college or university and to the nursing program. Once admitted, students may take tests to place out of courses in the program. For example, they may have had a genetics course and may not need to take a similar course in the nursing program. Tests also can be used to determine the appropriate level of a course, for example, which research methods course would be best for the student in a graduate nursing program. In many prelicensure nursing programs, students take tests as they progress through each level and at the end of the program to identify gaps in learning and assess their risk for not passing the National Council Licensure Examination for Registered Nurses (NCLEX-RN®). These tests provide feedback to students and faculty for developing a learning plan for students to be successful as they continue through the nursing program, improve their test-taking strategies, and prepare for the NCLEX-RN (Brodersen & Mills, 2014; Harding, 2012; Simon-Campbell & Phelan, 2016). Another use of tests is for evaluating student learning and performance at the end of a nursing program. Tests used in this way are for program evaluation and accreditation rather than indicating what students have learned in a particular course.

The NCLEX-RN and National Council Licensure Examination for Practical Nurses are tests used to validate nurses' knowledge and competencies to engage in safe and effective practice at the entry level. Certification examinations verify nurses' knowledge and competencies in a specialized area of practice.

There are many types of test items that can be used for assessment of learning in nursing courses. Chapter 13 describes different types of test items and principles for writing each of those items on a test.

PAPERS AND OTHER WRITTEN ASSIGNMENTS

Papers and other types of written assignments enable students to search for literature and resources, analyze theories and their application to practice, build their higher level thinking skills, analyze issues and situations in health care, and improve writing skills (Oermann & Gaberson, 2017). When written assignments are used for summative evaluation and are graded, they should provide assessment data for specific outcomes of the course. All too often students complete assignments that are not geared to any particular objective or goal of the course; these assignments may have been in a course for years but are no longer relevant for the aims of the current course. Papers and other types of writing assignments should be carefully selected based on the outcomes of the course. If an objective of a course is to identify resources for evidence-based practice, students could prepare a short paper on reputable websites such as the Agency for Healthcare Research and Quality and The Joanna Briggs Institute, journals such as *Evidence-Based Nursing* and *Worldviews on Evidence-Based Nursing*, and other sources of information they could use in the practice setting. In this way the paper is designed to assess if students can identify relevant resources for evidence-based practice in nursing.

Faculty members should periodically review the papers and other written assignments in courses to confirm that they are still relevant, meet specific outcomes of the course, are not "busywork," and are not too repetitive. While some repetition is important to develop knowledge and cognitive and writing skills, once students have mastered writing certain types of papers, the teacher might transition to a new assignment. Faculty in a school of nursing should periodically review assignments across courses to ensure that they build on one another.

FORMAL PAPERS

Students at all levels of nursing education need to write effectively (American Association of Colleges of Nursing, 2006, 2008, 2011). Term papers and other types of formal papers in a course, which include drafts and feedback from the teacher on the substance of the paper and the writing style and quality, enable students to develop their writing as a skill (Oermann, 2013). To improve writing ability, it is critical for students to prepare drafts of papers, get prompt and specific feedback on the content and writing, and rewrite the papers based on that feedback. Through this process students learn how to write "in the discipline" and communicate their ideas effectively to a professional audience (The Writing Across the Curriculum [WAC] Clearinghouse, 2017a).

Because formal papers are difficult for students to write, Luthy, Peterson, Lassetter, and Callister (2009) suggest dividing them into smaller assignments that build on one another and are more manageable for students. For example, one of the assignments might be a quality improvement paper related to the focus of the course. Students might first prepare a paper on a problem they identified in the clinical setting related to patient safety or quality care and data they examined to support that problem. The next assignment might be a literature review on the problem and related interventions that have been used to improve quality of care. The third assignment might be a proposal for a quality improvement project and how it would be implemented on the unit. This strategy of dividing term papers into smaller writing assignments is also valuable for the teacher because feedback can be given to students as they are thinking through the content of the paper and writing individual sections. Students can use the feedback in revising their drafts and writing the subsequent paper.

There are many types of formal papers students can write in a course, such as term papers, research proposals, integrative literature reviews, and papers analyzing theories and their application to patient care, among others. Exhibit 12.2 lists examples of formal papers for assessment in a nursing course.

EXHIBIT 12.2 Examples of Formal Papers for Assessment

- Term paper
- Research paper and development of research proposal
- Literature review and systematic review
- Evidence review (paper in which students critique and synthesize evidence and report on its application to clinical practice)
- Paper analyzing theories and their use in patient care
- Paper comparing different interventions and evidence base
- Concept analysis paper
- Critical analysis paper in which students analyze issues, compare options, and develop arguments for a position
- Case study analysis with written rationale

Source: Adapted from Oermann and Gaberson (2017, p. 146). Copyright 2017. Reproduced with the permission of Springer Publishing.

REFLECTIVE JOURNALS

Reflective journals encourage students to reflect on their experiences and think critically about them. Chan (2013) found that writing narratives and journaling had a positive effect on students' critical thinking and allowed teachers to assess difficulties students were experiencing. With reflective journals students gain an awareness of their environment and ability to self-assess (Schuessler, Wilder, & Byrd, 2012). Journals also provide an opportunity for faculty to give feedback to students (Lasater, 2011; Ruiz-López et al., 2015).

Davies, Reitmaier, Smith, and Mangan-Danckwart (2013) used reflective journals to assess student learning in an undergraduate gerontological nursing course. As part of the course, students visit older adults who share their life experiences with them. Students then write reflective journals based on these visits, which are evaluated in the course. Reflective journals also have been used effectively for assessment in service learning and study-abroad experiences as a way of encouraging students to think about the meaning of their experiences and for faculty members to provide feedback (Adamshick & August-Brady, 2012; Carpenter & Garcia, 2012; Lai et al., 2015). While some teachers assess journals for summative evaluation and grading, when the aim of the journal is to reflect on experiences and gain meaning from them, journals should be used for feedback purposes only.

SHORT PAPERS

Another type of written assignment for assessment is a short paper that focuses on a specific content area or outcome (Oermann et al., 2015; Oermann & Gaberson, 2017). For example, students might write a one-page paper that compares two similar patient problems and how to differentiate them in an assessment; a paragraph that describes using SBAR (Situation, Background, Assessment, and Recommendation) for bedside handoff; and a two-page paper that examines nursing interventions and supporting evidence for a patient with a particular health problem. Short assignments provide an opportunity for teachers to give quick feedback on students' knowledge, higher level thinking skills, and sometimes also writing skills. Short assignments can be completed by students individually or as a small group activity, and can be used for formative and summative evaluation.

CONCEPT MAPS

In a concept map, students illustrate how concepts relate to one another. In clinical practice, concept maps can help students plan their care for a patient, organize information, and visualize how the assessment data, problems, treatments, medications, and other information are interrelated. Students can develop a concept map as part of their planning for clinical practice and then revise the map after caring for the patient. Concept maps also enable students to apply theory to practice, gain new knowledge, and improve critical thinking (Jaafarpour, Aazami, & Mozafari, 2016; Lee et al., 2013; Mammen, 2016). An example of a concept map is in Figure 12.1.

Daley and Torre (2010) reviewed 35 studies on the use of concept maps in medical education and found that they promoted meaningful learning, were an additional resource for learning, provided feedback to students, and could be used for assessment of learning. With concept maps teachers can identify knowledge gaps and provide additional instruction (Torre, Durning, & Daley, 2013). While concept maps are typically assessed for formative purposes, they also can be graded, especially if students explain the relationships among concepts in the map.

WRITING-TO-LEARN ACTIVITIES

Writing activities in which students think about course content, reflect on their learning, and raise questions about the content are often referred to as writing-to-learn activities. These are short, informal, and frequently impromptu (Oermann, 2013; WAC Clearinghouse, 2017b). They can be used for assessment but should not be graded. For example, at the end of an online session or in-class presentation, the teacher may ask students to list content about which they have questions, summarize a key learning from the class or their readings, define a term they learned in class, or write a few sentences about how the class compared to their readings. With these short writing activities, students can self-assess where further learning is needed, and teachers can provide feedback to individual students and the class as a whole.

OTHER WRITTEN ASSIGNMENTS

There are many other written assignments that can be developed to assess student learning and writing ability. Students can prepare summaries of readings and their implications, analyze scenarios with a rationale supporting their analysis, prepare nursing care and teaching plans, develop discharge and follow-up plans, write up assessments, analyze quality and safety issues in the health care setting, and evaluate

FIGURE 12.1 Example of a concept map.

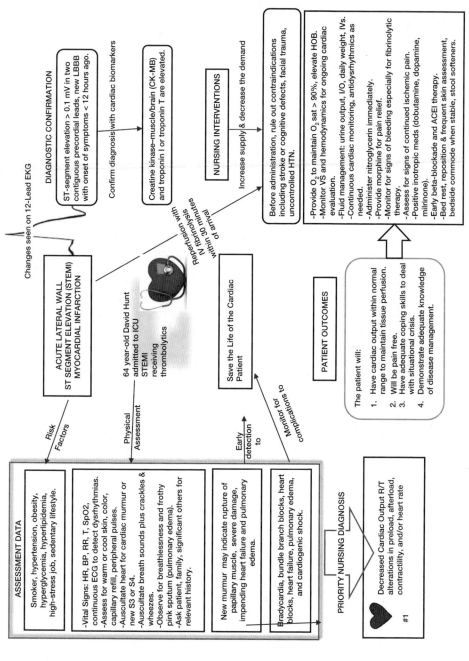

Developed by Deanne A. Blach, MSN, RN, 2017. Reprinted by permission of Deanne A. Blach.

interactions, among others. Depending on the type of assignment, they can be assessed formatively or graded.

ASSESSMENT OF PAPERS AND OTHER WRITTEN ASSIGNMENTS

For any written assignment, the teacher needs to have specific criteria for assessment, which should be shared with students prior to beginning the paper. The criteria depend on the type of assignment. For formal papers, the quality and comprehensiveness of the content, use of relevant and current literature, organization of the paper, writing style, and reference style would be considered. For other types of written assignments, some of these criteria would not be appropriate.

The teacher should develop a rubric for evaluating the paper. A rubric is a scoring guide, specifying the criteria to be assessed and points allotted to each criterion. Students should have the rubric ahead of time so they can prepare the paper accordingly. Brookhart and Nitko (2015) view a rubric as useful for both instructional purposes and assessment because it guides students in writing the paper and teachers in assessing it. Table 12.1 provides an example of a rubric for scoring a written assignment in a nursing course.

TABLE 12.1 Rubric for Scoring Written Assignment

Content		
Content relevant to purpose of paper, comprehensive	Content relevant to purpose of paper	Content not relevant to purpose of paper, no depth
5	3	1
No errors in content	Few errors in content	Many errors
3	2	1
Current evidence synthesized and integrated in paper	Relevant evidence in paper but not synthesized	Limited evidence in paper
7	4	1
Organization		
Content well organized	Organization understood but could be improved	Poorly organized
3	2	1
Multiple perspectives explored in paper	Some alternate perspectives explored	No alternate perspectives explored
3	2	1
Writing Style and Format		
Sentence structure clear, correct grammar and punctuation, no spelling errors	Sentence structure adequate; some grammar, punctuation, and spelling errors	Poor sentence structure; many errors in grammar, punctuation, and spelling
3	2	1
Format consistent with requirements	Parts of paper missing or not consistent with requirements	Missing sections, does not meet requirements
3	2	1

(continued)

TABLE 12.1 Rubric for Scoring Written Assignment (*continued*)

References current, no errors in APA style	References limited but current, some errors in APA style	Few and old references, errors in APA style
3	2	1

Total Points _____ (sum points for total score)

APA, American Psychological Association.

Source: Adapted from Oermann and Gaberson (2017, pp. 150–151). Copyright 2017. Reproduced with the permission of Springer Publishing.

Following are principles for assessing papers and other written assignments:

1. Written assignments should be planned to guide students in meeting specific outcomes of the course, and the criteria for assessment should address those outcomes.
2. The number of required papers in a course should be reasonable, based on the outcomes to be met, and consider the number of drafts to be submitted with teacher feedback.
3. Written assignments should foster students' higher level thinking about the content rather than summarizing what they have read.
4. The directions about the purpose and format of the paper should be clear, students should know the dates when drafts and the final paper are due, and they should have the rubric ahead of time.
5. In evaluating papers in which students analyze issues, the criteria should focus on the rationale for the position, not the specific position.
6. The teacher should read papers anonymously (to avoid potential bias); read each paper twice before scoring (to gain an overview of how students approached the topic, as the rubric may need to be modified if no students addressed a particular content area); and grade papers in random order (to avoid bias, as papers read first may be scored higher than those at the end).
7. If unsure about a grade on a paper or other assignment, the teacher should have a colleague read the paper, also anonymously (Oermann & Gaberson, 2017).

CASES

Integrative cases, unfolding cases, and case studies are strategies for teaching clinical judgment, problem solving, and decision making and helping students engage in higher level learning (Carmona, Cleveland, Paper, Solis, & Taylor, 2015; Harrison, 2012; Oermann, Shellenbarger & Gaberson, 2018). They also are appropriate for assessing those outcomes. Cases typically present a clinical scenario that integrates various concepts, followed by questions about that scenario. Often the scenarios are short to avoid directing students' thinking in advance (Oermann, 2008). Students analyze the case and might identify patient problems and possible interventions, apply theories and other knowledge to the case, and discuss it from different points of view. Questions can ask students what they noticed in the situation, to analyze the scenario and decide on actions that are appropriate or if no actions are needed, and to reflect on how patients might respond to those actions. With these types of questions, case discussions can improve students' clinical reasoning skills. Shellenbarger and Robb (2015) suggested adding podcasts, images, video clips, and other visuals to the scenario. This adds reality to the case and often engages students more in its analysis.

Unfolding cases simulate a changing scenario similar to what might occur in actual clinical practice. With this method the case unfolds to reveal new information about the situation. With unfolding cases students can make decisions about the relevance and meaning of the new information added to the case, and as a group or individually decide on actions to take. Case studies are longer and provide background information about the patient, family, community, or other context. In their analysis of a case study, students can describe the theories that guided their analysis, cite related literature, and provide a rationale for their analysis and any decisions they made.

Cases can be analyzed by students individually or in small groups in class, online, or in postclinical conferences. Discussions about the case expose students to other possible approaches and perspectives that they may not have identified themselves. With this method, the teacher can provide feedback on the content and thought process used by students to arrive at their answers. When grading cases, the teacher first establishes criteria for grading, develops a rubric, and scores answers to the questions using the rubric (Oermann & Gaberson, 2017). Cases are also useful in preparing students for thinking through higher level test items such as on the licensure examinations. Exhibit 12.3 provides an example of an integrative case, an unfolding case, and a case study.

EXHIBIT 12.3 Examples of Cases for Assessment

Case

Your patient fell at home and was admitted yesterday with a hip fracture. She is scheduled for surgery today. At shift report the nurse says the patient had lab work done on admission, but she does not know the results. Later you find that the patient's hemoglobin is 5.0 g/dL and hematocrit is 16%.

1. What were unsafe practices in this situation?
2. Which *National Patient Safety Goals* were not met? What are the implications of these to nursing practice?
3. What should have been done?

Unfolding Case

Your 93-year-old patient in a long-term care facility has a Stage I pressure ulcer at her sacrum. The patient is also coughing and tells you she is too weak to get out of bed for lunch.

1. Describe what the pressure ulcer should look like. What other data should you collect? Why?
2. Develop a plan of action for this patient, with a rationale.

    The following day the patient is coughing more, has shortness of breath, and is more fatigued. A nurse tells you in report it looks like the patient has a blister on her sacrum.

1. What does this new information mean?
2. What are possible problems of this patient? List them in priority and provide a rationale for your prioritization.
3. What will you report to the nurse at handoff?

(continued)

EXHIBIT 12.3 Examples of Cases for Assessment (*continued*)

> The patient's daughter comes to find you on the unit and tells you how angry she is that a nurse moved her mother to a chair.
>
> 1. What would you say to her? Why?
> 2. How can you provide patient-centered care in this situation?
> 3. Develop a new plan for this patient and family with a rationale for your approaches.
>
> **Case Study**
>
> A patient comes to the emergency department with severe abdominal pain and diarrhea. The patient has lost 12 pounds in the past 2 weeks and has no appetite. The nurse does not detect any masses, but there is abdominal tenderness and pain. The patient's wife indicates the patient has been healthy except for this "flu," which has lasted for 2 weeks. She says the patient travels frequently and was recently in Portugal and Canada. The patient does not smoke or drink alcohol. The wife explains that last year the patient was treated for depression but is fine now and has no prior health problems. They have two children, and the grandparents are currently watching them.
>
> 1. What are possible problems that the patient might have?
> 2. What assessment data would you collect from the medical record? Why is this information important to deciding what is wrong with the patient? List the two questions you would ask the wife next.
> 3. What laboratory tests would you expect to be ordered? Why?
> 4. Add laboratory values to the case and discuss with a peer how that information would influence decisions about the patient's problems.

MULTIMEDIA FOR ASSESSMENT

Short segments of a digital recording, a video from YouTube, and other media clips can also be used for assessment. Rather than describing a case in print form, the scenario can be visualized in a media clip. These can be used in class to explore if students can apply their learning to the scenario in the multimedia, placed online for student analysis individually or in groups, and used in place of a written case or case study. Media clips allow students to visualize the clinical situation and get a sense of what the experience is like for patients, families, and providers. Questions can be developed by the teacher related to the multimedia for students to answer, either for formative or summative purposes.

ELECTRONIC PORTFOLIO

In an electronic portfolio students collect materials they have developed in the course that provide documentation that they have met the course outcomes. For clinical courses the materials and projects in the portfolio demonstrate their clinical knowledge and competencies. Portfolios are valuable for assessment because they contain the evidence for judging if students have met the outcomes of the course.

Portfolios also are valuable for program evaluation: students can document their achievement of program outcomes in a portfolio. Portfolios developed for a course or nursing program can be used later for job applications and career development. Nurses can continue to add materials and documentation of their accomplishments to their portfolios. In this way the portfolio represents the continued development of the nurse's expertise over the years. Portfolios also are used for faculty members to present their accomplishments in teaching, research, and service as part of promotion reviews. Used in this way, the teaching portfolio is a collection of documents that demonstrate expertise in teaching, which would not be apparent on a curriculum vitae. A portfolio can also be developed to document the educator's most significant research accomplishments and contributions to service (Thomas et al., 2016).

There are two types of portfolios: best work and growth (Brookhart & Nitko, 2015). Best-work portfolios contain examples of students' "best" products of learning; when used for assessment, these products provide evidence that students have met the outcomes of the course. Growth portfolios are designed for formative evaluation. In a growth portfolio students collect evidence of their work with narrative reflections about each item in the portfolio (Holmboe, Davis, & Carraccio, 2008).

The contents of the portfolio depend on the course outcomes to be assessed. Students can select papers and projects they completed in the course, group projects, self-reflections on clinical and other experiences, and other products they developed that demonstrate their learning and achievement. Holmboe et al. (2008) suggested that when portfolios are used for summative evaluation and grading, the portfolio content should be standardized across students but also provide an opportunity for students to include products they believe reflect their professional development. The evaluation should be based on specific, measurable criteria, which are known to students. In some programs portfolios are presented at an oral defense; in those situations teachers can confirm their assessment of the content and the grade they assigned for the portfolio assignment (Holmboe et al., 2008).

Although portfolios can be prepared and submitted as hard copies, electronic portfolios can be updated, stored, and shared more easily with others. With electronic portfolios students can also include multimedia and links to show relationships among materials.

DISCUSSIONS AND CONFERENCES

Discussions are an exchange of ideas between two or more people (Oermann, Shellenbarger, & Gaberson, 2018). These are often informal but may also be planned discussions about a particular topic. In a discussion the teacher can assess students' knowledge of a topic, explore decisions made and the reasoning underlying those decisions, and provide feedback to learners. Open-ended questions rather than ones answered with a "yes–no" response encourage students' higher level thinking and promote discussion about alternate perspectives and approaches. Chan's (2013) systematic review of studies on critical thinking revealed that asking higher level questions, a sequence of questions from low to high level, and multiple questions rather than only one promoted critical thinking among nursing students. These questions are an effective method for assessing students' critical thinking because the teacher can ask students about other perspectives of the situation, possible options and implications of each, and a rationale for their thinking. Socratic questioning, which are guided questions to promote critical thinking about a topic and explore complex ideas, may also improve nursing students' moral reasoning and ethical decision making (Torabizadeh, Homayuni, & Moattari, 2016). These types of questions in a discussion provide a way for educators to assess students' moral reasoning and how they think through ethical issues particularly in clinical situations. The teacher should recognize, though, that students may answer questions in a discussion focused on ethics and values consistent with what is appropriate professionally, which may not reflect their true feelings and values.

Conferences are planned discussions on a topic. These include pre- and postclinical conferences, interprofessional conferences, and other types of seminars in which the student participates. In a conference students can develop their oral communication skills and ability to lead and engage others in discussing an issue or a problem and deciding on actions to take. Although most clinical conferences are face-to-face with the teacher or preceptor, Berkstresser (2016) recommended shifting these conferences to an asynchronous online postclinical conference. Online clinical conferences are more student-centered than teacher-centered face-to-face conferences. In an online conference, students have an opportunity for equal participation in the discussion and may be more willing to discuss issues they encountered in the clinical setting than in a face-to-face postclinical conference. In a project by Terry (2012), a patient created a digital story about his health care experience and then engaged in online discussions with students. These discussions enabled students to reflect more deeply on how nursing care is delivered and patients' perceptions than in a traditional clinical conference.

Assessment of student participation in a conference is typically best for formative evaluation because the teacher can provide feedback to students as a group and individually during the discussion. This feedback can encourage students to consider other points of views and think more broadly about a topic. The teacher also can clarify any misunderstandings and share how the teacher would analyze a situation and arrive at a decision. However, conferences can be evaluated for summative purposes, including how well a student led a conference and the quality of students' participation in it. If conferences are assessed for grading purposes, specific criteria need to be established and shared with students prior to their leading or participating in the conference. These criteria include how well the student led the group discussion, presented ideas to the group, encouraged critical thinking about the topic and consideration of alternate perspectives, and encouraged peers to participate in the discussion. The criteria should also address the leader's knowledge of the topic and preparation for the conference.

GROUP PROJECTS

Group projects encourage cooperative learning; development of skills in problem solving, teamwork, and collaboration; and engage students actively in learning (Monsivais & Robbins, 2017; Noonan, 2013). These outcomes are important to students' future practice where they will work in teams and need to collaborate with others. Monsivais and Robbins (2017) suggested that group projects allowed students to create final products that were more complex than an individual student might develop. Some group projects are short term with students meeting in class, online, or out of class for the time it takes to develop the product, such as a poster or group presentation. Other groups, however, are long term, for example the length of the course, for cooperative learning purposes. With either type of group, the group products and individual student participation in the group efforts can be assessed.

Group projects can be assessed in three ways. A group grade can be determined, and each student in the group receives that grade. The main issue with this approach is it does not account for individual student participation in the group work. A second method is for students to specify their contributions to the group product or complete a self-assessment of their participation in the group. The teacher can then evaluate and grade each student's contribution and provide a grade for the group or grade only the individual student's contributions. Students can also evaluate each other's participation in the group work. A third way of grading group projects is for students to prepare a group and an individual product, with both of these evaluated and graded.

When group projects are assessed, the teacher needs a rubric developed specifically for evaluating that project (Brookhart & Nitko, 2015). The rubric should include criteria related to the substance of the group project and also to the process of working as a team. Two examples are provided of rubrics for assessing group projects. The rubric in Exhibit 12.4 was designed to evaluate a group presentation of an assignment in which students explored the literature to answer a selected clinical question. The rubric includes criteria on the substance of the project, for example, the literature review and synthesis of the findings, the quality of the presentation, and how well the students actively engaged the audience in the discussion. The rubric in Exhibit 12.5 is a peer evaluation for a group project in which students critiqued research studies.

SIMULATIONS

Chapter 7 presents types of simulations in nursing, how to integrate and implement them in a nursing curriculum, evaluation using simulations, and debriefing. With simulations students can analyze scenarios, make decisions about problems and actions to take, carry out interventions, demonstrate techniques and skills, and evaluate the effects of their decisions. In simulations students can engage in the deliberate practice of skills, improving their performance.

Simulations are valuable not only for instructional purposes; they also can be developed for assessment of competencies. They can be used for both formative and summative evaluation. For formative evaluation, in the debriefing session, teachers can provide feedback to students to further develop their clinical judgment and reflective thinking skills (Chmil, Turk, Adamson, & Larew, 2015; Dreifuerst, 2012; Fey & Jenkins, 2015; Lasater, 2011). The debriefing provides an opportunity to explore different perceptions of what occurred in the simulation, link theory to the experience, examine actions taken or not taken and other possible approaches, and analyze each student's role. Debriefing is also an opportunity for the teacher to provide feedback to students for their continued learning.

When simulation is used for summative evaluation, the aim is to verify if the student can perform specific competencies and behaviors (Oermann & Gaberson, 2017; Oermann, Kardong-Edgren, & Rizzolo, 2016). For summative evaluation, there should be standardization across students so that there is consistency with the evaluation, and the tools must be valid and reliable. The teacher or other evaluator needs to be trained in the process, use of the tools, and scoring. If the evaluation will be used for making critical decisions about the student—for example, if it is high-stakes and students need to pass the evaluation to pass the course—more than one rater should be used (Oermann et al., 2016). These decisions are too important to be based on only one person's observations and judgment.

Principles for implementing simulation-based assessment for summative evaluation include:

- The simulation should be developed to assess particular course or program outcomes or competencies. The teacher begins with the outcomes or competencies and then determines the optional assessment method using simulation.
- The teacher should match the features and fidelity of the simulator to the competencies to be assessed. For example, a task trainer might be more appropriate for evaluation of a specific skill than use of a high-fidelity patient simulator.
- For some competencies a combination of simulation modalities (e.g., task trainer and standardized patient) is needed to best represent a real patient encounter. This decision should be based on the outcomes and competencies to be assessed.

EXHIBIT 12.4 Rubric for Evaluating a Group Presentation of an Assignment

Criteria	Failure (0)	Poor (10–15)	Fair (16–17)	Excellent (18–20)	Score
Organization	Presentation is highly disorganized. Some members lack contribution. Presentation is lacking in smooth transition and logical progression.	Presentation is disorganized. Presenters contribute at varying lengths and levels. Most members demonstrate lack of preparedness. Presentation is lacking in smooth transition or logical progression.	Presentation is fairly well organized. Presenters contribute at varying lengths or levels. Most members demonstrate preparedness. Presentation is mostly smooth and logical in progression.	Presentation is highly organized. Presenters contribute equitably and demonstrate preparedness. Presentation exhibits flow, and material is presented in a logical progression. Smooth transitions take place between presenters.	

Criteria	Failure (0)	Poor (25–39)	Fair (40–44)	Excellent (45–50)	Score
Content: synthesis of literature review	Content is inaccurate or unclear. Literature review is weak or incomplete.	Presents a poor review of the literature. Content is inaccurate at times. Conclusions are inaccurate at times. The area of exploration lacks clarity.	Presents a fair review of the literature. Lists findings. Content is mostly accurate. Conclusions are mostly accurate. A basic exploration of the area is presented.	Presents a thorough review of the literature. Synthesizes findings. Content is accurate. Conclusions are accurate. In-depth exploration of the area is presented with supportive evidence.	

(continued)

EXHIBIT 12.4 Rubric for Evaluating a Group Presentation of an Assignment (*continued*)

Criteria	Failure (0)	Poor (10–15)	Fair (16–17)	Excellent (18–20)	Score
Creativity and engagement	Gives a lecture only. Audience is not engaged. No evidence of creativity. Provides no activities, handouts, or supportive materials to educate peers.	Gives a lecture-type presentation using PowerPoint with supportive images. Audience is minimally engaged. Provides a handout to educate peers.	Engages audience at times. Demonstrates elements of creativity in the presentation. Provides an activity or handout to educate peers.	Actively engages audience through multiple means and creatively throughout the presentation. Provides appealing activities, handouts, or other relevant and supportive means to educate peers.	

Criteria	Failure (0)	Poor (10–15)	Fair (16–17)	Excellent (18–20)	Score
References and APA format	References are not mentioned or listed.	Reference list presented with many errors in APA 6th edition format. In-text citation missing. Uses fewer than five references, or references are outdated or lack credibility.	Reference list presented with few errors in APA 6th edition format or in-text citation missing. Uses fewer than 10 references that are current (< 5 years old) and reputable.	Reference list accurately presented in APA 6th edition format. In-text references cited appropriately. Uses 10 or more reputable references < 5 years old.	
				Total Score out of 100 points	

APA, American Psychological Association.

Source: Copyright by Cynthia Foronda. Reprinted by permission of Cynthia Foronda.

EXHIBIT 12.5 Rubric for Peer Evaluation of Group Project

Instructions: Rate each member, excluding yourself, on whether the member of your group met the criterion of a substantive and meaningful contribution to each of the areas indicated. After completing the rating, compare the score to the descriptions at the bottom of the document to see if your rating matched the description of the member's performance.

Use the following rate scale: 0 = No and 1 = Yes

	Member's Name	Member's Name	Member's Name	Member's Name	Member's Name	Member's Name
Participated in group discussions						
Contributed ideas during group meetings or by written means						
Participated according to agreed upon group role						
Assisted in problem resolution						
Positively challenged others in the group to deepen understanding of critique or apply research concepts correctly						
Supported other group members to encourage a sense of group cohesion						
Organized and influenced the logical flow of the group's writing						
Carried his or her share of the workload						
Met deadlines established by the group						
Submitted individual contributions of sufficient quality to be used by the group, including results of plagiarism reports						
Total Points: Add down each column for maximum score						
Comments:						

Note: Your individual ratings of each group member will be kept confidential by the instructor.

10—**Full Participation.** This individual was a true team player, committed to the totality of the project and who made significant content and process contributions. He or she may have contributed in one primary area, but he or she was clearly committed to making the whole project a success.

8—**Strong Selective Participation.** This individual made a significant contribution to the project, but within a clearly defined scope; he or she limited participation to a particular content or process role—and showed initiative in that area—but did not view the overall project as his or her responsibility.

6—**Weak Participation.** This individual did not cause any problems, but made little substantive contribution to content or process. He or she showed little initiative and contributed only what was specifically requested.

3—**Virtually Absent.** This individual was frequently not involved with the project; he or she often missed meetings or other important communications, was consistently unprepared, and/or contributed substandard work that required correction by fellow team members; this individual exhibited little effort and made minimal contribution to the project.

0—**Totally Absent.** This individual was totally absent from this project, and the end product in no way reflects a contribution on his or her part.

Source: Copyright by Karen H. Frith. Used with permission of Karen H. Frith.

- The testing situation needs to be the same for each student; that is, it has to be reproducible. Frequently standardized patients are used when there are high-stakes decisions to be made because they are trained to consistently simulate a condition or situation.

- The tool for rating performance in the simulation must be valid and reliable. Nursing faculty and educators in clinical settings should not use simulation for high-stakes decisions without assurance that the rating tool and process are valid and reliable based on carefully done studies.

- Evaluators need to be trained on the process and use of the tool. Parsons et al. (2012) developed a formal training program for faculty members to use their tool in assessing performance in simulation. As part of the training, the evaluators come to consensus on the minimum expectations of student performance in the simulation to indicate passing each competency on the tool. Findings suggested that training and dialogue about the use of the tool in assessing a particular scenario improve reliability.

STANDARDIZED PATIENTS

Standardized patients are actors trained to portray the role of a patient with a specific condition. With standardized patients, students can be assessed on interpersonal and communication skills, history and physical examination techniques, and other competencies. Standardized patients are often used for formative evaluation, as they are prepared to provide both written and oral feedback to students about their performance (McWilliam & Botwinski, 2012). However, because standardized patients recreate the same patient condition and clinical situation each time they are with a student, providing for consistency in the assessment, they can be used for summative evaluation and high-stakes decisions. Standardized patients are being used increasingly for assessment in nursing programs. Rutherford-Hemming and Jennrich (2013) indicated that standardized patients allow students to practice in a safe environment and receive feedback on their performance, preparing them for clinical practice.

OBJECTIVE STRUCTURED CLINICAL EXAMINATION

Another assessment method is an OSCE. With OSCEs students rotate through stations where they perform a skill or activity, analyze cases, or are tested on their knowledge and ability to apply that in scenarios, and interact with standardized patients. Because OSCEs have a high degree of standardization, they are effective for assessing skills in nursing (Mårtensson & Löfmark, 2013). At each station in the OSCE, students are evaluated on their performance, often with rating scales or checklists. If standardized patients are incorporated in the OSCE, they also can rate the performance. OSCEs are often used for assessment at the end of a semester or program (Kardong-Edgren, 2013).

Following are principles for setting up an OSCE for formative or summative evaluation:

- An examination blueprint should be developed that specifies the skills and other competencies to be assessed and types of scenarios to be used. Case scenarios should be written based on this blueprint and by faculty members who have expertise in the content and competencies.

- Multiple OSCE scenarios can be developed to provide more than one assessment of students' knowledge and performance.

- The content validity of the scenarios should be established prior to using them for an OSCE. The OSCE scenarios should be updated as needed.
- Standardized patients should be trained to portray the patient diagnosis or situation related to the skills of the student to be assessed.
- Rating scales, checklists, and other tools used for evaluation must be valid and reliable, including interrater reliability. The validity and reliability of the tools should be established prior to using them for summative evaluation.
- Evaluators, and standardized patients if their role includes giving feedback to students and rating their performance, need to be trained on the expected performance and proper use of the tools.
- If OSCEs are used for summative purposes, a standard needs to be set as to the score that differentiates students who pass from those who do not.

SELF-EVALUATION

An important outcome of a nursing education program at all levels is the ability of students to evaluate their own learning and performance. With this self-reflection, students can identify areas in which continued learning and development need to occur. Self-evaluation is a developmental process. With a positive teacher–student environment, students will be more likely to share reflections and own assessment with their teachers than in an environment that is punitive and viewed as not facilitating their learning. Self-evaluation is for formative evaluation only and not graded.

SUMMARY

Assessment is the collection of information about student learning and performance. It is critical to determining the student's grade in a course because assessment provides the data on which the grade is based. Assessment also reveals gaps in learning and performance and the need for further instruction. When the teacher adds a value judgment about the quality of learning and performance, the process is evaluation. Formative evaluation occurs throughout the instructional process and provides feedback to students. Summative evaluation "summarizes" what students have learned. This is evaluation at the end of a point in time, for example, midterm and the end of a course, for determining a course or clinical grade.

A grade is a symbol (A through F, pass–fail) that represents the student's achievement in a course and clinical practice. Grades are for summative evaluation, indicating how well the student performed in individual assignments, practice settings, and the course as a whole. Test scores and the scores resulting from other types of assessment can be interpreted using norm- or criterion-referenced standards. In norm-referenced interpretation, each student's score is compared to those of a norm group. In contrast, in criterion-referenced interpretation, students' tests and other scores from an assessment are compared to preset criteria, not to how well they performed in relation to other learners. Clinical courses can be graded with letter grades, such as A through F, or as pass–fail and other two-dimensional systems.

There are many methods teachers can use to assess students' learning in a course and performance skills. Tests are a common method in nursing education. Another assessment method used frequently in courses is written assignments. Students can prepare formal papers such as term papers. These types of papers enable students to search for literature and resources, analyze theories and their application to practice, build their higher level thinking skills, reflect on issues and situations in practice, and improve writing. When assignments are used for summative evaluation and are graded, they should be selected to provide assessment data for specific outcomes of a course. The teacher should use a scoring rubric for evaluating the paper. A rubric specifies the criteria to be used for assessing the paper and points allotted to each criterion.

Another type of written assignment is a reflective journal. A journal can be used to encourage students to think critically about clinical practice and decisions they have made in the practice setting, evaluate decisions, and become more self-aware. Short papers provide an opportunity for teachers to give quick feedback on students' thinking and judgments and sometimes also writing skill. For example, students might write a short paper that analyzes a safety issue they identified in clinical practice. Another type of written assignment is a concept map. In a concept map, students think about how concepts relate to one another and illustrate these relationships. Concept maps help students organize information about patients and other data and visualize how the assessment data, problems, treatments, medications, and other information relate to one another. There are many other written assignments that can be developed to assess student learning and writing ability.

Writing activities in which students think about course content, reflect on their learning, and raise questions about the content are often referred to as writing-to-learn activities. These are short, informal, and frequently impromptu. They can be used for giving feedback to learners but should not be graded.

With integrative cases, unfolding cases, and case studies, students can apply theory and other knowledge to practice situations and develop their higher level thinking skills. These are also appropriate for assessment. Cases typically present a clinical scenario that integrates various concepts followed by questions about that scenario. Students analyze the scenario and might identify patient problems, possible interventions, and alternate ways of approaching the situation; apply theories and other knowledge to the case; and discuss it from different points of view. Rather than describing the scenario in print form, short segments of a digital recording, a video from YouTube, and other media clips can also be used to present the scenario.

In an electronic portfolio, students collect materials they have developed in the course that provide documentation that they have met the course outcomes. Portfolios are valuable for assessment because they contain the evidence for judging if students have met the outcomes of the course.

Conferences are planned discussions about a topic. These include pre- and postclinical conferences, interprofessional conferences, and other types of seminars in which the student participates. In a conference, students can develop their oral communication skills and ability to lead and engage others in discussing an issue or a problem and deciding on actions to take.

Group projects encourage cooperative and active learning, teamwork, and communication, among other outcomes. Some group projects are short term, with students meeting in class, online, or out of class for the time it takes to develop the product such as a poster or group presentation. Other groups are long term, for example, the length of the course, for cooperative learning purposes. Group projects can be assessed in three ways: (a) a group grade can be determined, and each student in the group receives that grade; (b) students can specify their contributions to the final group product, complete a self-assessment of their participation, or evaluate each other's contributions, and the teacher can incorporate those contributions into the grade; or (c) students can prepare a group and an individual product, with both of these graded.

With simulations, students can analyze scenarios and make decisions about actions to take, demonstrate techniques and skills, and implement care. These activities and others completed in a simulation can be assessed for feedback to students and for summative evaluation. Standardized patients are actors trained to portray the role of a patient with a specific condition. With standardized patients, students can be assessed on interpersonal and communication skills, history and physical examination techniques, and other competencies. Another assessment method is an OSCE. With OSCEs students rotate through stations where they perform a skill or activity, analyze cases or are tested on their knowledge and ability to apply it in scenarios, and interact with standardized patients.

An important outcome of a nursing education program at all levels is the ability of students to evaluate their own learning and performance. With this self-reflection, students can identify areas in which further learning and development need to occur.

REFERENCES

Adamshick, P., & August-Brady, M. (2012). Reclaiming the essence of nursing: The meaning of an immersion experience in Honduras for RN to bachelor of science students. *Journal of Professional Nursing, 28*, 190–198. doi:10.1016/j.profnurs.2011.11.011

American Association of Colleges of Nursing. (2006). *The essentials of doctoral education for advanced nursing practice.* Washington, DC: Author.

American Association of Colleges of Nursing. (2008). *The essentials of baccalaureate education for professional nursing practice.* Washington, DC: Author.

American Association of Colleges of Nursing. (2011). *The essentials of master's education in nursing.* Washington, DC: Author.

Anderson, L. W., & Krathwohl, D. R. (Eds.). (2001). *A taxonomy for learning, teaching, and assessing: A revision of Bloom's taxonomy of educational objectives.* New York, NY: Longman.

Berkstresser, K. (2016). The use of online discussions for post-clinical conference. *Nurse Education in Practice, 16*(1), 27–32. doi:10.1016/j.nepr.2015.06.007

Bloom, B. S., Englehart, M. D., Furst, E. J., Hill, W. H., & Krathwohl, D. R. (1956). *Taxonomy of educational objectives: The classification of educational goals. Handbook I: Cognitive domain.* White Plains, NY: Longman.

Bourgault, A. M., Mundy, C., & Joshua, T. (2013). Comparison of audio vs. written feedback on clinical assignments of nursing students. *Nursing Education Perspectives, 34*, 43–46.

Brodersen, L. D., & Mills, A. C. (2014). A comparison of two nursing program exit exams that predict first-time NCLEX-RN outcome. *Computers, Informatics, Nursing, 32*, 404–412. doi:10.1097/CIN.0000000000000081

Brookhart, S. M., & Nitko, A. J. (2015). *Educational assessment of students* (6th ed.). Upper Saddle River, NJ: Pearson.

Carpenter, L. J., & Garcia, A. A. (2012). Assessing outcomes of a study abroad course for nursing students. *Nursing Education Perspectives, 33*, 85–89. doi:10.5480/1536-5026-33.2.85

Chan, Z. C. Y. (2013). A systematic review of critical thinking in nursing education. *Nurse Education Today, 33*, 236–240. doi:10.1016/j.nedt.2013.01.007

Chmil, J. V., Turk, M., Adamson, K., & Larew, C. (2015). Effects of an experiential learning simulation design on clinical nursing judgment development. *Nurse Educator, 40*, 228–232. doi:10.1097/NNE.0000000000000159

Cleveland, L. M., Carmona, E. V., Paper, B., Solis, L., & Taylor, B. (2015). Baby Boy Jones interactive case-based learning activity: A web-delivered teaching strategy. *Nurse Educator, 40*, 179–182. doi:10.1097/NNE.0000000000000129

Daley, B. J., & Torre, D. M. (2010). Concept maps in medical education: An analytical literature review. *Medical Education, 44*, 440–448. doi:10.1111/j.1365-2923.2010.03628.x

Davies, S. M., Reitmaier, A. B., Smith, L. R., & Mangan-Danckwart, D. (2013). Capturing intergenerativity: The use of student reflective journals to identify learning within an undergraduate course in gerontological nursing. *Journal of Nursing Education, 52*, 139–149. doi:10.3928/01484834-20120213-01

Dreifuerst, K. T. (2012). Using debriefing for meaningful learning to foster development of clinical reasoning in simulation. *Journal of Nursing Education, 51,* 326–333. doi:10.3928/01484834-20120409-02

Fey, M. K., & Jenkins, L. S. (2015). Debriefing practices in nursing education programs: Results from a
national study. *Nursing Education Perspectives, 36,* 361–366.

Harding, M. M. (2012). Efficacy of progression testing in predicting nursing student academic success.
Journal of Nursing Education and Practice, 2(2). doi:10.5430/jnep.v2n2p137

Harrison, E. (2012). How to develop well-written case studies. *Nurse Educator, 37,* 67–70. doi:10.1097/
NNE.0b013e3182461ba2

Holmboe, E. S., Davis, M. H., & Carraccio, C. (2008). Portfolios. In E. S. Holmboe & R. E. Hawkins (Eds.),
Practical guide to the evaluation of clinical competence (pp. 86–101). Philadelphia, PA: Mosby Elsevier.

Jaafarpour, M., Aazami, S., & Mozafari, M. (2016). Does concept mapping enhance learning outcome of
nursing students? *Nurse Education Today, 36,* 129–132. doi:10.1016/j.nedt.2015.08.029

Kardong-Edgren, S. (2013). A wake up call with an Objective Structured Clinical Examination. *Clinical
Simulation in Nursing, 9,* e3–e4. doi:10.1016/ j.ecns.2012.11.002

Lai, C. K., Chan, J. H., Wong, I. Y., Fung, J. T., Pang, P. C., Fung, K. H., & Kwok, C. P. (2015). Gains and
development of undergraduate nursing students during a 2-year community service program.
Journal of Nursing Education, 54(Suppl. 3), S21–S25. doi:10.3928/01484834-20150218-06

Lasater, K. (2011). Clinical judgment: The last frontier for evaluation. *Nurse Education in Practice, 11,*
86–92. doi:10.1016/j.nepr.2010.11.013

Lee, W., Chiang, C. H., Liao, I. C., Lee, M. L., Chen, S. L., & Liang, T. (2013). The longitudinal effect
of concept map teaching on critical thinking of nursing students. *Nurse Education Today, 33,*
1219–1223. doi:10.1016/j.nedt.2012.06.010

Luthy, K. E., Peterson, N. E., Lassetter, J. H., & Callister, L. C. (2009). Successfully incorporating writing
across the curriculum with advanced writing in nursing. *Journal of Nursing Education, 48,* 54–59.

Mammen, J. R. (2016). Computer-assisted concept mapping: Visual aids for knowledge construction.
Journal of Nursing Education, 55, 403–406. doi:10.3928/01484834-20160615-09

Mårtensson, G., & Löfmark, A. (2013). Implementation and student evaluation of clinical final
examination in nursing education. *Nurse Education Today, 33,* 1563–1568. doi:10.1016/
j.nedt.2013.01.003

McWilliam, P. L., & Botwinski, C. A. (2012). Identifying strengths and weaknesses in the utilization
of Objective Structured Clinical Examination (OSCE) in a nursing program. *Nursing Education
Perspectives, 33,* 35–39.

Miller, M. D., Linn, R. L., & Gronlund, N. E. (2013). *Measurement and assessment in teaching* (11th ed.).
Upper Saddle River, NJ: Prentice Hall.

Monsivais, D. B., & Robbins, L. K. (2017). Using evidence-based education to guide quality improvement in a graduate online nursing program: Group projects as an exemplar. *Nurse Educator, 42,*
65–66. doi:10.1097/NNE.0000000000000294

Noonan, M. (2013). The ethical considerations associated with group work assessments. *Nurse
Education Today, 33,* 1422–1427. doi:10.1016/j.nedt.2012.11.006

Oermann, M. H. (2008). Using short cases for teaching "thinking" in a nursing course. In N. Facione &
P. Facione (Eds.), *Critical thinking and clinical reasoning in the health sciences: An international multidisciplinary teaching anthology* (pp. 123–129). Millbrae, CA: California Academic Press.

Oermann, M. H. (2013). Enhancing writing in online education. In K. H. Frith & D. J. Clark (Eds.),
Distance education in nursing (3rd ed., pp. 145–162). New York, NY: Springer.

Oermann, M. H., & Gaberson, K. B. (2017). *Evaluation and testing in nursing education* (5th ed.). New York,
NY: Springer Publishing.

Oermann, M. H., Kardong-Edgren, S., & Rizzolo, M. A. (2016). Summative simulated-based assessment
in nursing programs. *Journal of Nursing Education, 55,* 323–328. doi:10.3928/01484834-20160516-04

Oermann, M. H., Leonardelli, A. K., Turner, K. M., Hawks, S. J., Derouin, A. L., & Hueckel, R. M. (2015).
Systematic review of educational programs and strategies for developing students' and nurses'
writing skills. *Journal of Nursing Education, 54,* 28–34. doi:10.3928/01484834-20141224-01

Oermann, M. H., Saewert, K. J., Charasika, M., & Yarbrough, S. S. (2009). Assessment and grading
practices in schools of nursing: National survey findings Part I. *Nursing Education Perspectives, 30,*
274–278.

Oermann, M. H., Shellenbarger, T. & Gaberson, K. B. (2018). *Clinical teaching strategies in nursing*
(5th ed.). New York, NY: Springer Publishing.

Parsons, M. E., Hawkins, K. S., Hercinger, M., Todd, M., Manz, J. A., & Fang, X. (2012). Improvement
in scoring consistency for the Creighton Simulation Evaluation Instrument. *Clinical Simulation in
Nursing, 8*(6), e233–e238.

Ruiz-López, M., Rodriguez-García, M., Villanueva, P. G., Márquez-Cava, M., García-Mateos, M., Ruiz-Ruiz, B., & Herrera-Sánchez, E. (2015). The use of reflective journaling as a learning strategy during the clinical rotations of students from the faculty of health sciences: An action-research study. *Nurse Education Today, 35*, e26–e31. doi:10.1016/j.nedt.2015.07.029

Rutherford-Hemming, T., & Jennrich, J. A. (2013). Using standardized patients to strengthen nurse practitioner competency in the clinical setting. *Nursing Education Perspectives, 34*, 118–121.

Scheckel, M. (2016). Designing courses and learning experiences. In D. M. Billings & J. A. Halstead (Eds.), *Teaching in nursing: A guide for faculty* (5th ed., pp. 159–185). St. Louis, MO: Elsevier.

Schmidt, R. A., & Lee, T. D. (2005). *Motor control and learning: A behavioral emphasis* (4th ed.). Champaign, IL: Human Kinetics.

Schuessler, J. B., Wilder, S., & Byrd, L. W. (2012). Reflective journaling and development of cultural humility in students. *Nursing Education Perspectives, 33*, 96–99.

Shellenbarger, T., & Robb, M. (2015). Technology-based strategies for promoting clinical reasoning skills in nursing education. *Nurse Educator, 40*, 79–82. doi:10.1097/NNE.0000000000000111

Simon-Campbell, E. L., & Phelan, J. (2016). Effectiveness of an Adaptive Quizzing System as an institutional-wide strategy to improve student learning and retention. *Nurse Educator, 41*, 246–251. doi:10.1097/NNE.0000000000000258

Terry, L. M. (2012). Service user involvement in nurse education: A report on using online discussions with a service user to augment his digital story. *Nurse Education Today, 32*, 161–166. doi:10.1016/j.nedt.2011.06.006

Thomas, J. V., Sanyal, R., O'Malley, J. P., Singh, S. P., Morgan, D. E., & Canon, C. L. (2016). A guide to writing academic portfolios for radiologists. *Academic Radiology, 23*, 1595–1603. doi:10.1016/j.acra.2016.08.015

Torabizadeh, C., Homayuni, L., & Moattari, M. (2016). Impacts of Socratic questioning on moral reasoning of nursing students. *Nursing Ethics*. doi:10.1177/0969733016667775

Torre, D. M., Durning, S. J., & Daley, B. J. (2013). Twelve tips for teaching with concept maps in medical education. *Medical Teacher, 35*, 201–208. doi:10.3109/0142159X.2013.759644

The Writing Across the Curriculum Clearinghouse. (2017a). *What is writing in the disciplines?* Retrieved from http://wac.colostate.edu/intro/pop2e.cfm

The Writing Across the Curriculum Clearinghouse. (2017b). *What is writing to learn?* Retrieved from http://wac.colostate.edu/intro/pop2d.cfm

13

Developing and Using Tests

KATHLEEN B. GABERSON

OBJECTIVES

- Explain how assessment validity and reliability affect test quality
- Describe general rules for writing test items to measure desired learning outcomes
- Apply specific rules for writing test items of various types
- Discuss test design and administration practices that may affect the reliability of test scores

---

A test is a measurement instrument, designed to assess learners' knowledge and cognitive abilities. Teachers use test results to make important educational judgments and decisions that affect learners, teachers, patients, future employers, and the educational program. Like every measurement instrument, a test must produce relevant and consistent results to form the basis for sound inferences about what learners know and can do. Good planning, careful test construction, proper administration, accurate scoring, and sound interpretation of scores are essential for producing useful test results. This chapter presents a brief discussion of assessment concepts that influence the quality of test results, and then describes the process of planning, constructing, administering, scoring, and analyzing tests.

ASSESSMENT QUALITY OF TESTS

Like any measurement instrument, a test should produce relevant, accurate results. A teacher who constructs a test or decides to use an existing test must be confident in its assessment quality. Two main considerations of the quality of a test are assessment validity and reliability.

ASSESSMENT VALIDITY

Older definitions of validity characterized it as a quality of the test itself; a test was considered to be valid to the extent that it measured the variable of interest. The current concept of validity focuses on the accuracy or appropriateness of inferences about test results and how those results are used. This understanding of assessment validity therefore focuses on the consequences of testing: Do teachers draw relevant, meaningful conclusions about learners' knowledge and abilities based on their test scores, and what are the intended and unintended consequences of those conclusions (Brookhart & Nitko, 2015; Miller, Linn, & Gronlund, 2013; Oermann & Gaberson, 2017)?

Validity is not an either/or condition; the degree of assessment validity for a test depends on the purpose of the test and how the results will be used in educational decision making. A test can be used for different purposes, and inferences about test results can have greater validity for one purpose than for another. For example, the results of a standardized achievement test in pediatric nursing might be highly valid for the purpose of evaluating the quality of the pediatric nursing course and the effectiveness of the teaching, but have low validity for the purpose of assigning final grades for students who completed the course (Oermann & Gaberson, 2017). Teachers can have greater confidence in the validity of their interpretation and use of test scores when they collect evidence of four major considerations for validation: content, construct, assessment-criterion relationships, and consequences (Miller et al., 2013).

The purpose of *content validation* is to determine the extent to which test items accurately represent a particular content domain. A test contains only a sample of all possible items about a content domain that could be written, but teachers usually want to generalize from that sample to the universe of items. Thus, if a student correctly answers 89% of items on a community health nursing test, the teacher usually infers that the student would answer correctly 89% of all items related to that content domain (Oermann & Gaberson, 2017). However, because desired learning outcomes in nursing education programs involve integration of complex abilities, it usually is not possible to make such specific generalizations (Miller et al., 2013). A process for generating test items that adequately represent the desired content domain, the construction of a test blueprint, will be described later in this chapter.

Construct validation concerns the extent to which it is possible to make inferences from test results to more general abilities and characteristics. A construct is a theoretical construction that can be inferred from an observed behavior (e.g., clinical reasoning). Construct validation involves two fundamental issues: construct representation and construct relevance (Miller et al., 2013). If test items do not adequately represent important elements of the construct, assessment validity is decreased. For instance, a test that requires students to solve problems defined only by the teacher is an inadequate representation of the construct of clinical problem solving, because a student's ability to identify clinical problems is an essential aspect of the construct (Oermann & Gaberson, 2017).

Tests that also measure abilities unrelated to the construct of interest, such as familiarity with cultural colloquialisms, spelling skill, or writing ability, also decrease assessment validity. Evidence of construct representation and relevance should be collected during the test development process by clearly defining the meaning of the construct. Other methods include comparing test results of groups known to possess different levels of the ability being measured, comparing test results before and after instruction, and correlating test results with other measures of the same construct (Miller et al., 2013).

Assessment-criterion relationship considerations focus on the extent to which test results (the assessment) predict performance on another assessment (the criterion measure), either in the future (predictive) or at the same time (concurrent). Nursing faculties often use scores from standardized comprehensive exams at the end of a program to predict performance on high-stakes tests such as National Council Licensure Examination (NCLEX®) and certification exams, but they rarely have use for concurrent validity evidence for teacher-made tests (Oermann & Gaberson, 2017).

Concern about the social consequences of testing leads to the need for *consideration of consequences*. All testing has both intended and unintended consequences. Use of standardized testing programs can have the intended effect of identifying students who are likely to pass licensure or certification exams, but the unintended effect might be to increase student anxiety (Oermann & Gaberson, 2017). Assessment validity must take into account both intended and unintended consequences of testing.

Multiple factors influence test validity. Some characteristics of the test itself, such as clerical errors, unclear directions, too few test items, and a noticeable pattern of correct responses, might decrease the validity of inferences made about the test scores. Student factors such as lack of motivation to perform well, test anxiety, illness, or an emotionally upsetting experience might also affect students' performance on tests and thereby decrease measurement validity. Finally, factors associated with the administration and scoring of tests can lower assessment reliability. Such factors include allowing insufficient time for testing, errors in scoring, variability in the amount of aid to students who ask questions during an exam, and failing to follow the protocol for administering a standardized test (Oermann & Gaberson, 2017).

ASSESSMENT RELIABILITY

Reliability concerns the consistency, stability, or reproducibility of test scores. Measurement reliability boosts the teacher's confidence in assessment results. However, perfect consistency is not possible due to the influence of many extraneous factors:

- Instability of the behavior being assessed (e.g., emotional or health status)
- Varying samples of tasks among different forms of the assessment
- Varying assessment conditions
- Inconsistent scoring procedures (Oermann & Gaberson, 2017)

Inconsistency introduces an unknown amount of error into every assessment result. Reliability estimates therefore gauge the amount of measurement error present under varying conditions. The smaller the measurement error, the greater the assessment reliability (Miller et al., 2013).

Assessment reliability is an essential condition for assessment validity. "Teachers cannot make valid inferences from inconsistent assessment results" (Oermann & Gaberson, 2017, p. 32). However, highly consistent results do not guarantee a high degree of validity, because the assessment might be reliably measuring the wrong construct. Assessment reliability only provides the consistency that makes valid inferences possible (Miller et al., 2013).

Because of different types of consistency, there are different methods of determining assessment reliability:

- Stability: consistency over time
- Equivalence: consistency among different forms of the assessment

- Internal consistency: consistency within the assessment itself
- Interrater reliability: consistency of judgments among different raters (Oermann & Gaberson, 2017)

For teacher-made tests, the most commonly used and appropriate method of estimating reliability is internal consistency, also known as the split-length or half-length method. This method shows the degree to which very similar results are obtained from both halves of the same test. Longer tests tend to yield higher reliability estimates because they sample the content domain more fully, so a split-half reliability estimate usually underestimates the true reliability of the whole test. However, this underestimate can be corrected statistically. It is important to remember that a reliability estimate is not a stable property of the test itself; it will fluctuate each time the test is used with different groups of students.

Various factors can affect assessment reliability, arising from three main sources:

- The test itself: test length, homogeneity, and technical quality of test items
- The test-taker: heterogeneity of student ability, test-taking skill, motivation
- Testing conditions: test security (prevention of cheating), adequacy of time (Oermann & Gaberson, 2017)

The degree of reliability desired depends on factors such as the importance of the decisions made, based on test scores; the consequences of such decisions; and whether it is possible to reverse the decision later. For most teacher-made tests, a reliability estimate of .60 to .85 is desirable (Miller et al., 2013).

TEST PLANNING

Too often, teachers spend too little time and effort preparing tests, and the result is a test with clerical errors and items that are ambiguous, irrelevant to the content domain, and too easy or too difficult. Adequate planning for test construction and careful critique of the completed test items are essential for tests to produce reliable results that can be used to make valid judgments about how much students know about a content domain. This section of the chapter will describe the steps involved in planning and constructing a test.

PURPOSE OF THE TEST AND STUDENTS TO BE TESTED

Decisions involved in planning a test should be based on the purpose of the test and characteristics of the students to be tested. Purpose relates to why the test is given, what it is supposed to assess, and how the results will be used. If a test is intended to measure the degree to which students have met course learning objectives, and the test score will be used to determine a grade, the purpose is summative. A test designed to provide feedback to staff nurses about how much they learned during a continuing education program has a formative purpose. Understanding the characteristics of the learners to be tested helps a teacher determine which test item formats to use, how many items to include, and how to score the test. Student factors that might influence these decisions include English language literacy, academic program level, and previous testing experience, among others (Oermann & Gaberson, 2017).

TEST LENGTH

The ideal length of a test (i.e., the number of test items or total possible points) depends on a number of variables, including the test's purpose, the ability level of the students, the available testing time, and the desired reliability of test results. As noted earlier, longer tests usually produce more reliable results because they sample the content domain more fully. Test length usually is limited by the length of a classroom period. The number of test items that can be completed in a fixed time period should take into account the nature of the assessment tasks. Items with complex assessment tasks, such as analyzing patient data, take more time to complete; therefore, fewer items of those types can be included on a test with a fixed administration time. The majority of students working at their normal pace should be able to complete a test of the appropriate length within the allotted time (Brookhart & Nitko, 2015; Miller et al., 2013).

DIFFICULTY AND DISCRIMINATION LEVEL

The expected difficulty of a test and its ability to distinguish among different levels of achievement are related to the purpose of the test and the way in which results will be interpreted and used. The difficulty of individual test items depends on the complexity of their assessment tasks, the ability of the students, and the quality of teaching. For tests with results that will be interpreted in a criterion-related way, as are most tests in nursing education programs, the ideal difficulty level correctly classifies students according to whether they met the criterion or not. That is, even if a test item is relatively easy, meaning that the majority of students answered it correctly, if students whose total scores met the criterion tended to answer that item correctly and students who failed to meet the criterion tended to answer incorrectly, the item difficulty is appropriate (Miller et al., 2013; Oermann & Gaberson, 2017).

Item difficulty can only be estimated in advance. Teachers with more experience in assessing the selected content domain and with greater knowledge of their students' abilities usually make more accurate estimates. After the test is administered and scored, a teacher can compute the actual item difficulty levels, compare them with the expected difficulty, and revise them for future use if they are much more or less difficult than anticipated.

The ability of each test item to distinguish between students who have greater knowledge of the content domain and those who have less knowledge is its discrimination power. In general, high discriminating power indicates better-quality test items, although this does not indicate item validity. Discrimination power is related to item difficulty. Items that are answered correctly or incorrectly by all students do not discriminate between knowledgeable and less knowledgeable students; items with moderate difficulty tend to have maximum discriminating power (Oermann & Gaberson, 2017).

ITEM FORMATS

Though some students might prefer multiple-choice items or believe that they do better on essay items, the desired learning outcomes, the specific competency to be assessed, and students' ability level should determine the teacher's choice of item formats. Despite common beliefs, no one item format is better than another for testing nursing students, and academic policies that mandate the use of a specific item format on tests do more harm than good. A test that contains several item formats gives students greater opportunity to demonstrate their competency than tests with only one item format (Brookhart & Nitko, 2015).

Each item format has advantages and disadvantages, as explained later in this chapter. Some desired learning outcomes are better measured with certain item formats. For example, a multiple-choice item would be inappropriate to measure a desired learning outcome such as "discuss the comparative advantages and disadvantages of wet-to-dry and autolytic dressings for Stage III pressure injuries"; an essay format would be more suitable. Students should have adequate practice with the item format types that a teacher will use on tests; this might be accomplished by using various item formats in classroom exercises.

Another common belief is that certain item types assess more objectively than others. Although true–false, multiple-choice, and matching items are often described as "objective," objectivity refers to the manner of scoring, not the format of the item (Miller et al., 2013). Objectively scored items will yield the same total score as long as the same answer key is used by multiple scorers or by the same scorer on repeated occasions. Subjectively scored items such as essay items require a scorer's judgment to determine the extent of correctness and produce more score variability.

SCORING PROCEDURES

The choice of item format affects the choice of test scoring procedures. Use of essay and short-answer items requires hand-scoring, whether the answers are recorded on the test itself or on a separate answer sheet. Answers to multiple-choice, true–false, and matching items are usually recorded on a separate answer sheet that can be hand-scored or, more frequently, electronically scanned. Electronic scoring has the advantage of speed as well as the ability to allow computer-generated test and item analysis reports. The teacher must decide whether available resources suggest the use of hand- or electronic scoring (Oermann & Gaberson, 2017).

TEST BLUEPRINT

The best way to ensure that a teacher will be able to make valid judgments about the meaning of test scores is to construct a test blueprint before beginning to choose or write test items. A test blueprint, also called a test plan or table of specifications, guides the teacher to write items at the appropriate level to test the desired content areas. Without a test blueprint, teachers often rely on ease of construction in writing items. This often results in tests with a limited sample of assessment tasks that might omit outcomes that are more important but more difficult to assess (Miller et al., 2013).

Essential elements of a test blueprint include (a) a list of major topics or learning outcomes that the test will assess, (b) the level of complexity of assessment tasks, and (c) the emphasis that each topic or learning outcome will have as indicated by the number or percentage of items or points (Oermann & Gaberson, 2017). Figure 13.1 is an example of a blueprint for a unit test on preoperative nursing care. The row headings along the left margin are the main topic areas to be tested; in this case, they comprise a general outline of content. A more detailed content outline, a list of relevant learning outcomes, or both can be used instead. The column headings across the top are selected from an updated taxonomy of cognitive objectives (Anderson & Krathwohl, 2001); the teacher who prepared this blueprint chose not to use all of the cognitive levels, but other teachers might use all levels or a different taxonomy.

FIGURE 13.1 Example of a test blueprint for a unit test on preoperative nursing care.

Content	Cognitive Level				Total Points
	R	U	Ap	An	
I. Preoperative nursing assessment		4	6	5	15
II. Patient safety	2	3	1	2	8
III. Legal and ethical issues		2	2	2	6
IV. Planning nursing care		3	2	3	8
V. Patient and family teaching		2	4		6
VI. Documentation	2	3	4	4	13
Total points	4	17	19	16	56

An, analyzing; Ap, applying; R, remembering; U, understanding.

The body of the blueprint is a grid formed by the intersections of topic areas and cognitive levels. The cells in the grid represent one or more test items to be developed related to that content area and cognitive level, and the numbers represent the number of points allotted to that cell. The teacher should judge the appropriate emphasis and balance of content areas and cognitive levels to determine which cells should be filled and by how many points; some cells can remain blank, as in this example (Oermann & Gaberson, 2017).

A test blueprint is a useful tool for guiding a teacher to select or write test items at the appropriate level to assess important content areas and learning outcomes. It also should be used to inform students about the nature of the test and how to prepare for it. Although they might have a general idea of what content areas will be tested, students often lack awareness of the cognitive levels at which they will be assessed. Although instructional objectives should inform students of the expected level of performance, they might not be able to interpret these objectives accurately. Some teachers worry that sharing the test blueprint with students will encourage them to study only the content areas that will be tested. This is not a harmful outcome: with knowledge of the content areas to be emphasized most heavily, students can focus their time and energy on studying those content areas and preparing for assessment tasks at the appropriate levels.

The beginning of the course or unit of study is the best time to share the test blueprint with students. Teachers might need to explain the blueprint and how students should use it to plan their test preparation. If the teacher must make modifications to the blueprint (e.g., because of a class cancellation due to weather emergency at the end of a semester), those changes should also be communicated to students (Brookhart & Nitko, 2015; Oermann & Gaberson, 2017).

WRITING THE TEST ITEMS

The teacher should select or write test items that correspond to each numbered cell in the test blueprint. Regardless of item format, teachers should consider the following general rules that contribute to the quality of test items:

1. *Every item should measure something important.* Some teachers include test items that test trivial or obscure content with the intent of determining which students have read all

of the assigned material. However, if this content is important, it will be represented as such on the test blueprint, and all students will be prepared to demonstrate the required competency. Others write filler items to meet a targeted number of items (most frequently, 100). There is no reason to set a fixed number of items or points on all tests, other than for ease of calculating a percentage score. It is better to have a smaller number of test items that assess knowledge of important content than to add meaningless items that serve only to increase test-taking time and that might make valid interpretation of scores more difficult (Oermann & Gaberson, 2017).

2. *Every item should have a correct answer.* "Correct" means that experts would agree on the answer (Miller et al., 2013). The teacher must follow the distinction between fact and belief; in some cases, the correct or best response to an item might be a matter of opinion. Citing a specific authority in the item, such as "according to the AORN Guidelines for Perioperative Practice," prevents students' justifiably arguing a response other than the one the teacher expected. Items that ask students to state an opinion on an issue and support that position with evidence should not be scored as correct or incorrect, but with variable credit based on the rationale given and soundness of reasoning (Oermann & Gaberson, 2017).

3. *Use simple, clear, concise, grammatically correct language.* Clear wording of test items is essential for students' understanding of the assessment task required. Using simple words and sentence structure is challenging when writing about complex, highly technical content. The goal is to include enough detail to communicate the intent of the test item but to avoid extraneous words and complex syntax that only increase reading time and that might confuse nonnative English speakers. Linguistic simplification includes using the active voice and simple, short sentences and avoiding negative forms and conditional and subordinate clauses (Bosher & Bowles, 2008). Because of current concerns that even native English speakers are entering postsecondary programs with low reading proficiency, linguistic simplification is likely to benefit all students.

4. *Avoid jargon, slang, and unnecessary abbreviations.* Although health care professionals frequently use jargon and acronyms informally in the practice environment, informal language in a test item might fail to communicate accurately the meaning of the item. Many students are at least somewhat anxious when taking tests, and they might not interpret an abbreviation correctly in terms of the context in which it is used. For example, does RA mean rheumatoid arthritis, right atrium, or right arm? If the desired learning outcome is to define commonly used health care abbreviations, it is appropriate to use the abbreviation in the item and to ask the student to select or supply the definition. As noted, slang, jargon, acronyms, and abbreviations contribute to linguistic complexity for nonnative English speakers. Also, given growing concern about health care errors attributed to poor communication, nurse educators should use only those abbreviations approved for use in clinical settings (Oermann & Gaberson, 2017).

5. *Use positive wording.* Avoid using words like *no, not,* and *except* in test items. Negative wording is particularly difficult for nonnative English speakers to understand, but test-anxious students also might not read such sentences accurately. Negative forms are particularly confusing in true–false items. Teachers should avoid asking students to identify the incorrect alternative as the correct response to the item, as in this example of a multiple-choice stem: "Which of the following is NOT an indication for high-level disinfection of surgical instruments and equipment?" This wording tends to reinforce the incorrect alternative, and it might cause confusion when students try later to recall the correct information (Oermann & Gaberson, 2017).

6. *Items should not contain irrelevant cues to correct answers.* Flaws in item construction can allow test-wise students to improve their chances of guessing the correct answer when they do not know it, interfering with valid interpretations of their scores. Irrelevant cues include

- A multiple-choice stem that is grammatically inconsistent with one or more alternatives.
- Repeating important words from the stem in only the correct answer.
- Using qualifiers such as "never" and "always" in incorrect alternatives.
- Having a consistent pattern of correct answers being longer than incorrect alternatives or true statements being longer than false statements.
- Using the same response position consistently for correct answers (Oermann & Gaberson, 2017).

7. *No item should depend on another item for meaning.* Items should not be linked such that students who answer one item incorrectly will likely answer the related item incorrectly. An example of such linking is:

   1. Which drug should be available in case of malignant hyperthermia? _____
   2. What solvent should be used to mix the drug in Item 1? _____

   However, a series of items that relate to a particular context such as a diagram, case study, or graph are called interpretive or context-dependent items. This is not a violation of the rule because the items relate to a common context, not to each other (Oermann & Gaberson, 2017).

8. *Eliminate unnecessary information.* Including fictitious patient names or initials in test items increases reading time unnecessarily, might be a distraction from the items' intent, and might introduce cultural bias. If the purpose of an item is to assess whether students can evaluate the relevance of clinical data and use only relevant information to arrive at the correct answer, extraneous data other than patient names can be included (Oermann & Gaberson, 2017).

9. *Request peer critique of the test item.* Colleagues who teach the same content or who are skilled in the technical aspects of item writing are the best critics of newly written test items. If these colleagues are not available for critique, the teacher should set the items aside and return to them in a few days with a fresh perspective to identify clerical errors or lack of clarity (Oermann & Gaberson, 2017).

10. *Prepare more test items than the test blueprint calls for.* This will permit replacement of items discarded in the critique process. Unused extra test items can be kept in a test item bank for future use (Oermann & Gaberson, 2017).

ITEM-WRITING PRINCIPLES FOR SPECIFIC ITEM FORMATS

In addition to the general item-writing rules previously described, there are specific principles for writing test items of each item format. The following discussion offers helpful suggestions for writing effective test items of various types. For a more in-depth discussion and specific guidelines for developing items of each type, see Oermann and Gaberson (2017).

TRUE–FALSE

A true–false item comprises a statement that the student must judge as true or false. Variations of this format include requiring students to explain why the statement is true or false, or to correct false statements. True–false items are most effective for testing recall of specific information or for understanding of a principle or concept. They are not useful for testing complex thinking and reasoning (Musial, Nieminen, Thomas, & Burke, 2009). Because these items require relatively little time to read, students can respond to a large number of them in a short period of time, allowing the teacher to sample a broad content area. The main disadvantage of true–false items is the 50% probability of guessing the correct answer. However, this probability pertains to a single test item; on a test with many items, the probability of obtaining an adequate score through guessing alone is small (Brookhart & Nitko, 2015).

Examples of true–false items are in Exhibit 13.1. Important principles to follow when constructing these items are (Oermann & Gaberson, 2017):

- Avoid testing recall of trivial information.
- Each statement should be unconditionally true or false without qualification.
- Avoid words such as *usually* and *often*, which typically occur in true statements, and *never, always, all,* or *none*, which are usually in false statements (Miller et al., 2013).
- Each item should include only one idea to be tested; multiple ideas often result in part of the statement being true and part being false.
- Avoid the use of negative wording, particularly in statements that are intended to be false.
- Attempt to make all true–false items similar in length. True items tend to be longer than false items because they often include more precise language.
- Use approximately the same number of true statements and false statements, or include slightly more false than true items, because false statements tend to have higher discrimination power (Waugh & Gronlund, 2013).
- Avoid ordering true–false items in a noticeable pattern, such as TTFF or TFTF.
- For variations in which students are expected to correct false items or supply an explanation for their judgment, award an additional point for correctly changing the wording or providing a satisfactory rationale.

EXHIBIT 13.1 Examples of True–False Items

- T F According to the AORN Guideline for Surgical Attire, the scrub top should be donned before the cap. (F)
- T F The circulating nurse should check the position of the patient's feet before surgical drapes are applied. (T)
- T F The ordered preoperative antibiotic dose should be repeated if the procedure lasts 2 hours or more. (T)

AORN, Association of periOperative Registered Nurses.

MATCHING EXERCISES

Matching exercises comprise a series of homogeneous items (premises) with the same set of responses. They are most appropriate for assessing students' ability to classify and categorize information such as definitions of terms, generic and trade names of medications, or pharmacologic classifications (Miller et al., 2013). Important principles to follow when constructing matching exercises are listed here. A sample matching exercise is in Exhibit 13.2.

- Write unequal numbers of premises and responses to avoid giving a clue to the final match. Usually the list of responses is longer, but the use of a scannable answer sheet can limit the number of responses. In that case, the list of premises should be longer.

- Keep the lists of premises and responses short. Miller et al. (2013) recommended four to seven items in each column.

- Place premises on the left and responses on the right. Premises usually are longer; students must read each premise and then search the responses for the correct match. The list of the responses therefore is read repeatedly, so short responses help students to find the correct answer quickly.

- Directions for each matching exercise should state the basis on which premises and responses should be matched, and whether each response can be used once, more than once, or not at all (Oermann & Gaberson, 2017).

EXHIBIT 13.2 Sample Matching Exercise

Directions: For each description of a pressure injury in Column A, select the appropriate stage from Column B. Responses in Column B can be used once, more than once, or not at all.

Column A	Column B
(e) 1. Base of the lesion is covered by slough or eschar or both	a. Stage I
(d) 2. Exposed bone or tendons are visible or directly palpable	b. Stage II
(b) 3. Shiny or dry shallow lesion without sloughing or bruising	c. Stage III
(c) 4. Visible subcutaneous fat without exposure of bone or muscle	d. Stage IV
	e. Unstageable

MULTIPLE CHOICE AND MULTIPLE RESPONSE

Multiple-choice items can be used to assess many types of desired learning outcomes at various levels of the cognitive taxonomy, especially application and analysis. Well-written multiple-choice items include new information in the stem and require students to apply concepts and principles or use analytical thinking to respond to the item. Nursing students need to have experience with multiple-choice testing because they will encounter many of these items on licensure, certification, and other published tests (Oermann & Gaberson, 2017). However, as stated previously, this is not a good reason to use *only* multiple-choice items on nursing tests.

Each multiple-choice item comprises three parts: stem, correct answer, and distractors. The stem is a question or incomplete sentence that must be answered or completed by one of the alternatives. The alternatives or options include the correct answer and a number of distractors. The correct or best answer is also called the keyed response because it is the alternative marked on the answer key. Distractors are incorrect alternatives that appear plausible to students who are unsure of the correct answer. Specific guidelines for writing each of these components are discussed next.

Whether the stem is a question or incomplete statement, it must communicate clearly the intent of the item. The stem should present a problem or issue that relates to an important learning outcome. The student should be able to read the stem and know what type of response the teacher expects (Brookhart & Nitko, 2015). Guidelines for writing the stem include (Oermann & Gaberson, 2017):

- Clearly present sufficient information for the problem to be solved. As a test of clarity and completeness, the item writer should cover the alternatives and judge whether the stem alone specifies what to look for in the alternatives.
- Avoid including extraneous information unless the purpose of the item is to assess students' ability to differentiate relevant from irrelevant data. Humorous content should be avoided because it can be confusing to nonnative English speakers.
- Do not use the stem to teach. The goal of testing is to assess learning, not to teach or reinforce information.
- Eliminate key words from the stem that would provide a cue to the correct answer, such as a word in the stem that can relate to the same concept as a word used in the answer; for example, *aging* and *elderly*.
- Avoid negative wording; ask for the correct or best answer rather than the only incorrect response, as previously discussed. If there is no acceptable alternative wording, consider revising the stem to a true–false, completion, or multiple-response format.
- Avoid ending a stem in the form of an incomplete sentence with "a" or "an" because these words provide clues as to whether the correct answer begins with a consonant or a vowel. Ending the stem with "a/an" is not a good remedy because students then must read each alternative with "a" and then again with "an."
- If the stem is an incomplete sentence, the alternatives should complete the statement at the end of the sentence. A blank in the middle of the sentence, which the correct answer is supposed to fill, acts as a barrier to reading comprehension (Brookhart & Nitko, 2015).

Alternatives are listed under the stem and can vary in number. The more options, the more discriminating the item, as long as all options are plausible. Most standardized tests use four alternatives, but for teacher-made tests, it is not necessary to have the same number of alternatives for every item. Most scannable answer sheets allow up to five alternatives, which reduces the chance of guessing the correct answer to 20%; however, it is challenging to write four plausible distractors. If the teacher can construct only two plausible distractors for one correct answer, a three-option item is certainly acceptable (Popham, 2012; Rodriguez, 2005; Tarrant & Ware, 2012). Guidelines for writing good alternatives include:

- Make all alternatives similar in length, detail, and complexity. The correct answer frequently is the longest because the teacher tends to include more details, which testwise students might recognize.
- Each alternative should contain the same number of parts. If the correct answer contains two parts (e.g., specific pieces of information), and each distractor contains only one part, this provides a cue to the testwise student.
- Alternatives should be grammatically consistent with each other and with the stem (if it is an incomplete sentence).
- All alternatives should sample the same content domain, such as nursing interventions, diagnostic test results, or assessment findings. Avoid including opposite responses in the alternatives because this often is a clue that the correct answer is one of the opposites.
- If words are repeated in each alternative, move them to the stem to decrease reading time. If alternatives contain several parts, such as clinical manifestations of a

postoperative complication, and the same word or phrase appears in each alternative, that word or phrase should be moved to the stem.

- If the stem is a complete sentence or question, end it with the appropriate terminal punctuation and begin each alternative with a capital letter. If the alternatives complete an incomplete sentence in the stem, end the stem with a comma or colon as appropriate, begin each alternative with a lower-case letter, and use terminal punctuation at the end.
- Alternatives with ranges of numerical values should not overlap each other. If a portion of the range of values in one distractor is within the range of the correct answer, students might argue that there is more than one correct answer.
- Place each alternative on a separate line and all lines in one column under the stem. Usually items are numbered, and alternatives are lettered; this format helps students avoid making clerical errors when they use a separate answer sheet.
- Avoid using *none of the above* and *all of the above* as alternatives. If a student knows that at least one of the other options is true, *none of the above* can be eliminated; likewise, if one option is known to be incorrect, *all of the above* is obviously incorrect. Teachers often use *all of the above* when they have difficulty constructing enough plausible distractors, but it is better to use three options (the correct answer and two plausible distractors) or a multiple-response format, to be described later in this chapter.
- If students are required to choose the best rather than the correct answer, the best answer should be supported by consistency among expert practitioners and in the scientific evidence (Oermann & Gaberson, 2017).

Multiple-response items allow students to select one or more options as the correct or best answer. These items might be in combined-response form (also known as multiple-multiple-choice, or complex multiple-choice), or they might simply allow students to indicate every correct alternative (if that option is provided by the electronic scanning software used). Because this item format is used on licensure, certification, and other types of standardized tests, students should have experience with the format during their educational programs. Guidelines for writing items of this variation include:

- In combined-response items, group the options logically rather than randomly to avoid combinations that are internally contradictory.
- Use options an equal number of times in each combination of alternatives. If one of the options appears in every combination, add this information to the stem. Limited use of one option can be a cue to the correct answer for the testwise student (Oermann & Gaberson, 2017).

Examples of multiple-choice and multiple-response items are in Exhibit 13.3.

EXHIBIT 13.3 Examples of Multiple-Choice and Multiple-Response Items

1. According to the Surgical Care Improvement Project, prophylactic antibiotics other than vancomycin should be administered:
   a. for at least 24 hours preoperatively.
   b. for at least 72 hours postoperatively.
   c. up to 2 hours before incision.
   d. within 1 hour of incision.

(continued)

EXHIBIT 13.3 Examples of Multiple-Choice and Multiple-Response Items (*continued*)

2. Common adverse medication reactions in elderly surgical patients include:
   1. confusion.
   2. dry mouth.
   3. headache.
   4. nausea and vomiting.
   5. respiratory depression.
       a. 1, 3
       b. 2, 5
       c. 1, 2, 4
       d. 3, 4, 5
       e. 1, 2, 3, 4, 5

SHORT-ANSWER

Short-answer items require a word, phrase, or number as an answer. These occur in two formats: question and completion (also known as fill-in-the-blank). These items are best used to assess recall of specific information and ability to perform calculations. Short-answer items might ask students to label a diagram, identify specific items, or provide correct abbreviations for medical terms. A variation, ordered-response items, requires students to place a list of responses in the proper order. Completion items consist of a statement with a key word or phrase missing; the student must supply the missing material.

Examples of short-answer items are in Exhibit 13.4. Guidelines for writing these items include:

- Do not use verbatim material from textbooks and other readings; doing so can result in assessing only recall of information without comprehension.
- Construct the item so that only one unique word, phrase, or number will correctly complete it.
- Write items that are specific enough that they can be answered briefly. Think of the correct answer first and then write a question or statement to elicit that response. If more than one response could be correct, list all possible correct answers on the answer key.
- Items requiring mathematical calculations should specify the nature of the desired response and degree of specificity.
- For fill-in-the-blank items, place the blank at or near the end of the statement to make it easier for students to discern the intent of the item after reading it only once. Avoid giving grammatical clues such as "a" or "an" and singular or plural forms just before the blank. If more than one blank is used, blanks should be equal in length to avoid giving a clue to desired length of response. More than two blanks might not leave enough of a context for students to grasp the intent of the item.
- Direct students where to record their answers. Instead of filling in blanks within or at the end of the items, students can be asked to write their answers in blanks arranged in a column to the left or right of the item to facilitate scoring (Oermann & Gaberson, 2017).

EXHIBIT 13.4 Examples of Short-Answer Items

1. A patient weighs 220 lbs. You need to prepare an initial dose of 2.5 mg/kg of dantrolene sodium. What is the correct dose in milligrams? _____ Show your work:

2. According to Spaulding classification, what level of items should receive a minimum of high-level disinfection? _____

ESSAY

Essay items call for a more lengthy response than short-answer ones. They are useful for assessing complex learning outcomes and higher levels of learning. Essay items are appropriate for assessing students' abilities to analyze (patient data, clinical situations, ethical issues); critique (scientific evidence, approaches to solving a problem); and develop (teaching plans, protocols, arguments for and against a position or decision). Although responses to essay items require students to compose and write responses, the quality of their writing should not enter into the evaluation of their responses.

Limitations in using essay items include:

- Essay items do not provide a broad sample of a content domain. Because of the amount of time needed for students to organize and write their responses to essay items, teachers usually can include only a few of them on a test.

- Essay responses tend to be scored differently by different teachers (Miller et al., 2013) and by the same teacher at different times. Essay items that are highly structured and focused tend to produce greater reliability in scoring.

- Scoring essay responses might produce a carryover effect in which the teacher develops an impression about the student's knowledge and ability from one answer and tends to expect the same quality of response for the next essay item. For this reason, it is best to evaluate all student responses to one essay item before reading responses to the next one.

- Teachers can have the tendency to be influenced by general impressions of or by feelings about students when evaluating essay responses. These impressions and feelings create a halo effect that might influence the teacher's score. For this reason, the identity of the student who wrote each response should be masked until all responses are scored. Students' essay responses can be identified by assigned or selected numbers that are then matched to their names when scoring is complete.

- The teacher's judgment of essay responses often is affected by students' writing abilities. As previously mentioned, teachers should focus on the substance of essay responses and attempt to ignore writing style, grammar, and spelling (Brookhart & Nitko, 2015; Waugh & Gronlund, 2013).

- The first essay responses read in a scoring session tend to be scored higher than those read near the end, due to teacher fatigue and time constraints. This problem is called "rater drift." To prevent rater drift, teachers should read essay responses in random order, rearrange the order before scoring another item, and read each response twice before computing a score.

- Some teachers allow students to choose a subset of essay items to respond to. For example, from a set of six essay items, students are allowed to choose which four they want to answer. Miller et al. (2013) advised against this practice because, when students choose which items to answer, they actually are taking different tests, which affects measurement validity.

In writing essay items, the teacher should: (a) develop items that require analysis, integration, and synthesis rather than summary of the content; (b) use clear wording to direct students to the intended response; (c) prepare students for an essay test by asking questions in class, clinical practice, and online that require clinical reasoning, synthesis of content from various sources, critique of opposing views, and comparison of approaches; (d) indicate the point value of each essay item, an approximate amount of time students should allot to answering it, or both; and (e) write an ideal answer to each essay item while drafting it to determine whether it is clearly stated and could be answered in a reasonable timeframe. The teacher can save this ideal response to use when constructing a scoring rubric. Examples of essay items are in Exhibit 13.5.

EXHIBIT 13.5 Examples of Essay Items

1. Give three examples of circumstances in which perioperative personnel should wear personal protective equipment when handling used instruments and equipment. (3 points)
2. Critique arguments for and against the practice of suspending Do Not Resuscitate status when patients undergo surgery. Based on your critique, state which position you believe is the strongest and provide a rationale supporting your choice. (7 points)

Essay items can be scored by two methods, holistic and analytic. *Holistic scoring* involves reading the entire response and judging its overall quality. This can be done by comparing each student's response with those of other students and ranking them by degrees of quality. Answers are read to assess the overall quality of response (sometimes by comparing them to a model answer), and then sorted into piles representing different degrees of quality; each pile then receives a particular score. For *analytic scoring*, the teacher identifies the content that should be included in the answer and assigns a number of possible points for each content area. A scoring rubric can be developed that describes how points should be assigned for various degrees of completeness, logic, organization, and accuracy. Use of an analytic rubric also provides feedback to students about the quality of their essay responses (Oermann & Gaberson, 2017).

CONTEXT-DEPENDENT ITEM SETS

A context-dependent item set (also known as an interpretive exercise) is a group of test items that relate to the same introductory material. The introductory material might be a description of a clinical situation, a set of patient assessment findings or laboratory test results; a diagram; a graph; a table; a photograph; or excerpts from health care records, textbooks, or research reports. Students read, interpret, and analyze the introductory material and then respond to each test item related to it. The test items in the interpretive exercise can be in any item format, but all items in the same set should be the same format.

Context-dependent item sets are most appropriate for assessing higher level learning outcomes such as application of knowledge to novel situations, solving problems, making decisions, synthesizing information, and creating or developing new approaches.

Interpretive items are also included on licensure, certification, and other standardized tests, so students should have some experience with this type of test item during their academic programs.

A sample context-dependent item set is provided in Exhibit 13.6. Suggestions for developing these item sets are:

- The introductory material or context should provide enough information for analysis without limiting or directing students' thinking or creativity. One approach is to draft the test items first and then construct introductory material that includes the essential information needed to respond to the items.

- The introductory material can include irrelevant as well as relevant information if the intent of the exercise is to assess the student's ability to select relevant data on which to base judgments. All information included, however, should appear logical and pertinent to the situation.

- All items in the set should relate directly to the introductory material; students should not be able to arrive at a correct or best answer without reading and analyzing the context.

- The length of the context should correspond to the number of items that relate to it. It is a waste of students' time to read a lengthy scenario before responding to only two test items related to it.

- Arrange the context-dependent item set so that it is clear to the students which items relate to the introductory material. Use a heading to indicate the item numbers in the set (e.g., "Items 34–38 relate to the following patient assessment findings") and consider centering the introductory material horizontally on the page so that it is more visible. If possible, place the context and all items related to it on the same page (Oermann & Gaberson, 2017)

EXHIBIT 13.6 Sample Context-Dependent Item Set

Items 1 to 4 relate to the following situation:

An 82-year-old woman is scheduled for an open reduction and internal fixation of her right femur. She rates her pain at 4 on a 1 to 10 scale and has not received any preoperative sedation. Three days ago, on admission, an indwelling urinary catheter was inserted and it is now draining clear, light yellow urine. While transferring the patient to the OR bed, the perioperative RN notices a reddened area on her sacrum, approximately the size and shape of a silver dollar; the skin is intact with no blistering apparent, and it feels warm to touch. The patient is positioned supine on the fracture OR bed with the left leg supported in a padded stirrup. Her right arm is positioned over her chest in a sling and the left arm is on a padded arm board.

T F 1. According to the National Pressure Ulcer Advisory Panel definitions of pressure injuries, the perioperative RN should document the lesion on the patient's sacrum as Stage I.

T F 2. This patient is at an increased risk for inability to give informed consent for the surgical procedure.

T F 3. The patient's position on the OR bed increases her risk of compression and stretch injury to the left sciatic nerve.

T F 4. According to the National Guideline Clearinghouse guideline for prevention of catheter-associated urinary tract infections, this patient has an increased risk of such an infection.

OR, operating room.

ASSEMBLING THE TEST

The final appearance of a test and the way in which it is administered can affect measurement validity. Confusing directions, haphazard arrangement of components, and clerical errors all contribute to measurement error. Teachers can avoid such errors by following certain test design rules.

ARRANGE ITEMS IN A LOGICAL SEQUENCE

There are various methods for arranging items on the test: by order of expected difficulty, according to the sequence in which the content was learned, and a combination of the two. If using two or more item types, the teacher should first group items of each type together. This allows students to maintain the mental set required to respond to each type of item and prevents errors caused by frequent task changes (Oermann & Gaberson, 2017). Miller et al. (2013) recommended the following order of item formats on a test, from simplest to most complex:

1. True–false
2. Matching
3. Short-answer or completion
4. Multiple-choice
5. Context-dependent item sets
6. Essay items

Using all item formats on a single test is not necessary nor recommended, but the longer the test, the greater variety of item formats can be included. If the test is to contain complex item formats requiring more reading and processing time, they should be combined with only one or two additional item types.

Within each item format, items can be arranged according to the order in which the content was presented in the course, which can help students recall essential information more easily. Finally, in the combination of item format and content sequencing, items can be arranged in order of expected difficulty, easiest items first. Beginning each section with easier items can help anxious students relax so that they can demonstrate their best performance (Miller et al., 2013; Oermann & Gaberson, 2017).

WRITE DIRECTIONS

The teacher should write a set of clear general directions for the test, including such information as:

- How and where to record responses
- Whether students may write on the test booklet
- The amount of time permitted
- Whether students may ask questions during the test

Each section (according to item format) should begin with a set of directions that specify the assessment tasks. For example, for multiple-choice items, students need to know whether to select the correct or best response.

USE A COVER PAGE

A cover page serves to keep the test items concealed during the distribution of test materials so that the first students to receive the test will not have more time to complete it than students who receive their copies later. If a separate answer sheet is used, the cover page can be numbered to help maintain test security. Students are asked to record their numbers in a specified location on their answer sheets, and when test materials are returned, teachers can identify any missing test booklets. The general directions for the test can be printed on the cover page, allowing the teacher to review them with the students before anyone begins reading and responding to test items.

AVOID CROWDING

Teachers should allow enough space between and around test elements so that each test item is distinct from the others. Tightly packing words on a page might minimize the amount of paper used, but it can also interfere with students' maximum performance by contributing to reading and clerical errors.

KEEP RELATED MATERIAL TOGETHER

In addition to grouping items of the same format together, the teacher should ensure that all parts of a test item appear on the same page, such as the stem and alternatives of a multiple-choice item and the directions and both columns of a matching exercise. As previously mentioned, the introductory material and all related context-dependent items should appear on the same page, if possible (Miller et al., 2013).

FACILITATE SCORING

If the teacher will be hand-scoring the test, the test or answer sheet layout should facilitate quick, accurate scoring. If students record their answers on the test booklet itself, items should be formatted with scoring in mind. For example, arrange true–false items with columns of Ts and Fs at the left margin and ask students to circle their responses, as in this example:

T F 1. A clean mastectomy incision primarily closed and with a Jackson-Pratt drain should be categorized as a Class II wound.

T F 2. A 10% bleach solution should be used for environmental cleaning of patient care areas for patients infected with *C. difficile*.

T F 3. Contact precautions should be used when caring for patients infected with seasonal influenza.

NUMBER ITEMS CONTINUOUSLY

Although test items should be grouped according to format, the teacher should number them continuously from the beginning to the end of the test instead of starting each item format section with item number 1. This technique helps to prevent clerical errors when students record their answers on a separate answer sheet and helps students to recognize items they have skipped.

PROOFREAD

To ensure optimum measurement reliability and validity, the test should be free of spelling, grammatical, and typing errors. The test designer often does not recognize his or her own errors, so a colleague who is familiar with the content should be asked to proofread a copy of the test before it is duplicated. Spell-check and grammar-check features of computer software are insufficient because they do not always recognize words that are spelled correctly but used in the wrong context, or structural errors such as giving two test items the same number.

PREPARE AN ANSWER KEY

For both hand scoring and electronic scoring, the teacher should prepare an accurate scoring key to provide a final check on the accuracy of the test items. This answer key should also be proofread by someone who did not prepare it, verifying that it is accurate. The teacher should also prepare ideal responses to short-answer items and prepare scoring rubrics for essay items.

REPRODUCING THE TEST

Obviously, the teacher must provide a copy of the test for each student, but it is wise to make extra copies for proctors or to replace defective copies that might have been distributed to students. The original copy of the test should be produced on a laser or other high-quality printer, and the copies should be made on a machine that has sufficient toner to produce crisp, dark print without artifacts.

The test should be printed on only one side of each sheet of paper to prevent students from inadvertently skipping items by failing to notice the printing on the back of a page. If students are to record their answers on the test itself, printing on only one side makes hand-scoring easier.

Teachers are responsible for maintaining the security of tests by protecting them from unauthorized access. Dishonest students who gain access to test materials can use them to obtain higher scores than they deserve, contributing to measurement error. Printed tests should be stored in locked areas, and computer files should be password protected or encrypted. Printed drafts and old copies of used tests should be shredded. In some schools tests are taken online, with its own set of principles. Learning management systems should have appropriate protections to prohibit unauthorized access of test files.

PREPARING STUDENTS TO TAKE TESTS

Teachers should create conditions under which students will be able to demonstrate their best performance on tests. One of these conditions involves adequate preparation of students to take tests (Miller et al., 2013; Brookhart & Nitko, 2015).

INFORMATION NEEDS

Students need information about the test to prepare effectively for it. They should have sufficient time to prepare, so the date and time of the test should be announced well in advance. Although many teachers believe that unannounced or pop tests motivate students to study, no credible evidence supports this belief. Students also need to know about the testing conditions, including how much time will be provided, whether they will be able to use resources such as a calculator, number and type of test items, and whether any items, such as cell phones, books, and papers, will not be permitted in the testing room.

Students need to know which content domains will be assessed, the cognitive level at which they will be expected to perform, and the relative weights assigned to each content area. As previously discussed, teachers can communicate this information by sharing and discussing the test blueprint with students.

TEST-TAKING SKILLS

Students need adequate test-taking skills for the type of test to be administered. Skill in test-taking is often called testwiseness, but this term more appropriately refers to the ability to use test-taking skills and experience along with clues from poorly constructed test items to achieve a score higher than a student's true knowledge would predict. All students need adequate test-taking skills so that they are not at a disadvantage when their scores are compared with those of testwise students. Some of these skills are:

- Following test directions
- Reading and understanding test items
- Recording responses accurately
- Using testing time wisely
- Checking answers for clerical errors
- Distributing test preparation and getting adequate rest before a test (Oermann & Gaberson, 2017)

A common misconception is that students should not change their answers to test items because their first response is usually correct. Students should be encouraged to change answers any time they have a good reason for the change, such as later recalling necessary information or getting a clue from another item.

TEST ANXIETY

Teachers should prepare students to approach a test with helpful attitudes. Anxiety is a common response in testing situations, but excessive anxiety is likely to interfere with a student's performance (Miller et al., 2013). Test anxiety is a trait with physical, emotional, and cognitive components. Research evidence demonstrates an interaction among these components: negative thoughts about testing can produce negative feelings that interfere with performance (Poorman, Mastorovich, & Molcan, 2007). Physical feelings and reactions associated with test anxiety relate to autonomic reactivity, producing symptoms of perspiration, increased heart rate, and gastrointestinal upset, although not all test-anxious students have these reactions.

Students whose text anxiety interferes with their test performance can benefit from treatment that addresses the negative emotions (e.g., worry) and thoughts (e.g., distractibility, difficulty concentrating) as well as improvement of test-taking skills. Teachers who identify students who are affected by test anxiety should refer those students for treatment.

TEST ADMINISTRATION

Administering the test is usually the easiest step in the testing process. However, common problems associated with test administration can affect the reliability of test scores and the validity of inferences made about the scores. Careful planning can help teachers prevent or minimize those problems by using such strategies as scheduling the test in a classroom that minimizes potential distractions such as noise and interruptions.

Teachers should distribute test materials efficiently; with large groups of students, several proctors can assist with this process. If a cover page is used, as previously recommended, students should be instructed not to turn to the first page of test items until they are told to start. If there is no cover page, distribute the tests face down and instruct students not to turn them over until told to do so. General instructions about the testing procedures should be given before students are permitted to begin taking the test.

How to respond to student questions during a test is a challenge for most teachers. Some teachers do not answer any questions related to the content of the test items, even to clarify their meaning. In this case, the teacher should provide students with an opportunity to record their questions and concerns on a separate piece of paper to be reviewed later. Teachers who do answer questions during the test should do so quietly and briefly, avoid giving cues to the correct answer, and ensure careful proctoring of the group while answering one student's question.

Cheating during tests is a common concern. No matter how widespread the practice might be, teachers should protect the security of test materials throughout the testing process so that honest students are not at a disadvantage when their scores are compared with those of students who cheat. A number of methods have been proposed to deter cheating during a test, but the single most effective method is careful proctoring. There should be enough proctors to allow one to respond to student questions or a student emergency during the test. Proctors should devote their full attention to proctoring and not use this time to grade papers, read, or check e-mail. Because of the variety of creative ways in which students can access unauthorized information during a test, it is wise to also prohibit students from bringing certain items into the testing room, including backpacks, caps with bills, facial tissues, water bottles, cell phones, earbuds, and the like (Oermann & Gaberson, 2017).

TEST AND ITEM ANALYSIS

Computer software for scoring scannable answer sheets and analyzing test results is widely available. These applications provide useful information about how well the test as a whole functioned as a measurement instrument and about the effectiveness of each test item.

Test statistics usually include the range and distribution of scores, measures of central tendency (i.e., the average or typical score), measures of variability (e.g., standard deviation), and reliability estimates. These test characteristics help teachers to interpret the test results and make appropriate inferences about them.

To determine the effectiveness of each test item, teachers should review their difficulty and discrimination indexes. Item difficulty (or p-value) is calculated as the percentage of students who responded correctly to that item; values range from 0 to 1.00. The difficulty level is commonly understood to mean that the higher the percentage, the easier the item. However, difficulty is not an intrinsic characteristic of a test item; different p-values can be obtained on the same item by students with more or less ability or by students who were taught by more- or less-effective teachers. Difficulty level is also related to the probability of students' guessing the correct response. Thus, the probability of guessing the correct response to a true–false item is .50, whereas the probability of correctly guessing the answer to a five-option multiple-choice item is .20. Moderately difficult test items have p-values approximately halfway between the chance of blind-guessing and 1.00.

The discrimination index, *D*, indicates how effectively each test item measures what the entire test measures (Miller et al., 2013). *D*-values range from –1.00 to + 1.00. Negative values indicate that the item was answered correctly more often by students with low total test scores than by high-scoring students. A *D*-value of 0.00 means that the item has no discriminating power because equal numbers of high- and low-scoring students answered it correctly. Positive *D*-values mean that high-scoring students tended to answer the item correctly more often than low-scoring students.

Students often argue that if all or most of them answered an item incorrectly, that item should be deleted from the test, or that students who answered incorrectly should receive an extra point. Difficulty index alone is an insufficient basis on which to delete a test item from scoring: the teacher should carefully review the item in question, and if it measures important content, was expected to be difficult for many students, and is not seriously flawed, it should remain. If there is a fatal flaw, such as omission of the correct answer from a multiple-choice item, that item should be eliminated and the test rescored without it. Review of the discrimination index should help teachers determine whether a very difficult item effectively distinguished between high-scoring and low-scoring groups of students; if so, that item should be retained (Oermann & Gaberson, 2017).

SUMMARY

A test is a measurement instrument for assessing learners' knowledge and cognitive abilities. Test results allow teachers to make important educational decisions that affect learners, teachers, patients, future employers, and the educational program. A test must produce relevant and consistent results to form the basis for sound inferences about what learners know and can do. Good planning, careful test construction, proper administration, accurate scoring, and sound interpretation of scores are essential for producing useful test results. This chapter discussed assessment concepts that influence the quality of test results, and the process of planning, constructing, administering, scoring, and analyzing tests. Guidelines were presented for writing true–false, matching, multiple-choice, multiple-response, short answer, and essay items, and context-dependent item sets.

REFERENCES

Anderson, L. W., & Krathwohl, D. R. (Eds.). (2001). *A taxonomy for learning, teaching, and assessing: A revision of Bloom's taxonomy of educational objectives.* New York, NY: Longman.

Bosher, S., & Bowles, M. (2008). The effects of linguistic modification on ESL students' comprehension of nursing course test items. *Nursing Education Perspectives, 29,* 165–172.

Brookhart, S. M., & Nitko, A. J. (2015). *Educational assessment of students* (7th ed.). Upper Saddle River, NJ: Pearson.

Miller, M. D., Linn, R. L., & Gronlund, N. E. (2013). *Measurement and assessment in teaching* (11th ed.). Upper Saddle River, NJ: Prentice Hall.

Musial, D., Nieminen, G., Thomas, J., & Burke, K. (2009). *Foundations of educational measurement.* Boston, MA: McGraw-Hill.

Oermann, M. H., & Gaberson, K. B. (2017). *Evaluation and testing in nursing education* (5th ed.). New York, NY: Springer Publishing.

Poorman, S. G., Mastorovich, M. L., & Molcan, K. L. (2007). *A good thinking approach to the NCLEX and other nursing exams* (2nd ed.). Pittsburgh, PA: STAT Nursing Consultants.

Popham, W. J. (2012). *Selected-response tests: Building and bettering* (Vol. 12). Boston, MA: Pearson.

Rodriguez, M. C. (2005). Three options are optimal for multiple-choice items: A meta-analysis of 80 years of research. *Educational Measurement: Issues and Practice, 24*(2), 3–13. doi:10.1111/j.1745-3992.2005.00006.x

Tarrant, M., & Ware, J. (2012). A framework for improving the quality of multiple-choice assessment. *Nurse Educator, 37,* 98–104. doi:10.1097/NNE.0b013e31825041d0

Waugh, C. K., & Gronlund, N. E. (2013). *Assessment of student achievement* (10th ed.). Upper Saddle River, NJ: Pearson.

14

Clinical Evaluation

MARILYN H. OERMANN

OBJECTIVES

- Describe the clinical evaluation process, differences between formative and summative clinical evaluation, and guidelines for evaluating student performance
- Describe methods for evaluating students in the clinical setting and guidelines for their use

As students learn about nursing, they develop their knowledge base, higher level thinking skills, and a wide range of practice competencies essential for patient care. Learning concepts in a classroom or an online environment is not sufficient: students need to apply those concepts and other knowledge to clinical situations and be proficient in carrying out care. Teachers guide student learning in the clinical setting and evaluate their performance in practice. This chapter describes the clinical evaluation process, the importance of giving prompt and specific feedback to students as they are learning, principles that are important when observing and rating performance, and grading clinical practice.

WHAT OUTCOMES AND COMPETENCIES SHOULD BE EVALUATED?

Each school of nursing establishes its own program and course outcomes, or objectives, consistent with a range of factors that are described in Chapter 15. Some of those course outcomes relate to care of patients, families, and communities and are best met through clinical practice experiences. In these experiences students learn to apply their knowledge to clinical situations, transfer skills acquired in other settings to patient care, gain essential competencies for practice, and develop their clinical reasoning skills. Students use the nursing process to deliver holistic and patient-focused care (American Nurses Association, 2013). They search for and use evidence to guide decisions, enabling them to learn about evidence-based practice and how it is implemented in patient care.

They also learn about quality care and the nurse's role in improving health care quality and patient safety (Cronenwett et al., 2007; Dolansky & Moore, 2013; Drenkard, 2015; Phillips, Stalter, Dolansky, & Lopez, 2016; Sherwood, 2012).

Other outcomes of clinical practice are to develop psychomotor skills; gain informatics competencies (Flood, Gasiewicz, & Delpier, 2010; Committee on the Robert Wood Johnson Foundation Initiative on the Future of Nursing at the Institute of Medicine, 2011; Tellez, 2012); develop ability to use technology; learn to collaborate with nurses and other health professionals and function on interprofessional teams (Horsley et al., 2016; Interprofessional Education Collaborative, 2016); become culturally competent (Blanchet Garneau, 2016; Giddens, North, Carlson-Sabelli, Rogers, & Fogg, 2012; Hawala-Druy & Hill, 2012); and develop professional values and competencies in patient-centered care (McKeon, Norris, Cardell, & Britt, 2009; Sherwood & Barnsteiner, 2012). In clinical courses, students learn to accept responsibility for their own actions and become self-directed learners. Depending on the course, intended learning outcomes for students can also include gaining leadership and management skills.

These outcomes, and others in a nursing program, can be stated as outcomes or objectives to be met in a clinical course or as clinical competencies to be developed by students. Regardless of the format, these outcomes, objectives, or competencies provide the framework for the teacher to plan clinical activities for students and for assessing their performance. These outcomes are listed in Exhibit 14.1. Not all of the outcomes are relevant to each clinical course, but generally as students progress through a curriculum, they will meet these outcomes and develop related competencies.

EXHIBIT 14.1 Areas of Outcomes or Competencies for Clinical Evaluation

1. Apply concepts and other knowledge in patient, family, community, and global health care
2. Develop higher level thinking and clinical judgment skills
3. Deliver holistic and patient-centered care (nursing process)
4. Use evidence in clinical practice
5. Gain knowledge, skills, and values for improving the quality and safety of care
6. Develop psychomotor, technological, and informatics skills
7. Develop communication skills with patients, families, the interprofessional team, and others with whom the nurse interacts
8. Develop values and cultural competencies essential for care of culturally and ethnically diverse patients
9. Accept responsibility and accountability for own actions and decisions
10. Become a self-directed learner
11. Develop leadership and management skills

CLINICAL EVALUATION PROCESS

In clinical evaluation, the teacher makes judgments about the quality of the students' performance in practice. These judgments indicate whether the student is meeting or has met the outcomes or objectives of the clinical course, and can perform the competencies to be developed in it. Clinical evaluation involves observing students' performance; assessing their understanding of the clinical situation through questions, discussions, and assignments completed by students; and collecting other data about student learning and performance. The teacher then uses these data to determine whether the student is progressing in the course, or at the end, has met each of the outcomes or objectives and can perform the competencies.

Clinical evaluation is a judgmental process (Oermann & Gaberson, 2017). The teacher's judgment influences the data collected through observations of students and other sources, and what those data mean, that is, decisions about the quality of the performance. First, in any clinical situation teachers can make varied observations of performance and collect different types of data on which to base the evaluation. For example, if two teachers observe a student in practice, one might collect information on how well the student interacted with the patient during a procedure, whereas the other focuses mainly on procedural skills, resulting in varied observations on which to judge the performance. Second, teachers can have different interpretations of how well the student performed. For this reason it is important to have multiple sources of data and to collect data over a period of time before arriving at a conclusion about the quality of the student's performance.

Another issue is that the teacher's personal values, attitudes, beliefs, and biases can influence the observations made and decisions about the quality of the performance (Oermann & Gaberson, 2017). Teachers need to be aware of these when evaluating students' performance. For example, a teacher who prefers working with students who are outgoing and initiate conversation can be biased when assessing the performance of a beginning student who is quiet and needs guidance in interacting with patients. Issues with interactions can affect the communication competencies on the clinical evaluation tool, but they should not influence the assessment of other unrelated competencies. As students are learning, it is the teacher's responsibility to guide their development. In this situation, the teacher's goal should be to help this student develop skills and confidence in communication. The teacher's main role is teaching students to gain competencies for practice, not only to evaluate their performance.

FORMATIVE AND SUMMATIVE CLINICAL EVALUATION

The teacher can evaluate students' performance to provide feedback for improving it (formative evaluation) or to indicate the outcomes met and competencies achieved in the clinical practicum (summative evaluation). In formative evaluation, the teacher provides feedback to students about their progress in the clinical practicum and how to improve performance. Feedback enables students to reflect on their performance, identify continued learning needs, and decide how to meet them (Bonnel, 2008). This is good teaching: the nurse educator identifies gaps in learning and performance and provides specific and instructional feedback to resolve those gaps. Altmiller (2016) emphasized that feedback about the student's clinical performance should be unbiased and should reflect specific observations made by the teacher. Students, though, need to reflect on the information provided to them and incorporate the feedback into their own learning (Bonnel, 2008). Formative evaluation is diagnostic, and it should not be graded (Brookhart & Nitko, 2015).

At periodic intervals, the teacher summarizes the extent of learning achieved in the course. This is done in relation to the outcomes or objectives to be met, or the expected competencies to be learned, answering questions such as: What outcomes have been met by the student? What is the student's current level of performance? Summative clinical evaluation is typically done at midterm and the end of the clinical practicum to decide on the student's grade. Summative evaluation is for grading—it usually comes too late for students to have an opportunity to improve their performance (Oermann & Gaberson, 2017).

FOCUS ON FORMATIVE EVALUATION

The teacher should focus on giving prompt and continuous feedback to students (formative evaluation) because the feedback will enable them to improve their performance. For feedback to guide student learning and improve performance, it should be:

1. *Precise, specific, and instructional.* Saying to a student, "Your organization needs to improve," or writing on a paper that the "content lacks depth" does not specify the problem with organization of care and the paper's content or how to improve. Instead, the teacher should indicate the specific skills and knowledge that are lacking and provide suggestions about what to do next to gain those missing skills. By incorporating guidance on how to improve, feedback is instructional and leads to improved performance.

2. *Delivered using varied and relevant modes.* With oral feedback, the teacher describes the observations made of performance, explains what to do differently, and shares other ways of thinking about the clinical situation. Some of the best learning occurs when students and teachers engage in dialogue about the feedback. For procedures and psychomotor skills, feedback should be oral (explaining the errors in performance and how the skill should be performed) and visual (demonstrating the correct procedure). The student can then practice the skill under the guidance of the teacher or someone else with expertise. Written comments on students' papers and other assignments provide another mode of feedback and should meet the same criteria: be precise, specific, and instructional.

3. *Prompt.* Feedback needs to be given at the time of learning or shortly thereafter. The longer the time between the performance and feedback, the less effective the feedback is, because students cannot recall the specifics of their performance to be modified.

4. *Individualized*, based on the needs of the student. Students need varying degrees of feedback and positive reinforcement as they are learning, especially in the clinical setting. As they become more clinically competent, they are better able to assess their own performance, but with new experiences they still need feedback on their thinking and judgment as well as skills.

5. *Given in private.* No one likes to be told in public and for others to hear about improvements needed in his or her care. The teacher should be sensitive to the setting in which feedback is delivered: it should be communicated in a private setting, with the goal of guiding students in their learning.

Gigante, Dell, and Sharkey (2011) outlined a five-step process for giving feedback to students that reflects the important principles of good feedback. First, the teacher should review the outcomes, objectives, or competencies students need to achieve in the course. These specify what is expected of students in the clinical practicum. Second, the teacher should set the stage for students to receive the feedback, for example, by beginning with this statement: "I am giving you feedback." Then it is clear to students that the information from the teacher is intended to guide their learning and performance. Third, the teacher should have students reflect on their performance and assess its quality— what went well, and what needs improvement from their point of view. Fourth, the teacher should share specific observations of performance with examples and areas for improvement. The last step in this process is for the teacher to recommend specific ways to improve performance.

SUPPORT OF STUDENTS IN THE EVALUATION PROCESS

Being evaluated is stressful, especially in the clinical setting, where patients, family members, other nursing students, nurses, and others can be observing the student provide care and teachers assess performance. Clinical practice in and of itself is stressful for students, and being evaluated adds to that stress. Students need a supportive learning environment where they are comfortable asking for help and seeking feedback from the teacher. Both teachers and nursing staff need to support students in their learning and be cognizant of the stress students experience in clinical practice. To reduce some of this stress, Dearmon et al. (2013) provided a 2-day, simulation-based orientation for students prior to their first clinical experience. In the simulation, students interacted with standardized patients in realistic clinical situations. Findings indicated that students increased their knowledge and confidence and experienced a decrease in anxiety following the simulation.

SELECTION OF CLINICAL EVALUATION METHODS

Clinical evaluation should be based on the outcomes, objectives, or competencies of the clinical course or practicum. These indicate the expectations for performance and areas to be assessed. The learning activities planned for students, including patient assignments, should enable students to meet these outcomes and become proficient in the identified competencies—the teacher's observations and subsequent assessment should focus on whether the desired outcomes were achieved.

There are different clinical evaluation methods that can be used to assess performance. Using multiple methods takes into consideration individual student needs, abilities, and characteristics and avoids relying on one source of information about student learning (Oermann & Gaberson, 2017). Most often the methods provide data for assessing more than one outcome or objective. For example, an observation of the student completing a health history of an elderly patient would provide data related to assessment, interviewing, communication, developmental needs, and others. In deciding on the evaluation methods for a clinical course, the teacher should review the outcomes or competencies and select methods for assessing them. In this way the methods are geared to the learning expected of students.

The clinical evaluation methods planned for a course should be realistic, considering the types of experiences available in the setting or through simulation, and both student and teacher time. Planning for an evaluation method that depends on a certain type of patient in the clinical setting is not realistic; such an evaluation would be better done with simulation or standardized patients. Some methods are not feasible because they might not be available for all of the students or take too much time. Weekly writing assignments might provide data on a number of the course outcomes but require too much time for students considering other course and clinical requirements and demand too much of the teacher's time to review them and give prompt feedback. In such cases, an alternate assessment method might be used, such as a group project or discussions with students, or the teacher might use fewer papers but focused on specific outcomes to be assessed. Bourgault, Mundy, and Joshua (2013) examined the use of audio recordings for providing feedback on weekly clinical assignments rather than written feedback. Students reported that the audio feedback was more personal, contained more positive and constructive feedback, and was easier to understand than written feedback. However, it did not save the faculty time.

CLINICAL EVALUATION METHODS

OBSERVATION OF PERFORMANCE

Oermann, Yarbrough, Ard, Saewert, and Charasika (2009) found in a survey of 1,573 faculty members teaching in prelicensure nursing programs that the main strategy they used to evaluate students' clinical performance was by observing them in the clinical setting. Observations of performance provide data about student achievement of the outcomes and their proficiency in the clinical competencies to be demonstrated. These guide the teacher on *what* to observe. Observations over a period of time in different clinical situations provide more reliable data on student performance than a one-time observation.

Teachers should share their observations with students and be willing to include student perceptions of their performance. The teacher might have had an incorrect impression; for example, deciding that a student lacked knowledge of a patient's problem, when in fact the student did not understand the teacher's question. Teachers should discuss their observations with students and be willing to modify their judgments about performance.

NOTES ABOUT STUDENTS' PERFORMANCE

Observations of performance should be recorded, because otherwise the teacher cannot recall details about the performance and the clinical context. Teachers should develop a strategy for documenting their observations in the clinical setting. Some educators use anecdotal notes, which are narrative descriptions of observations, with or without a judgment about how well the student performed (Di Leonardi Case & Oermann, 2010). Hall, Daly, and Madigan (2010) found in a survey of clinical teachers in six schools of nursing that most (97%) used anecdotal notes. In a study by Hall (2013), faculty identified a variety of uses for anecdotal notes: the most common reason was bringing attention to patient safety concerns. Qualitative findings indicated that anecdotal notes were important for providing accurate feedback to students for formative evaluation.

These notes can be handwritten in the clinical setting or recorded using devices such as smartphones, tablets, or other types of portable devices. With this technology teachers can keep a running record for each student. Zurmehly (2010) suggested that using technologies results in more accurate clinical evaluation because the observations can be recorded in real time. In a study by Swan et al. (2013), the use of tablets by teachers in the clinical setting was hampered by the lack of an Internet connection at some of the sites. At other clinical sites, faculty members were not able to use school of nursing tablets because of privacy concerns.

CHECKLISTS

For assessment of procedures, skills, and implementation of technology, checklists are typically used. A checklist includes a list of specific actions or steps in a procedure to be observed and a place for marking if the student performed them correctly (Brookhart & Nitko, 2015). Checklists also allow learners to self-assess their performance before it is evaluated by the teacher. They are commonly used for assessing skills in learning laboratories and simulation. Checklists are often used when skills are assessed in an Objective Structured Clinical Examination or by a standardized patient. In using checklists to assess performance of skills, it is important to focus on the ability of students to perform the skill safely; when there are different ways of carrying out the skill, the teacher should give students this flexibility.

CLINICAL EVALUATION TOOLS (RATING SCALES)

Clinical evaluation tools, which are types of rating scales, are more comprehensive than checklists. They typically list the outcomes or objectives to be met, or competencies to be demonstrated, at the end of the clinical practicum, with a scale for rating their performance. Clinical evaluation tools are intended for summative evaluation. At midterm the teacher can rate how well the student is performing at that point in time, and then at the end of the semester can indicate the outcomes or competencies that were achieved. Rating scales also are used to assess the quality of student performance of particular activities in clinical practice, such as leading a conference, in simulation, and in Objective Structured Clinical Examinations, among other uses.

Rating scales used for clinical evaluation can be pass–fail or satisfactory–unsatisfactory, or they can include multiple levels for rating performance, such as 1 to 4, or below average to exceptional. A pass–fail scale requires only two levels of judgment: did the student achieve the outcome or perform the competency at a satisfactory level to indicate a pass? In a survey of nursing faculty, 83% ($n = 1{,}116$) used pass–fail rating forms for clinical evaluation (Oermann et al., 2009).

With a system that has multiple levels, the teacher needs to judge the quality of the performance and decide which level it represents on the tool. Brookhart and Nitko (2015) suggested that for this type of instrument, a short description should be included with each number or level for each of the outcomes or competencies to improve consistency across teachers. For example, for the competency "Collects relevant data from patients," the descriptions for each level might be:

4: Collects significant data from patients and other sources, differentiates relevant from irrelevant data, analyzes data from multiple sources to identify additional information needed
3: Collects significant data from patients, uses multiple sources of data
2: Collects data from patients related to main problems
1: Does not collect significant data and misses important cues in data

With the goal of preparing students with the knowledge and skills for improving the quality of care, many faculty are incorporating quality and safety competencies into their clinical evaluation instruments. Exhibit 14.2 provides an example of a clinical evaluation tool that incorporates the Quality and Safety Education for Nurses (QSEN) competencies (QSEN, 2014; Walsh, Jairath, Paterson, & Grandjean, 2010). The Clinical Performance Evaluation Tool in Exhibit 14.2 is a generic tool used in all clinical courses for assessing student performance related to the QSEN competencies. In addition to this tool, each clinical course has its own key with competencies specific to that course. An example of the key that accompanies the first adult health nursing course is in Exhibit 14.3. Guidelines for grading clinical performance for all of the clinical courses in the nursing program are provided in Exhibit 14.4.

Another approach to clinical evaluation developed by Caputi (Appendix C) examines student learning outcomes performed in the clinical setting with learning activities tied directly to the behaviors on the clinical evaluation tool. These behaviors reflect the course outcomes and competencies. Caputi's approach is to also include activities

EXHIBIT 14.2 Example of Clinical Evaluation Tool Integrating QSEN Competencies

CUA   The Catholic University of America School of Nursing
Clinical Performance Evaluation Tool
[date]

Student Name _____ Faculty _____ Facility _____
Date _____ Midterm
Date _____ Final Evaluation
Student must obtain a Satisfactory "S" grade in all competencies at the final evaluation to pass the course.

Core Competencies	Midterm			Final	
	S	NI	U	S	U
Provides Patient-Centered Care					
• Values					
• Caring/Human Dignity					
• Spirituality					
• Ethics					
• Utilizes and Performs Nursing Process					
Exhibits Teamwork and Collaboration					
• Communication					
• Personnel (Faculty, Staff, Patients, Peers, Family)					
• Oral (Nonverbal)					
• Written (Documentation)					
Incorporates Evidence-Based Practice Into Clinical					
• Exhibits Critical Thinking					
Understands and Applies Quality Improvement Methods					
• Promote Healing					
Promotes Safety					
• Technical Skills					
• Safe Medication Administration					
• Timeliness					
Understands and Utilizes Informatics					
• Appropriate decision making based on core competencies above and implemented with informatics support					

Midterm Comments (Address Strengths and Weaknesses)
by Instructor
by Student
Final Comments (Address Strengths and Weaknesses)
by Instructor
By Student
Student Signature _____ **Date** _____
Faculty Signature _____ **Date** _____

QSEN, Quality and Safety Education for Nurses.

Source: From the School of Nursing, The Catholic University of America, Washington, DC. Copyright 2017.
Reprinted by permission of the School of Nursing, The Catholic University of America, Washington, DC, 2017.

EXHIBIT 14.3 Key With Clinical Competencies for Adult Health Nursing Course

 The Catholic University of America School of Nursing
Clinical Evaluation Tool—**KEY**
[date]
N275-Performance I[a]

1. Patient Centered

   a. Elicit patient values, preferences, and their expressed needs as part of the clinical interview, while performing within the process of assessment, planning, intervention, and evaluation in the implementation of the plan of care.

   b. Communicate patient values, preferences, and expressed needs to other members of health care team.

   c. Assess presence and extent of pain and suffering.

   d. Assess levels of physical and emotional comfort.

2. Teamwork and Collaboration

   a. Demonstrate awareness of own strengths and limitations as a team member.

   b. Function competently within own scope of practice as a member of the health care team.

   c. Initiate requests for help when appropriate to situation.

   d. Communicate effectively and appropriately in nonverbal, verbal, and written forms with other team members, while adapting one's own style of communication. Adapt communication styles to meet the needs of the client, team, clinical instructor, and situation.

3. Evidence-Based Practice

   a. Demonstrate knowledge of basic scientific methods and processes.

   b. Differentiate clinical opinion from research and evidence summaries.

   c. Base individualized care plan on patient values, clinical expertise, and evidence.

   d. Read original research and evidence reports related to area of practice.

4. Quality Improvement

   a. Describe strategies for learning about the outcomes of care in the setting in which one is engaged in clinical practice.

   b. Recognize that nursing and other health profession students are parts of systems of care and care processes that affect outcomes for patients and families.

   c. Give examples of the tension between professional autonomy and system functioning.

   d. Explain the importance of variation and measurement in assessing quality of care.

   e. Describe approaches for changing processes of care.

5. Safety

   a. Demonstrate effective use of technology and standardized practices that support safety and quality (medication administration).

   b. Demonstrate effective use of strategies to reduce risk of harm to self or others.

   c. Use appropriate strategies to reduce reliance on memory (such as checklists).

   d. Communicate observations or concerns related to hazards and errors to patients, families, and the health care team.

6. Informatics

   a. Explain why information and technology skills are essential for safe patient care.

   b. Navigate the electronic health record.

(continued)

EXHIBIT 14.3 Key With Clinical Competencies for Adult Health Nursing Course (*continued*)

> c. Document and plan patient care in an electronic health record.
> d. Recognize the time, effort, and skill required for computers, databases, and other technologies to become reliable and effective tools for patient care.
> e. Maintain safety and confidentiality in informatics.

Source: From the School of Nursing, The Catholic University of America, Washington, DC. Copyright 2017. Reprinted by permission of the School of Nursing, The Catholic University of America, Washington, DC, 2017.

[a] Competencies for N275 Adults in Health and Illness. Each clinical course has its own key with competencies specific to that course based on QSEN outcomes.

EXHIBIT 14.4 Guidelines for Grading Performance

 The Catholic University of America School of Nursing

Clinical Evaluation Tool Guidelines
[date]

Tool Guidelines

- Each student will fill out an evaluation at (1) midterm (2) final.
- Each faculty member will fill out an evaluation at (1) midterm (2) final.
- Each row item (boxes) must be checked at (1) midterm (2) final.
- The Clinical Score will be completed by the Clinical Faculty by placing a √ or an x in the appropriate box for each student.
- The Clinical Score will be completed by the Student by placing a √ or an x in the appropriate box for each student.
- The score for Clinical Evaluation will be either *PASS* or *FAIL*.
- A passing grade will be assigned only if *all* the items are checked *S* at the time of the final evaluation.

Core Competency Key

- Each core competency (as outlined in BOLD) has a template or key, which specifies individual guidelines and examples for each.
- The keys are based on level of matriculation in each clinical course.

Grading Guidelines—Entire Course

- The score for each student in the course will be the numeric grade received for the course based on all of the didactic work required in the syllabus.
- Clinical Performance will be evaluated with a Clinical Performance Tool, and will be scored either *PASS* or *FAIL*.
- Every student must receive a score of *PASS* on the Clinical Performance Tool to pass the course.
- A student who receives a *FAIL* on the Clinical Performance Tool will receive *FAIL* for the course and receive a grade of *F* for the course.

Source: From the School of Nursing, The Catholic University of America, Washington, DC. Copyright 2017. Reprinted by permission of the School of Nursing, The Catholic University of America, Washington, DC, 2017.

students are required to complete during the clinical experience. A description of this approach with examples is provided in Appendix C.

Regardless of the outcomes or competencies on the tool, the areas rated and the rating scale must be understood by all involved in the process. Teachers, students, preceptors, and others should understand what is meant by each competency to be rated and how to use the scale (Oermann & Gaberson, 2017). In addition, teachers should be able to identify examples of performance that reflect a pass or fail or at each level in the scale. For example, what is passing performance for "collects comprehensive data from patients?" If there are multiple levels in the scale, what is the difference in the collection of data at each level? Teachers should discuss as a group the meaning of each outcome or competency on the tool and acceptable performance. These discussions enable educators to come to consensus about behaviors that demonstrate competency for each of the items on the instrument (Parsons et al., 2012; Oermann & Gaberson, 2017). Teachers, adjunct faculty members, and preceptors can practice using the tool to assess the performance of students in digitally recorded simulations or video clips. Discussing their ratings and rationale improves use of the tool and its reliability. In addition, teachers should review the instrument with students, explaining each outcome and competency and expected performance. Other important principles for using a clinical evaluation tool are listed in Exhibit 14.5.

EXHIBIT 14.5 Guidelines for Using Clinical Evaluation Tools (Rating Scales)

1. Be alert to the possible influence of your own values, attitudes, and biases in observing performance and making judgments about its quality.

2. Use the outcomes, objectives, or competencies to focus your observations. Give students feedback on other observations made about their performance.

3. Collect sufficient data on students' performance before arriving at conclusions and judgments about the quality of the performance.

4. Observe students more than one time before rating performance. Rating scales for clinical evaluation should represent a pattern of the student's performance over a period of time.

5. Observe students' performance in different clinical situations or in simulation, or use additional methods for evaluation.

6. Do not rely on first impressions; these might not be accurate.

7. Always discuss observations with students, have students reflect on their performance and obtain their perceptions, and be willing to modify your own judgments and ratings when new data are presented.

8. Collect data on students' performance as it relates to the outcomes or competencies on the tool. These indicate the expectations for learning and performance and *what* should be evaluated in the clinical setting.

9. Avoid using the clinical evaluation tool as the only source of data about a student's performance—use multiple methods for evaluating clinical practice.

10. Rate each outcome or competency on the tool separately based on your observations of performance and other data you have collected. If you have insufficient information to rate a particular outcome or competency, leave it blank.

11. Rate students' performance based on the data. Do not let your general impressions of the student or personal biases influence the ratings.

12. If the clinical evaluation tool is not effective for judging student performance in your clinical course, revise it. Consider these questions: Does use of the tool yield

(continued)

EXHIBIT 14.5 Guidelines for Using Clinical Evaluation Tools (Rating Scales) (*continued*)

> data for making valid decisions about students' competence? Does it yield reliable, stable data? Is it easy to use? Is it realistic for the types of learning activities students complete and that are available in clinical and simulation settings? Is there consistency across faculty members in their use of the tool.
>
> 13. Discuss as a group (with other educators and preceptors involved in the evaluation) each competency on the clinical evaluation tool. Come to agreement as to the meaning of the competencies and what a student's performance would look like for a pass or fail and at each rating level in your tool. Share examples of performance, how you would rate them, and your rationale. As a group exercise, observe a digital recording or simulation of a student's performance, rate it with the tool, and come to agreement as to the rating. Exercises and discussions such as these should be held before the course begins and periodically to ensure reliability across teachers and settings.
> 14. Review the clinical evaluation tool at least annually and modify as needed.

Source: Adapted from Oermann and Gaberson (2017). Copyright 2017. Reproduced with the permission of Springer Publishing.

OTHER CLINICAL EVALUATION METHODS

Observations of students, summarizing observations in anecdotal notes, using checklists to assess skills, and rating how well students performed the expected clinical competencies are not the only methods for evaluating clinical practice. Other methods are listed in Exhibit 14.6. These methods, which are also described in Chapter 12, provide additional data about student achievement of the outcomes of the clinical course.

EXHIBIT 14.6 Clinical Evaluation Methods

- Observation
- Notes on student's performance
- Checklist
- Clinical evaluation tool (rating form)
- Formal (term) paper
- Short paper
- Reflective journal and other types of journals
- Nursing care plan
- Concept map
- Analysis of interactions in clinical setting and simulation
- Case including unfolding case and case study
- Media clip
- Electronic portfolio
- Discussion and clinical conference

(*continued*)

EXHIBIT 14.6 Clinical Evaluation Methods (*continued*)

- Group project
- Game
- Simulation
- Standardized patient
- Objective structured clinical examination
- Self-evaluation

GRADING CLINICAL COURSES

Clinical courses can be graded as pass–fail or satisfactory–unsatisfactory, or with letter grades such as A through F. Based on a survey of nursing programs, pass–fail appears to be the most common method of grading clinical nursing courses (Oermann et al., 2009). When using pass–fail grading, faculty can specify that the student must pass all of the competencies to pass the course or can identify critical behaviors for passing. When letter grades are used, the grade can be determined according to the number of outcomes or competencies achieved by the student. For example, an A might be assigned if all of the competencies were met and a B if the critical ones and half of the others were achieved (Oermann & Gaberson, 2017). The grade can also incorporate other evaluation methods used in the course. For example, the rating on the clinical evaluation tool can count for 50% of the clinical grade, with the other 50% determined by grades on written assignments, a portfolio, and a conference presentation. Or, the grade might be computed based only on the grades on assignments and other clinical evaluation methods used in the course, with the requirement that students receive a pass on the evaluation tool. In some schools, the clinical assignments and other evaluation methods provide data for determining whether students achieved the outcomes and competencies, but they are not evaluated and graded separately.

There are important principles for the teacher to be aware of related to grading clinical practice. First, the teacher should understand the outcomes to be met in the course, expectations of performance, and the specific evaluation methods used in the course. This information should be communicated in writing to students and reviewed with them. Second, students need to understand how the course is graded. For example, if students must pass the clinical course to progress in the program, no matter what grade they have in the course overall, this information should be in the course syllabus and school policies and should also be reviewed with students. Third, it is important to share all of the evaluation data with students and to consider their feedback on performance. Students should sign any evaluation documents and summaries of performance. Signing does not mean they agree with the evaluation, but it confirms that they had an opportunity to read what was written about their performance. Fourth, the most important role of the teacher in clinical practice is to provide continuous feedback to students on their performance and to help them improve. If the teacher identifies problems with performance, it is critical to discuss these with students and to prepare a learning plan with strategies mapped out for the student to correct deficiencies and further develop competencies (Oermann & Gaberson, 2017). Fifth, the teacher should document observations of performance as the course proceeds, discussing those with students so they are aware of their progress. All nurse educators need to be aware of the policies of the nursing program on unsafe clinical performance and failing a clinical course and to follow those precisely.

SUMMARY

Clinical evaluation is a process in which the teacher collects data through observations of performance and other assessment methods and, based on those data, makes judgments about the quality of the students' performance in practice. These judgments indicate whether the student is meeting or has met the outcomes or objectives of the course, or can perform the competencies expected in the course. Through formative evaluation the teacher provides feedback to students about their progress in the clinical practicum and specifically how to improve their performance. Feedback should be prompt, specific, and instructional; continuous during the learning process; and given in private. Formative evaluation is diagnostic and is not graded. At periodic intervals, such as at midterm and at the end of the clinical practicum, the teacher summarizes the extent of learning and performance. This process is referred to as summative evaluation.

Being evaluated is stressful, especially in the clinical setting where patients and others observe the student providing care and teachers assess performance. Both teachers and nursing staff need to provide a supportive and caring environment for students to learn and for the evaluation process to be less stressful.

Clinical evaluation methods should be selected based on the outcomes or competencies of the clinical course. These indicate the expectations for performance and areas to be assessed. Observations of performance provide data about student achievement of the outcomes and their proficiency in the clinical competencies to be demonstrated. Observations over a period of time in different clinical situations provide more reliable data on student performance than a one-time observation. When assessing a skill or procedure, the teacher might use a checklist, which includes the specific steps to perform the skill or carry out the procedure and a place for marking if the student performed each step correctly and in the right order. Clinical evaluation tools, which are rating scales, are more comprehensive than checklists. They typically list the outcomes or competencies to be demonstrated at the end of the clinical practicum with a scale for rating their performance. Clinical evaluation tools are intended for summative evaluation. Based on a survey of nursing programs, pass–fail appears to be the most common method of grading clinical nursing courses.

REFERENCES

Altmiller, G. (2016). Strategies for providing constructive feedback to students. *Nurse Educator, 41,* 118–119. doi:10.1097/NNE.0000000000000227

American Nurses Association. (2013). *The nursing process.* Retrieved from http://www.nursingworld .org/EspeciallyForYou/What-is-Nursing/Tools-You-Need/Thenursingprocess.html

Blanchet Garneau, A. (2016). Critical reflection in cultural competence development: A framework for undergraduate nursing education. *Journal of Nursing Education, 55,* 125–132. doi:10.3928/01484834 -20160216-02

Bonnel, W. (2008). Improving feedback to students in online courses. *Nursing Education Perspectives, 29,* 290–294.

Bourgault, A. M., Mundy, C., & Joshua, T. (2013). Comparison of audio vs. written feedback on clinical assignments of nursing students. *Nursing Education Perspectives, 34,* 43–46.

Brookhart, S. M., & Nitko, A. J. (2015). *Educational assessment of students* (7th ed.). Upper Saddle River, NJ: Pearson.

Cronenwett, L., Sherwood, G., Barnsteiner, J., Disch, J., Johnson, J., Mitchell, P., & Warren, J. (2007). Quality and safety education for nurses. *Nursing Outlook, 55,* 122–131. doi:10.1016/j.outlook.2007.02.006

Committee on the Robert Wood Johnson Foundation Initiative on the Future of Nursing at the Institute of Medicine. (2011). *The future of nursing: Leading change, advancing health.* Washington, DC: National Academies Press.

Dearmon, V., Graves, R. J., Hayden, S., Mulekar, M. S., Lawrence, S. M., Jones, L., & Farmer, J. E. (2013). Effectiveness of simulation-based orientation of baccalaureate nursing students preparing for their first clinical experience. *Journal of Nursing Education, 52,* 29–38. doi:10.3928/01484834-20121212-02

Di Leonardi Case, B., & Oermann, M. H. (2010). Clinical teaching and evaluation. In L. Caputi (Ed.), *Teaching nursing: The art and science* (2nd ed., pp. 82–141). Glen Ellyn, IL: College of DuPage.

Dolansky, M. A., & Moore, S. M. (2013). Quality and Safety Education for Nurses (QSEN): The key is systems thinking. *Online Journal of Issues in Nursing, 18*(3), Manuscript 1. doi:10.3912/OJIN.Vol18No03Man01

Drenkard, K. N. (2015). The power of alignment: Educating nurses in quality and safety. *Nursing Administration Quarterly, 39,* 272–277. doi:10.1097/NAQ.0000000000000112

Flood, L. S., Gasiewicz, N., & Delpier, T. (2010). Integrating information literacy across a BSN curriculum. *Journal of Nursing Education, 49,* 101–104. doi:10.3928/01484834-20091023-01

Giddens, J. F., North, S., Carlson-Sabelli, L., Rogers, E., & Fogg, L. (2012). Using a virtual community to enhance cultural awareness. *Journal of Transcultural Nursing, 23,* 198–204. doi:10.1177/1043659611434061

Gigante, J., Dell, M., & Sharkey, A. (2011). Getting beyond "good job": How to give effective feedback. *Pediatrics, 127,* 205–207. doi:10.1542/peds.2010-3351

Hall, M. A. (2013). An expanded look at evaluating clinical performance: Faculty use of anecdotal notes in the U.S. and Canada. *Nurse Education in Practice, 13,* 271–276.

Hall, M. A., Daly, B. J., & Madigan, E. A. (2010). Use of anecdotal notes by clinical nursing faculty: A descriptive study. *Journal of Nursing Education, 49,* 156–159. doi:10.3928/01484834-20090915-03

Hawala-Druy, S., & Hill, M. H. (2012). Interdisciplinary: Cultural competency and culturally congruent education for millennials in health professions. *Nurse Education Today, 32,* 772–778. doi:10.1016/j.nedt.2012.05.002

Horsley, T. L., Reed, T., Muccino, K., Quinones, D., Siddall, V. J., & McCarthy, J. (2016). Developing a foundation for interprofessional education within nursing and medical curricula. *Nurse Educator, 41,* 234–238.

Interprofessional Education Collaborative. (2016). *Core competencies for interprofessional collaborative practice: 2016 update.* Washington, DC: Author.

McKeon, L. M., Norris, T., Cardell, B., & Britt, T. (2009). Developing patient-centered care competencies among prelicensure nursing students using simulation. *Journal of Nursing Education, 48,* 711–715. doi:10.3928/01484834-20091113-06

Oermann, M. H., & Gaberson, K. B. (2017). *Evaluation and testing in nursing education* (5th ed.). New York, NY: Springer Publishing.

Oermann, M. H., Yarbrough, S. S., Ard, N., Saewert, K. J., & Charasika, M. (2009). Clinical evaluation and grading practices in schools of nursing: National survey findings Part II. *Nursing Education Perspectives, 30,* 352–357.

Parsons, M. E., Hawkins, K. S., Hercinger, M., Todd, M., Manz, J. A., & Fang, X. (2012). Improvement in scoring consistency for the Creighton Simulation Evaluation Instrument. *Clinical Simulation in Nursing, 8*(6), e233–e238.

Phillips, J. M., Stalter, A. M., Dolansky, M. A., & Lopez, G. M. (2016). Fostering future leadership in quality and safety in health care through systems thinking. *Journal of Professional Nursing, 32,* 15–24. doi:10.1016/j.profnurs.2015.06.003

Quality and Safety Education for Nurses Institute. (2014). Competencies. Retrieved from http://qsen.org/competencies

Sherwood, G. (2012). Driving forces for quality and safety: Changing mindsets to improve health care. In G. Sherwood & J. Barnsteiner (Eds.), *Quality and safety in nursing: A competency approach to improving outcomes* (pp. 3–22). Oxford, UK: Wiley.

Sherwood, G., & Barnsteiner, J. (Eds.). (2012). *Quality and safety in nursing: A competency approach to improving outcomes.* Oxford, UK: Wiley.

Swan, B. A., Smith, K. A., Frisby, A., Shaffer, K., Hanson-Zalot, M., & Becker, J. (2013). Enhancing tablet technology in an undergraduate nursing program. *Nursing Education Perspectives, 34,* 192–193.

Tellez, M. (2012). Nursing informatics education past, present, and future. *Computers, Informatics, Nursing, 30,* 229–233. doi:10.1097/NXN.0b013e3182569f42

Walsh, T., Jairath, N., Paterson, M., & Grandjean, C. (2010). Quality and safety education for nurses clinical evaluation tool. *Journal of Nursing Education, 49,* 517–522. doi:10.3928/01484834-20100630-06

Zurmehly, J. (2010). Personal digital assistants (PDAs): Review and evaluation. *Nursing Education Perspectives, 31,* 179–182.

Curriculum Development and
Evaluation of Nursing Program

The Context in Which Teaching Takes Place: The Curriculum

SARAH B. KEATING

OBJECTIVES

- Analyze the processes of curriculum development and revision and related role of the nurse educator
- Evaluate the major components of an existing curriculum, their interrelationships, and how they influence the implementation and evaluation of the curriculum
- Consider the role of the nurse educator in securing and managing resources for the provision of a quality educational program

It is vital that nurse educators take into account the context in which teaching takes place. The curriculum provides that context with an overview of the mission or purpose of the program, its vision for the future, the values or philosophy that relate to its mission, and the ultimate goals for the program. Nurse educators and learners participating in the program should be familiar with the curriculum to appreciate the end goal and ensure the integrity of its mission.

Over the past decade, nursing education is changing in response to newer trends in health care and education, including the Affordable Care Act (ACA; U.S. Department of Health & Human Services, 2014), emphasis on patient-centered care that includes quality and safety, interprofessional collaboration, a focus on learner-centered strategies, and the influences of technology and simulated learning experiences. These forces call for curriculum transformation to change from the traditional content-laden program to concept-based frameworks for the preparation of professionals capable of critical thinking when providing competent and compassionate care. Phillips et al. (2013) studied schools of nursing, representing a variety of types of educational institutions including private, public, small, and large, that identified themselves as having innovative curricula. Based on the study's findings, the authors presented a model for curriculum transformation that incorporates some of the newer trends in education and health care, including evidence-based practice, a focus on quality and safety, and professional competency. The model includes recommendations from the Institute of Medicine (Committee on the Robert Wood Johnson Foundation Initiative on the Future of Nursing at the Institute of Medicine, 2011) report and standards from various professional organizations.

Often, rather than focusing on concept-based teaching and learning strategies, both new and experienced teachers focus on the specific content of the classes or sessions they teach and lose sight of the course objectives and how they relate to the overall program and curriculum. The temptation is to adjust the course objectives and content to the individual teacher's personal interests and expertise. Such changes can result in the loss of the program's intent and planned student learning outcomes. If a teacher identifies the need to update the content of a class and thus the objectives, it is important to compare the proposed change to the overall curriculum to discover its impact on the total program. Such changes can involve revision of the curriculum and, depending on the setting, include other members of the educational team. In the case of major changes, approval processes for the revisions might be necessary through the hierarchial structures in the involved nursing program or health care setting. These processes focus on curriculum revision. However, if the need is for a new curriculum or educational program, the processes become that of curriculum development.

This chapter describes the components and processes for curriculum development or revision for schools of nursing and for educational programs related to patient education and staff development in health care settings. To determine whether a curriculum needs revision or if a new program is proposed, a needs assessment is necessary to document the need. This chapter reviews the factors that influence educational programs and curricula and provides educators with guidelines for collecting and analyzing data to make informed decisions about revising or developing curricula.

To gain an appreciation of the connection of teaching to the curriculum or educational program, the components of the curriculum are described. The influence of the components on the teacher, student/learner, courses or classes, and related learning activities are considered. The importance of program and student learning outcomes and how they direct subsequent instructional strategies and ongoing evaluation of the program are also discussed. Though the setting can vary according to the type of educational program (e.g., schools of nursing or health care agencies), the same processes and components of the curriculum apply. Budget considerations are reviewed briefly as they apply to curriculum development and revision.

NEEDS ASSESSMENT

Developing a new educational program or revising an existing one calls for a needs assessment; that is, there must be compelling factors to cause the change or to create a new one. For the purposes of this text, a brief review of possible factors that influence change or the development of new programs in academic or health care settings is discussed as they apply to nurse educators who teach in these programs. Keating (2015) discusses in detail the external and internal frame factors that influence curriculum development and offers outlines for collecting and analyzing relevant data for making decisions related to this activity. Figures 15.1 and 15.2 present models of these external and internal factors.

FIGURE 15.1 External frame factors for a needs assessment for curriculum development in nursing.

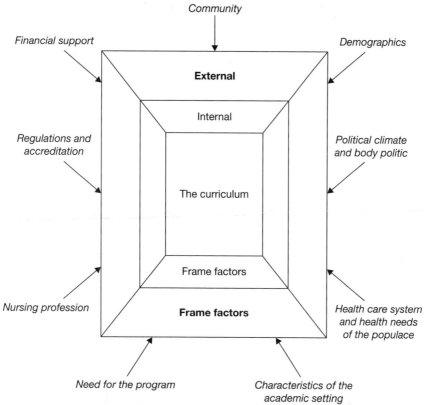

Source: Adapted from Johnson (1977). From Keating (2015). Reproduced with the permission of Springer Publishing.

Faculty members in the academic setting often see the need for revision or development of new programs within their schools of nursing. While the major functions of faculty may be those of teaching, research, and scholarly activities, service to the institution and community are also expectations. Service to the institution includes membership on curriculum committees and participation in level and course meetings that may lead to revision of the program. Members of committees, level and course coordinators, teachers, and administrators may identify the need for change to bring the curriculum up to date or to adjust learning objectives to improve student learning outcomes. All of these educators may also be aware of changes in nursing education or the health care system that call for new programs to meet the demands of the profession and needs of the population. In such instances, a new program is indicated.

Nursing educators in health care settings experience the same indicators for the need to change educational programs or create new ones in either staff development or patient education. While their central role may be teaching staff or patients, at the same time, they often recognize the need for new programs to update staff knowledge and skills or to educate patients on the newest treatment protocols and preventive health care strategies. The organizational structure is different from academic settings, but nurse educators in health care agencies also revise or create new programs and consult with other members of the organization, such as nurse administrators and managers, and other members of the multidisciplinary team.

FIGURE 15.2 Internal frame factors for a needs assessment for curriculum development in nursing.

Source: Adapted from Johnson (1977). From Keating (2015). Reproduced with the permission of Springer Publishing.

EXTERNAL FRAME FACTORS

No matter what the setting, the need for creation of new programs or revision of existing ones, the process for change is much the same. There are factors that influence the educational program and curriculum and indicate that a needs assessment is in order. External frame factors are those that are outside of the parent institution in which the program is housed, for example, the health care system and changes, nursing profession, community and population served by the institution, competitive schools or agencies, government and political bodies, and accrediting and program approval agencies. Table 15.1 provides examples of external frame factors influencing educational programs in academic and health care settings.

INTERNAL FRAME FACTORS

Internal frame factors are those that come from within the institution in which the educational program is housed. Like external frame factors, these influence the need for change or the creation of new programs. Nurse educators in academic setting, as contributing members to the school of nursing, participate on curriculum committees and other governance bodies within the school and the various levels of the institutional organization such as division or department curriculum or university-wide committees. Even faculty senates have influence and approval powers for curricula and their creation, revision, and/or discontinuance. The administrators of the institution also have influence; these persons include the president, vice president(s), provost, dean, associate deans, and chairs or directors of academic programs. All new programs must go through the appropriate echelons of approval bodies from the school or department faculty to the chief administrative officer. Major revisions experience the same approval processes as new programs. However, depending on the extent of the revision, such

TABLE 15.1 Sample External Frame Factors Influencing Educational Programs in Academic and Health Care Settings

External Frame Factor	Academic Settings	Health Care Settings
Health care system and changes in it	New technologies Changes in delivery of care (primary, acute, chronic care)	New technologies Health care demands: primary, secondary, tertiary
Nursing profession	Institute of Medicine calls for higher education Certification for advanced practice and leadership roles	Orientation needs Skills updates Continuing education requirements Role of nurse educators in patient education
Community and population served	Role of school of nursing in providing nursing workforce locally, regionally, and nationally Population health care needs, e.g., geriatrics, major causes of morbidity and mortality, health promotion and maintenance, etc.	Rural, suburban, urban Type of services (acute, tertiary, extended care, nursing home, rehabilitation, public health, home care, hospice, etc.) Population health care needs, e.g., geriatrics, major causes of morbidity and mortality, prevention, etc.
Competitive schools or agencies	Levels of nursing programs in direct competition Possibilities of collaboration Programs articulating with each other (e.g., associate degree leading into baccalaureate or master's programs)	Competitive agencies in the region Specialty units Possibilities for collaboration
Government and political bodies	Involvement in political activities that support higher education Awareness of financial programs that support student financial aid, program development, and research	Regulations governing health care services at state and national levels Medicare and Medicaid reimbursement policies Health insurance and other payers for health care services Regulations affecting professional practice
Accrediting and program approval agencies	Commission on Collegiate Nursing Education, Accreditation Commission for Education in Nursing, or Commission for Nursing Education Accreditation Regional accreditation Specialty accreditation Board of nursing approval	The Joint Commission Community-based accreditation and by specialty Board approval Government regulations

as minor changes to course objectives, approval at higher levels may not be necessary; only the curriculum committee in the school and/or faculty approval may be required. Internal frame factors in the academic setting include organizational and administrative structures, physical plant and resources, budget, faculty and staff numbers and qualifications, faculty governance, and the student body and characteristics.

Internal frame factors that influence health care settings are similar to those in academic settings. The cost and benefits of educational programs for patients and staff development influence the creation and revision of the curricula. Other factors are the type of organization (e.g., public or private, religion-based or nonsectarian, profit or nonprofit); administrative structure; physical plant; budget; nature of the staff, both professional and nonprofessional; governance; and characteristics of the population served. Table 15.2 provides examples of internal frame factors influencing academic and health care settings.

TABLE 15.2 Sample Internal Frame Factors Influencing Educational Programs in Academic and Health Care Settings

Internal Frame Factor	Academic Settings	Health Care Settings
Organizational and administrative structures (public or private; religion based or nonsectarian)	Place of nursing program within the institution (layers of decision making) Sources of funding (e.g., state, tuition, endowments, etc.)	Place of education within agency, power structure, person(s) to whom the educator reports Agency structure (e.g., independent, part of a health care system, governmental agency, etc.) Funding sources
Physical plant and resources	Faculty offices, classroom, labs, conference rooms, media supplies, and services Library and other support	Audiovisual materials, learning labs, classrooms, conference rooms, Internet access and support Supplies and services
Budget	Control for forecasting needs and expenditures External funding resources Scholarship and research support	Cost of program and benefit analysis Control for forecasting needs and expenditures
Governance	Faculty involvement Student representation	Place of educational program in the agency Educator involvement in governance
Nature of the staff both professional and nonprofessional	Faculty numbers and qualifications Support staff adequacy	Qualifications and experience of educators Staff support adequacy
Characteristics of the population served	Student body Community served by the students and faculty	Patient population Staff: nursing and other providers of care
Internal program approval	Periodic review by institution: frequency	Administrators Advisory Board

Nurse educators should be aware of the environment in which they teach. As educational programs are implemented and the need for new ones is identified, persons who teach in the programs must be part of the processes for conducting a needs assessment and developing curriculum. While teaching dominates their activities, educators' involvement in the assessment contributes to dynamic, evolving, and quality programs.

COMPONENTS OF THE CURRICULUM

The following discussion describes the classical components of the curriculum that apply to both schools of nursing and health care agencies' educational programs. When developing or revising curricula, the importance of involving key stakeholders in the process so that schools and health agencies respond to the health care needs of the community cannot be overemphasized. Four major statements—the mission, vision, values (philosophy), and goals—provide an overview of the educational program and directions for its implementation. The process comes full cycle by using the content in the statements as guidelines for continuous quality improvement and summative evaluation on how well the program is performing. Gurley, Peters, Collins, and Fifolt (2015) reviewed the literature related to the mission, vision, values, and goals of an educational program. Their review produced clear definitions of the four guiding statements of the curriculum that are useful to faculty in the process of revision or development.

Briefly, the four major statements are:

1. The *mission statement* declares the purpose of the program.
2. The *vision statement* encompasses the future expectations of the graduates of the school or the health care agency's role in health care.
3. The *values (philosophy) statement* describes the faculty/educators' philosophy about teaching and learning, health care, the profession, diversity, social justice, and so on.
4. The *end-of-program goals* describe the final product (graduate) of the program based on the mission, vision, and values of the program.

A conceptual or organizational framework follows the four statements; integrates the beliefs, theories, and concepts described in the statements; and delineates the learning outcomes to meet the specified program goals. The learning outcomes are stated in measurable objectives that lead to an implementation plan that includes a list of courses or learning sessions. These courses or sessions start with objectives that serve as guidelines to measure learning outcomes derived from the goals of the program. To implement the curriculum, teachers further develop the courses and sessions into course content, learning activities, and assessment and evaluation activities to measure learning outcomes according to the objectives.

MISSION AND VISION STATEMENTS

MISSION

The mission or purpose of the curriculum or educational program must align with the mission and vision of the parent institution. Therefore, educators should evaluate how congruent the mission of their program is with the parent's. Nursing programs in academic settings may be within institutions that are private or state supported, research extensive or intensive, liberal arts or professional focus, secular or nonsecular, or academic health science centers. Levi (2012) examined the three major roles of faculty—teaching, scholarship/research, and service—and compared them to the missions of institutions according to their purpose. The roles of faculty differ across the type and mission of the institution. For example, the research mission and faculty's role in research and scholarship have more emphasis in health sciences institutions than in associate degree programs, where the teaching mission and faculty role as teachers have greater emphasis.

The nature of the parent institution and therefore that of nursing will determine the mission of the program. Usually, the institutional mission is broad enough for professional programs to fit under its rubric. For example, a state university might have as its mission "To provide excellent teaching, research, and service." It explains further each of these three areas and includes its definition of "excellent." A school of nursing in such an institution has wide latitude in interpreting and applying these three areas to nursing. It might have a mission statement such as: "To provide a high quality education that prepares professional, scholarly nurses to serve the health care needs of the population." A health care system might have as its mission "Patient care, research, education, and service." Again, nursing education in this institution can focus on any one or all four of these elements depending on the purpose of the educational program. An example of a mission of the education department in such an agency is: "The education program promotes safe and high quality health care services for its patients through well-prepared professional and ancillary staff, patient education, and interprofessional scholarship and research."

VISION

The vision statement presents the institution's aspirations for the future and is based on the stakeholders' reflections about what they believe is the institution's role in education or health care services and its relationship to the health care system. Using the previous examples of mission statements, the vision statement for the school of nursing might be: "Graduates of the nursing program contribute to the improvement of the health care system through the provision of knowledgeable, safe, compassionate, and high quality patient care." The education department in the health care agency's vision might state: "The education department contributes to the agency's vision through state-of-the-art, safe, and high quality patient care services by assuring well qualified and knowledgeable staff."

When developing or revising mission and vision statements, educators should examine trends in the health care system, higher education, and the needs of populations they serve, both students and patients. Several articles from the literature discuss these trends, their effect on current programs, and the need to respond to them in order to offer programs that are state-of-the art and look to the future. Not responding to changes can result in antiquated educational programs that fail to meet the needs of those they serve.

Washington, Coye, and Feinberg (2013) describe the need for academic health science centers to respond to trends in the health care system. Through reflection and leadership, they advise that missions can be reconfigured to include patient-centered care and population health. Additionally, they point out that there is a need to use the mass of health data generated from new information systems for research and the development of new models of health care. Khatri (2014) discusses the impact of the health care system's transformation as a result of the ACA on the need for health care agencies to have missions that are comprehensive, are team-based, and provide coordinated, accessible, and quality care for patients.

PHILOSOPHY AND VALUES

As with mission and vision statements, a philosophy or values statement describes the beliefs of the members of the institution and significance of these beliefs toward reaching the final goal. The statements contain additional theories and concepts that guide the development of the curriculum or education program. In schools of nursing, central theories and concepts can include faculty's beliefs about teaching and learning, social justice, diversity, health and illness, and professional values, among others. Health care agencies develop philosophy or values statements that expound on their missions and visions to further explain the rationale and purpose for their services to the community and what is unique about them. Conger, Knuth, and McDonald (2014) describe a health care system that created a culture for values measurement to shape the mission and goals of the institution. In addition, an executive dashboard was developed that serves to assess agency performance on goals that promote a high level of quality care and are part of its mission.

Nurse educators are essential to the development of philosophy and value statements and their realization. Educators meet to discuss their personal beliefs about the educational program and come to consensus to produce a statement that reflects their values and ethics and the critical concepts and theories used in the program to deliver the program or curriculum. Nurses considering education positions or those in current teaching positions should review the philosophy/values statements of their institutions to ensure congruence with their personal and professional beliefs and values. If conflict is discovered, the issues should be discussed with others to possibly review the statement, or if incongruity exists and cannot be changed, the individual should consider finding a position in a program that holds similar values and beliefs.

OVERALL PROGRAM GOALS AND PURPOSE

Based on the mission and/or vision, the philosophy/values statements, the purpose of the program, and an overall goal(s) set the stage for defining the specific student learning outcomes, objectives, or competencies that the curriculum or educational program purports to achieve. The literature has many terms for signifying educational goals or aims, objectives, and the steps for completing them. Most nurse educators express the steps toward achieving desired learning outcomes in behaviorally stated objectives. The advantage to this format is the ability to measure the outcomes and therefore, assess and evaluate the success of the program. For the purposes of this chapter, goals are identified as the overall aims or purpose of the program, and program learning outcomes are a description of the product of the program, that is, what the graduate or participant in the program will achieve and in nursing terms, practice.

ORGANIZATIONAL/CONCEPTUAL FRAMEWORK

When developing or revising a program, participants in the change process should review the philosophy/values statement to assure that it includes current beliefs and that the major concepts and theories that apply to the program are present. From the mission, vision, philosophy, and purpose/goals statements, an organizational framework serves as the scaffolding for the curriculum. The framework is essential to integration of the theories and concepts in the statements and serves as an outline upon which to build the learning outcomes, objectives, courses or sessions, and content into a plan for delivering the program. Professional and accreditation standards often serve as frameworks. Examples in health care agencies might include standards defined by The Joint Commission, state regulations, and professional organizations. Another example in health care for patient education is the American Cancer Society's (2016) Guidelines on Nutrition and Physical Activity for Cancer Prevention.

Some schools of nursing use accreditation standards as organizational frameworks. These include the Accreditation Commission for Education in Nursing (ACEN; 2016), Commission on Collegiate Nursing Education (CCNE; American Association of College of Nursing [AACN], 2017a), or Commission for Nursing Education Accreditation (CNEA; National League for Nursing, 2015) standards and criteria. Many baccalaureate and higher degree programs integrate the AACN's Essentials of Baccalaureate Education for Professional Nursing Practice, of Master's Education in Nursing, and Doctoral Education for Advanced Nursing Practice as frameworks (AACN, 2017b).

Both schools of nursing and health care agencies sometimes use nursing and health-related models or theories as a framework on which to organize the program; for example, systems theory, health-belief models, stress and adaptation, and health-illness continuum. McCovery and Matusitz (2014) used Systems Theory to analyze U.S. health care delivery. Their work illustrates how a theory can be applied to an organization to assess its functioning and the components that contribute to its functioning and overall purpose. Their analysis serves as an example for how theory can serve as a framework for an educational program. Tables 15.3 and 15.4 are examples of organizational frameworks in a health care setting and a school of nursing.

Organizational frameworks, in addition to providing guidelines for the program, also provide a framework for assessment of student learning outcomes and evaluation of the program. For example, educators can return to the framework to ascertain the presence of certain concepts; find their location in the program; identify the objectives, content, and learning activities associated with them; and analyze the level of achievement that students reach in meeting the relevant objectives.

TABLE 15.3 Organizational Framework for a Health Care Agency Educational Program for Cancer Prevention: Target Population, Grades Kindergarten to Sixth (K–6) Grade

ACS Guideline	End-of-Program Goal	Patient Education Objectives
Achieve and maintain a healthy weight throughout life	The majority of children (80%) in grades K–6 will achieve and maintain recommended weight for age and height.	Children will: Describe the benefits of healthy weight over a lifetime. Exhibit healthy eating behaviors. Achieve recommended weight for age and height.
Be physically active	Children in grades K–6 will participate in daily physical activities.	Children will: Describe the benefits of daily physical activity. Participate in physical activities in school, at home, and in the community.
Eat a healthy diet with an emphasis on plant foods	At least 80% of children in grades K–6 will consume healthy diets in the home, school, and community environments.	Children will: Describe healthy diets by listing healthy foods with an emphasis on plant foods.

(continued)

TABLE 15.3 Organizational Framework for a Health Care Agency Educational Program for Cancer Prevention: Target Population, Grades Kindergarten to Sixth (K–6) Grade (*continued*)

ACS Guideline	End-of-Program Goal	Patient Education Objectives
		Children will be provided with healthy foods at school and during community events.
		Parents of children K–6 will attend nutrition classes sponsored by the school.
Public, private, and community organizations work together to apply policy and environmental changes that promote cancer prevention behaviors	Schools, parent–teacher organizations, the local health department, and ACS will work together to apply policy and environmental changes that promote cancer prevention behaviors.	A community advisory board will be organized to initiate healthy eating and physical activities for school-aged children.
		The advisory board will collaborate with the health care agency in implementing multipronged educational programs in the community to promote healthy eating and physical activity for school-aged children.

ACS, American Cancer Society.

Source: Adapted from American Cancer Society (2016).

TABLE 15.4 Organizational Framework for an Associate Degree Nursing Program Curriculum Based on ACEN Accreditation Standards 4.1 and 4.5

Standard	End-of-Program Objective	Year 1 Objectives	Year 2 Objectives
4.1 Consistent with cotemporary practice, the curriculum incorporates established professional standards, guidelines, and competencies, and has clearly articulated student learning and program outcomes	The graduate will incorporate ethical, professional standards and competencies in the provision of nursing care.	The student will analyze professional nursing standards and their relationship to ethical nursing care.	The graduate will incorporate ethical, professional standards and competencies in the provision of nursing care.

(continued)

TABLE 15.4 Organizational Framework for an Associate Degree Nursing Program Curriculum Based on ACEN Accreditation Standards 4.1 and 4.5 (*continued*)

Standard	End-of-Program Objective	Year 1 Objectives	Year 2 Objectives
4.5 The curriculum includes cultural, ethnic, and socially diverse concepts and may also include experiences from regional, national, or global perspectives.	The graduate will provide culturally competent nursing care for ethnically and socially diverse populations.	The student will: Analyze ethically, culturally, and socially characteristics in the patient population served by nursing. Recognize differences in populations served. Adapt nursing care according to the cultural needs of the patients served.	The graduate will provide culturally competent nursing care for ethnically and socially diverse populations.

ACEN, Accreditation Commission for Education in Nursing.
Source: Adapted from ACEN (2016).

IMPLEMENTATION PLAN

PROGRAM, LEVEL, AND STUDENT LEARNING OUTCOMES

To carry out the educational program or the curriculum, an implementation plan must be organized according to the program goals and program learning outcomes. To reach these outcomes, a series of steps is necessary to assist the learner to progress through the program and reach the ultimate goals. Learning outcomes are the objectives or steps the learner takes to reach the outcomes and goals of the program. Multiple texts and articles in the literature provide educators with steps for developing objectives or student learning outcomes.

Dickerson (2016) discusses the recent changes taking place in nursing credentialing regarding a focus from behaviorally stated objectives to learning outcomes. She argues that outcomes should pose the question as to what is expected of the learner. The taxonomies are still useful in determining the level of learning that takes place and its impact on practice; for example, understanding/comprehension of a clinical situation leading to analysis, critical thinking, and application for the provision of individualized patient care. An example of the utilization of core competencies and standards for the development of learning outcomes/objectives is presented by Herr et al. (2015). The authors give examples of how core competencies and other organizational and accreditation standards for pain management can be integrated into prelicensure curricula in the form of learning outcomes and objectives.

For a school of nursing, the curriculum may be divided into segments according to the level of progress toward the final year such as the sophomore, junior, and senior years. For a health care agency, the program may be self-contained and consist of only one session or multiple sessions depending upon the target audience. For example, in staff development, an orientation program may consist of guiding new employees in learning about the organization's mission and philosophy, familiarizing them with policies and procedures, reviewing the necessary skills to assure the employees' competency and patient safety, and assigning them to mentors. In these examples, the program learning outcomes are listed and filter down to the various levels of the program. Table 15.5 provides an example of a program learning outcome in a baccalaureate curriculum as it is tracked from the end of the program, through the senior, junior, and sophomore levels to course objectives at each level.

TABLE 15.5 Sample Tracking of a Program Learning Outcome in a Baccalaureate Nursing Program

Student Learning Outcomes (SLOs)	Relevant Course Number and SLOs
Senior-Level SLO	**N400 Community Health Nursing:**
Provide evidence-based therapeutic nursing interventions for culturally diverse patients and families in a wide variety of health care and community settings.	Demonstrate evidence-based practice in nursing interventions for patients, families, and communities. Apply culturally competent nursing care concepts to the care of patients, families, and communities in the community setting.
Junior-Level SLO	**N300 Nursing Care of Adults in Acute Care:**
Integrate evidence-based therapeutic nursing interventions into the care of ethnically and culturally diverse patients and families.	Analyze evidence-based concepts into the nursing process and the delivery of therapeutic nursing interventions for patients and families. Implement culturally competent nursing care in the acute care setting.
Sophomore-Level SLO	**N200 Introduction to Professional Nursing:**
Develop nursing care plans that reflect evidence-based practice and therapeutic interventions in the care of ethnically and culturally diverse patients.	Describe the concept of evidence-based practice. Describe the nursing process and therapeutic nursing interventions. Compare ethnically and culturally diverse patient groups and their health care needs.

Program Learning Outcome: The graduate will provide evidence-based therapeutic nursing interventions for culturally diverse patients and families in a wide variety of health care and community settings.

A familiarity with educational taxonomies is helpful when assessing or developing objectives to fit the level of learner as illustrated in the table. Note that the novice learner objectives use terms such as "describes," the intermediate "integrates," and the senior "provides." Once the level objectives are identified, course or session objectives with their sequencing fall into place. This becomes the "plan of study." Exhibit 15.1 is an example of a program of study for a master's nursing program, and Exhibit 15.2 is a sample staff orientation program.

The final step in curriculum development following the plan and sequencing of courses or sessions is to develop outlines for the course or session. Briefly, the classic components for a course description in an academic setting usually include a number with a prefix that indicates its discipline (e.g., NURS 100 for a nursing course). Following the identifier, the title of the course introduces the major concepts taught in the course (e.g., NURS100 Introduction to Professional Nursing). A brief description is listed, typically comprised of no more than three sentences, which captures the essence of the course. For example, the description of

EXHIBIT 15.1 Sample Program of Study for a Master of Science in Nursing Administration Program

Year 1	
Fall Semester	**Spring Semester**
• Theoretical and Scientific Foundations of Nursing (3) • Introduction to Quantitative and Qualitative Statistics (3) • Research in Nursing (3)	• Analysis of Health Care Organizations (3) • Health Care Policy and Political Action (3) Nursing Leadership Strategies (3)

Year 2	
Fall Semester	**Spring Semester**
• Informatics and Technology in Health Care Systems (3) • Health Care Economics (3) • Administration Role Development and Practicum I (2) • Nursing Project or Thesis Proposal (1)	• Human Resources and Budget Management (3) Administration Role Development and Practicum II (2) • Nursing Project or Thesis Defense (4)

Total Credits: 36

EXHIBIT 15.2 Sample Program of Study for a 6-Month Staff Orientation Program in an Acute Care Hospital With Responsible Parties

Month 1

- *Week 1:* Class: Description of mentoring program and assignment to mentor for observational experiences: educator and mentors
- *Week 2:* Class: Mission, vision, and philosophy of the agency: chief executive officer, chief nursing officer, chief operations officer

Patient care assignments to continue throughout the 6 months with the assigned mentor

- *Week 3:* Class: Agency personnel policies: human resources staff
- *Week 4:* Class: General agency policies and procedure: educator

Month 2

- *Weeks 1 and 2:* Class and lab practice: Skills competencies assessment and updating: educator
- *Weeks 3 and 4:* Class: Policies and procedures specific to assigned unit: educator and mentor

Month 3

- *Weeks 1 and 2:* Class and lab practice: Skills competencies assessment and updating: educator
- *Weeks 3 and 4:* Meeting: Performance assessment for probationary period: educator and mentor

(continued)

EXHIBIT 15.2 Sample Program of Study for a 6-Month Staff Orientation Program in an Acute Care Hospital With Responsible Parties (*continued*)

Month 4

- *Weeks 1 and 2:* Class and lab practice: Skills remediation and updating: educator
- *Weeks 3 and 4:* Staff governance participation: educator

Month 5

- *Weeks 1 and 2:* Class: Review of agency and unit policies and evaluation of orientation program: educator. (Weeks 3 and 4: patient care assignment)

Month 6

- *Weeks 1 and 2:* Meeting: Final performance assessment for probationary period: educator and mentor

NURS100 is: "Describes nursing as a profession, its history, and its role in the inter-disciplinary health care system." Course objectives follow and should align with level and program student learning outcomes. Using NURS100 as an exemplar, one objec-tive might be: "Compares the profession of nursing to the definition of a profession." A content outline follows that contains the topics specific to the objectives and time-frames when they are introduced, discussed, and assessed. The learning activities associated with the objectives and content accompany the topical outline and include such strategies as discussion, lecture, group activities, role-play, and assignments. The methods for measuring student progress toward meeting the learning outcomes are provided, and their contributions to the course grade are listed. These include quiz-zes, tests, essays, and participation in discussions, among others. Finally, statements on academic dishonesty and provisions for disability are reiterated according to aca-demic polices.

Parallel descriptions for courses and sessions apply to the health care setting. At the very least, the session should include the title for the session, a brief description, the expected learning outcomes/objectives, a topical outline, the timeframe, and a descrip-tion of the learning activities such as demonstration, practice, lecture, group work, and so on. A statement on how the outcomes and effectiveness of the session will be mea-sured should be mentioned, such as a quiz or ratings of the session according to objec-tives and teaching effectiveness.

CONCEPT OR CONTENT MAPPING

It is helpful for educators to review the curriculum or program as-a-whole to ensure that certain concepts or content critical to delivering the program are covered in the imple-mentation of the program. To accomplish this task, it is useful to create content or concept maps that trace the concept throughout the program. Levin, Swider, Breakwell, Cowell, and Reising (2013) present an example of a cross-mapping process to assess a curricu-lum for community-based nursing in home health, school health, occupational health, and environmental health according to competencies, standards, and scope of practice as defined by professional organizations. Their work led to the development of a compe-tency-based, advanced practice public health nursing doctoral program.

Novak and Cañas (2016) provide an extensive discussion on the purpose of concept maps, the theory underlying them, and how to construct them. Figure 15.3 provides an example of a simplified concept map that traces the concept of social justice in a nursing curriculum.

FIGURE 15.3 Sample concept map of social justice content in a baccalaureate nursing curriculum.

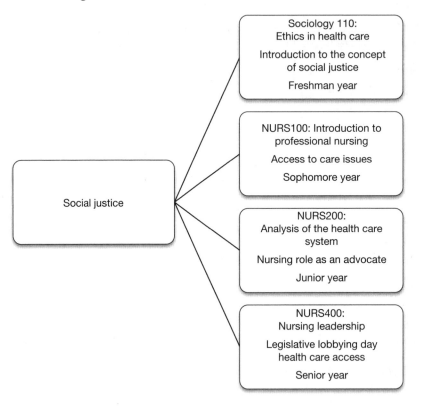

BUDGET CONSIDERATIONS

BUDGETS IN THE ACADEMIC SETTING

While teachers are not directly involved in the process of budget planning or management, they should have an appreciation for its place in developing and revising educational programs and curricula. In an academic setting, the dean or director of the school, college, or department of nursing usually has control over budget development and requests for funds to run the program. The dean or director also estimates additional budget items to supplement normal expenditures. The everyday costs to implement a curriculum include faculty and staff salaries; equipment and supplies; technology; computer hardware and software for faculty, staff, and classroom support; simulation and other skills lab equipment and supplies; faculty development activities, including research, scholarly activities, and travel; and the physical facilities such as offices, classrooms, conference rooms, labs, and so on. Additional funding beyond the usual includes the costs associated with program development and revision, such as released time for faculty members involved in the process and additional office supplies to support the development activities. Periodic program approval and accreditation expenses are part of the budget as well, including accreditation fees and, similar to program approval, release time for faculty and staff and the additional associated materials. These costs are some examples of the costs for maintaining a nursing program in the academic setting and are not necessarily complete.

Forecasting budget needs for the future, as well as decisions about the expenditures and maintenance of the budget, is usually within the dean's or director's prerogative; however, these functions can differ according to the organizational structure and political climate of the institution within which the program is housed. Size of the program also influences how the budget is administered; for example, in small programs the dean or director may be solely responsible for planning, requesting, expending, maintaining, and reporting on the budget. Larger programs may have an administrative assistant or staff to whom the dean delegates budget responsibilities.

Sources of funding are critical to the life of the program and the assurance of the quality of the program. In large multipurpose colleges and universities, nursing programs are often targeted as expensive owing to the clinical nature of the program and the low student-to-faculty ratio required for safe clinical supervision of students. Nursing's reply to these challenges usually points out that nursing students and their prerequisites from the sciences and liberal arts provide many full-time equivalents (FTEs) for the other disciplines.

Funding for the program is dependent on the nature of the parent institution: for example, income from general funds and tuition if state-supported, or tuition and endowment funds for private schools. All programs, whether state-funded or private, cannot rely solely on these sources of funds and thus, grants, donations in the form of endowments and scholarships, and some revenue-generating opportunities are sought. Faculty members are involved in these activities such as grant writing, with release time for research and program development as rewards if the grants are funded. Revenue-generating programs include faculty practice clinics with Medicare, Medicaid, and health care insurance reimbursement funding. Charging student laboratory fees to cover costs and special tuition rates through continuing education are additional sources of funds to pay for the cost of supplies and services and faculty and staff salaries.

All of these factors point out the need for faculty members to be aware of the sources of funding and the costs to run the educational program. Many deans and directors share budget planning and spending with faculty to involve them in the process and seek their input on cost savings and revenue generation. Such activities contribute to an appreciation of the budget and its influence on the implementation and quality of the program.

BUDGETS IN THE HEALTH CARE SETTING

Financial support for staff development and/or patient education varies widely in health care agencies. Depending on the size of the institution, its purpose, and its sources of funding, the budget for educational services may be set aside separately or as part of another department within the agency. Large medical centers and academic health science centers usually have an educational department staffed by nurse and other educators who have expertise in developing programs and teaching. Services include staff development, orientation of new staff, and patient education. A nurse or health educator may serve as the educator and also as coordinator for the programs with staff nurses, physicians, and other health care professionals teaching in the program. The budget for this type of structure is usually within the agency's overall budget or set aside to target specific educational services. In larger institutions, the education department may be composed of several staff members and coordinated by a manager who has administrative support staff. Budget responsibilities fall to the manager of the program, who accounts for staff salaries and benefits, office supplies and services, media and computer hardware and software, and associated facilities such as conference rooms, classrooms, and laboratories.

The educator's role is to make the case for educational needs in the agency and the associated costs for their delivery. Cost savings realized by the implementation of educational programs for staff and patients provide a significant rationale for the existence of the program. Larger institutions may have several educators on staff with administrative assistant support. Smaller institutions must depend upon an individual staff member's identification of educational needs, development of programs, and program implementation. Costs associated with these activities are absorbed into the time spent in delivering the services as a part of the care provided. Health departments and other governmental agencies use general funds to pay for educational programs. Again, depending on size, there may be dedicated nurse or health educators to provide patient education services and staff development/orientation as indicated. If it is a large department within the agency, the chief coordinator of the education department is responsible for the budget, while smaller agencies may depend upon separate requests to the agency administrator for the educational program. Nonprofit agencies in the community also provide patient education services. These agencies rely upon donations, endowments, and, to some extent, fees for services. The agencies may employ nurses or health educators or integrate the services into the specific care services that they provide.

As with academic settings, it is necessary for the nurse educator to document the need for education, justify its expense, and manage the funds that are provided. While educational services in health care settings are vital to maintain a competent staff and provide preventive and health maintenance educational services for patients, the importance of education is often lost. Nurses in these settings have a responsibility to bring the need to the attention of the administrators and public so that budgets for the services can be developed that are reasonable in cost, justify their need, result in cost savings and quality of patient care, and are sustainable over time.

SUMMARY

Chapter 15 reviewed the role of educators in schools of nursing and health care agencies in the context of the educational programs in which they teach. It compared the differences between curriculum development and revision and pointed out the necessity for examining the external and internal frame factors that influence change or the creation of new program. The chapter examined the major components of the curriculum, their interrelationships, and the implementation of the curriculum and its evaluation. Concept and content maps illustrate how nurse educators can track concepts or content throughout the curriculum to ensure their presence in levels of the program. The chapter also included brief overviews of the budget process for programs in both academic and health care settings.

REFERENCES

Accreditation Commission for Education in Nursing. (2016). *Accreditation manual: 2017 standards and criteria, associate. Standard 4.1 and 4.5.* Retrieved from http://www.acenursing.org/accreditation-manual

American Association of Colleges of Nursing. (2017a). *CCNE accreditation.* Retrieved from http://www.aacn.nche.edu/ccne-accreditation

American Association of Colleges of Nursing. (2017b). *Essentials series*. Retrieved from http://www .aacn.nche.edu/education-resources/essential-series

American Cancer Society. (2016). *Stay healthy: ACS guidelines on nutrition and physical activity for cancer prevention*. Retrieved from http://www.cancer.org/Healthy/EatHealthyGetActive/ ACSGuidelinesonNutritionPhysicalActivityforCancerPrevention/index

Conger, M., Knuth, M., & McDonald, J. (2014). Creating a culture for value measurement. *Health Care Financial Management, 68*, 54–62.

Committee on the Robert Wood Johnson Foundation Initiative on the Future of Nursing at the Institute of Medicine. (2011). *The future of nursing: Leading change, advancing health*. Washington, DC: National Academies Press.

Dickerson, P. S. (2016). Ditch the verb list? *Journal of Continuing Education in Nursing, 47*, 101–102. doi:10.3928/00220124-20160218-02

Gurley, D. K., Peters, G. B., Collins, L., & Fifolt, M. (2105). Mission, vision, values, and goals: An exploration of key organizational statements and daily practice in schools. *Journal of Educational Change, 16*, 217–242.

Herr, K., Marie, B. S., Gordon, D. B., Paice, J. A., Watt-Watson, J., Stevens, B. J., . . . Young, H. M. (2015). An interprofessional consensus of core competencies for prelicensure education in pain management: Curriculum application for nursing. *Journal of Nursing Education, 54*, 317–327. doi:10.3928/01484834-20150515-02

Johnson, M. (1977). *Intentionality in education*. Albany, NY: Center for Curriculum Research and Services.

Keating, S. B. (2015). *Curriculum development and evaluation in nursing* (3rd ed.). New York, NY: Springer Publishing.

Khatri, P. (2014). Health care reform, 2014: No matter what the question, mission is the answer. *Families, Systems, & Health, 32*, 253–255. doi:10.1037/fsh0000037

Levi, J. G. (2012). Three faculty communities. *Academe, 98*(1), 40–43.

Levin, P. F., Swider, S. M., Breakwell, S., Cowell, J. M., & Reising, V. (2013). Embracing a competency-based specialty curriculum for community-based nursing roles. *Public Health Nursing, 30*, 557–565. doi:10.1111/phn.12042

McCovery, J., & Matusitz, J. (2014). Assessment of collaboration in U.S. health care delivery: A perspective from systems theory. *Social Work and Public Health, 29*, 451–461. doi:10.1080/19371918.2013 .865109

National League for Nursing. (2015). CNEA mission and values. Retrieved from http://www.nln.org/ accreditation-services/the-nln-commission-for-nursing-education-accreditation-%28cnea%29

Novak, J. D., & Cañas. A. J. (2016). *The theory behind concept maps and how to construct them*. Retrieved from http://cmap.ihmc.us/publications/researchpapers/theorycmaps/theoryunderlyingconceptmaps.htm

Phillips, J. M., Resnick, J., Boni, P., Bradley, P., Grady, J. L., Ruland, J. P., & Stuever, N. L. (2013). Voices of innovation: Building a model for curriculum transformation. *International Journal of Nursing Education Scholarship, 10*. pii. doi:10.1515/ijnes-2012-0008

U.S. Department of Health & Human Services. (2014). *Key features of the Affordable Care Act*. Retrieved from http://www.hhs.gov/healthcare/facts-and-features/key-features-of-aca/index.html#

Washington, A. E., Coye, M. J., & Feinberg, D. T. (2013). Academic health centers and the evolution of the health care system. *Journal of the American Medical Association, 310*, 1929–1930. doi:10.1001/ jama.2013.282012

16
Curriculum Models and Development

THERESA M. "TERRY" VALIGA

OBJECTIVES

- Analyze the advantages, disadvantages, and implications of selected curriculum models for prelicensure nursing programs
- Interrelate the components of a curriculum to achieve internal consistency
- Examine how a course syllabus can be used to enhance student learning

Anyone who teaches in a nursing program is expected to implement the curriculum that has been approved by faculty, and in some instances faculty groups have the opportunity to engage in major revisions of a curriculum, the end result of which is the creation of a new "journey" to be experienced by students and faculty alike. This chapter is designed to help faculty consider various models for curriculum design, appreciate how essential it is for the curriculum to be internally consistent if students are to be successful in achieving stated program outcomes, and appreciate the significance of a course syllabus.

CURRICULUM MODELS

When starting the process of curriculum review, revision, and/or redesign, it is important for educators to consider a variety of models so that the decisions made are most appropriate for students served by the program, the context in which the program exists, the resources available to support implementation of the program, and the values expressed in the school's philosophy. The three basic models to consider are the parallel, building, and progressive, each of which is explored in terms of its advantages, disadvantages, and implications.

The *Parallel Model* (Figure 16.1) is designed so that students enroll in nursing and general education/support courses throughout their course of study. Although the figure suggests that the number of credits devoted to nursing and to general education/support courses are equal in each year of the program, that is not required;

in reality, the number of credits allotted to each category is likely to differ from year to year while remaining relatively balanced. The advantages of this model are that students are introduced to and engaged in nursing courses from the very beginning of the program, and they remain connected with nonnursing students, faculty, and concepts throughout their learning, rather than completing those requirements and never being challenged to think about or engage with them again. Disadvantages to this model are that unique nursing faculty resources are needed over a longer period of time, four cohorts of students are enrolled in nursing courses at any given time, and the realities of schedules for nonnursing courses may present challenges for students in the last 2 years as their clinical experiences are likely to increase. One significant implication of this model is that it challenges both faculty and students in nursing to continually reflect on why they are taking general education/support courses and how learning from those courses can be used to enhance learning of nursing concepts.

FIGURE 16.1 Parallel Curriculum Model for a 4-year baccalaureate program in nursing.

Year 1	Nursing Courses ↕	General Education & Support Courses ↕
Year 2		
Year 3		
Year 4		

The *Building Model* (Figure 16.2) is common in nursing programs today. It is designed so that students complete all their general education/support courses prior to starting nursing, and nursing courses are concentrated in the upper division (i.e., the junior and senior years). Advantages to this model are that all foundational courses in the biological and social sciences are completed before students begin nursing courses, and nursing faculty have the opportunity to be flexible about course schedules and clinical experiences because there is no need to accommodate other courses students might be taking. Despite these positives, the Building Model has disadvantages, including the fact that students learn foundational knowledge in isolation of nursing and, as a result, often do not see its relevance for the major they wish to pursue; students invest a great deal of time, effort, and money into building a foundation for a major they may decide is not for them; and finally, once students move into the junior year, they become somewhat isolated from students and faculty in nonnursing areas. When using this model, faculty may find that they need to review foundational knowledge (or provide students with resources to help them review relevant material on their own). Additionally, students often enroll in more than one clinical course each semester, which creates a "heavy load" for students and, often, difficulty in finding quality placements for those clinical experiences.

FIGURE 16.2 Building Curriculum Model for a 4-year baccalaureate program in nursing.

Year 1	General Education & Support Courses
Year 2	
Year 3	Nursing Courses
Year 4	

Finally, the *Progressive Model* (Figure 16.3) begins and ends the curriculum with both nursing and general education/support courses; however, the number of credits allocated to nursing increases over time, while those allocated to nonnursing courses decrease over time. This model introduces students to nursing early on, provides more time for students to learn nursing and address affective domain learning (which takes more time than cognitive or psychomotor learning), and keeps students "connected" with those outside the field, albeit to a decreasing extent over time. It also, however, requires careful planning, coordination with those in other departments, and precise course scheduling from beginning to end. In addition, nursing faculty resources need to be allocated over a larger number of courses and years. Similar to the Parallel Model, faculty involved with a Progressive Model are challenged to plan for and help students see the connections between what they are learning in nursing and what they are learning in other disciplines.

FIGURE 16.3 Progressive Curriculum Model for a 4-year baccalaureate program in nursing.

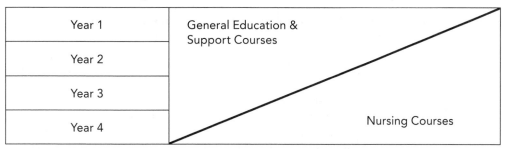

Some of the continua that faculty may choose to use to organize the nursing major include the following: concrete to abstract; experiences close to students' lives to those in the larger community; individual to group and community; simple to complex; and dependence to independence to interdependence. Such continua make sense and are familiar to many nursing faculty; however, we should question if they limit our creativity. For example, could it be appropriate for beginning students to have clinical experiences in an intensive care unit (ICU)? They would not be expected to provide patient care or take responsibility for any aspect of it, but they could carefully observe how nurses set priorities and make decisions, how the team functions, how the family is or is not involved, what the sounds are like, what the pace is like, what needs to be documented, what kinds of medications are used, how the patient's status is monitored, how the patient's emotional needs are addressed, and so on. Such an experience might serve to lay as strong a foundation for future learning and practice as does a clinical experience in a long-term care facility where students take vital signs, help one elderly resident with morning care, and learn about the resident's life history.

Regardless of the Curriculum Model chosen or the rationale used to organize it, it is critical that all components of the curriculum—from philosophy to conceptual framework to program outcomes and specific learning experiences in individual courses—are interrelated, logically organized, and internally consistent. Failing to do so can result in expressions of values and beliefs that are ignored, complex learning outcomes that are addressed only partially, core concepts that are attended to only haphazardly, repetition/duplication of topics addressed, and gaps in what students should be learning.

INTERRELATION AMONG CURRICULUM COMPONENTS

As noted in Chapter 15, curriculum design or revision takes place in a complex context that includes parent institution expectations, accreditation standards, available resources, regulatory requirements and professional standards, and student and faculty characteristics. Faculty often have no control or influence over many of these factors, but faculty *are* the ones who articulate the beliefs and values that guide the development of the curriculum, policies, student–teacher and student–student interactions, learning experiences, and so forth. Such beliefs and values are expressed in the school's statement of *philosophy*, a document that typically addresses what the faculty believe about human beings, health, society and the environment, the role of the nurse, and teaching/learning (Valiga, 2012). This is a critical document, not merely something that is written to please external evaluators and then allowed to "sit on a shelf." Instead, the philosophy should be reviewed, referenced, and reflected on often, as noted in the seminal work by Dickoff and James (1970), and appreciated for its significance in creating an evidence-based, context-relevant, unified curriculum (Iwasiw & Goldenberg, 2015). For example, if the philosophy indicates that faculty believe human beings are unique, want input to decisions that affect them, have potential, and are to be valued and respected regardless of their characteristics, faculty may need to remind themselves that students are human beings, as are faculty, and the uniqueness of each needs to be respected, each should be involved in decisions that affect them (such as course assignments, topics to be addressed in a course, or promotion and tenure criteria), and all have potential to grow and succeed.

Ideas expressed in the philosophy should highlight the core concepts that faculty will integrate throughout the curriculum: concepts which then serve as the *framework* for continued curriculum work. The curriculum framework might reflect a particular theory (e.g., stress/adaptation) or a particular nursing model (e.g., Orem's Self-Care Model), and a visual representing the framework might be rather complex (Boland, 2012). The framework, however, might also be a collection of core concepts expressed in the philosophy and depicted through a relatively simple visual representation. Figure 16.4 is an example of a visual depiction of one school's curriculum framework.

Once the core curriculum concepts are identified and defined by the school's faculty, they become the basis for formulating *program outcome*s, statements of what students are expected to know, be able to do, and value or appreciate on completion of the entire program and that serve as the basis for determining the effectiveness of the curriculum (Morin & Bellack, 2015; Payne & Mullen, 2014), as discussed in depth in Chapter 17. Since these statements reflect integration of learning throughout the program, they should be complex, multi-faceted, and comprehensive, not focused and specific as is the case for course objectives. Examples of prelicensure program outcomes are as follows:

> Make judgments in practice that synthesize nursing science and knowledge from other disciplines to provide safe, quality care; promote the health of diverse patients, families, and communities; and assist them to continually progress toward fulfillment of human capability.
>
> Use basic skills of negotiation, conflict resolution, team building, leadership and communication to engage in positive working relationships within an interprofessional healthcare team, and contribute a unique nursing perspective to care delivery.
>
> (Duke University School of Nursing, 2017. Reprinted with permission.)

Clarifying what the intended program outcomes are then allows faculty to formulate what are referred to as *level outcomes/objectives*. While program outcomes might

FIGURE 16.4 Visual representation of one school's curriculum framework.

Source: Duke University School of Nursing. Reprinted with permission.

be thought of as the final destination, level outcomes/objectives can be thought of as signposts or checkpoints along the way to that final destination. In other words, each level outcome/objective is focused, articulates what students are expected to have learned as a result of all the nursing courses taken in a particular level, and clarifies the progression of growth from beginning to end. Using the first program outcome noted earlier, the following level outcomes/objectives provide an example of signposts along the students' journey toward it:

Level I: Provide safe, quality care to diverse individuals who are essentially healthy or experiencing minor deviations in health.

Level II: Provide evidence-based, culturally-sensitive, and developmentally-appropriate care to diverse individuals and their families, as those individuals experience acute or chronic health deviations and strive to progress toward fulfillment of their human capability.

Level III: Collaborate with members of the health care team—including the patient and his family—to plan, implement, and evaluate the effectiveness of health promotion and disease management care provided to patients with complex health problems.

Level IV: Provide leadership within the nursing care team to plan, implement, and evaluate the effectiveness of care provided to groups of patients and their families. (Duke University School of Nursing, 2017. Reprinted with permission.)

A level is defined by the faculty in a particular school. It can be a semester, a year, three semesters, a 2-year block, or any other designation that makes sense to faculty. The important principle to keep in mind when defining a level is that the collection of courses and learning experiences in a particular level need to have some central theme or connection to one another that enables students to integrate what they are learning.

Using the previous example, the focus of Level I related to the core curriculum concept of Care Management is on safety and caring for essentially healthy individuals; students take courses in wellness, assessment, and homeostasis. In Level II, the focus is on individuals with acute or chronic illness, and students are expected to be more comprehensive in their approach to care by attending to evidence, cultural relevance, and developmental relevance in addition to safety; they take courses related to caring for women and children, pathophysiology, pharmacology, and evidence-based practice. Students in Level III focus on caring for patients with complex care needs and do that in collaboration with the health care team, which includes the patient/family. The collection of courses they take continues to address pathophysiology and pharmacology, caring for adults and elderly with complex health situations, and team collaboration. Finally, in Level IV, students are expected to provide some degree of leadership in their care settings to ensure quality care for groups and communities as well as for individuals. In addition to diverse clinical experiences, they take courses related to leadership and transition to practice.

Finally, it is important to emphasize that each course in a level does not need to address every core curriculum concept; if multiple concepts are addressed in a given course, the emphasis of each concept does not need to be equal to the emphasis on the others. For example, a clinical course is likely to emphasize concepts related to care management and collaboration. It also may address the concept of scholarship as students are challenged to consider the evidence that underlies their practice, but it is in the evidence-based practice course itself that students learn more details related to the concept of scholarship. In essence, then, it is critical to ensure that the *collection* of courses students take in a given level will help them meet the level outcomes/objectives.

Having identified the level outcomes/objectives, faculty then develop individual *courses*. The objectives for each course should clearly relate to the appropriate level outcome(s)/objective(s), reflect the foundational knowledge and skills that are identified as prerequisites, and serve to clearly distinguish one course from another. The *learning experiences* incorporated into each course should be appropriate to the nature of its objectives, and they should be varied to meet the diverse learning preferences of the student population (Billings, 2012). For example, the objectives for a course with a clinical component should not reflect only cognitive domain learning; instead, they also should reflect learning in the affective and psychomotor domains. Additionally, lecture should not be the only strategy used to facilitate learning, and multiple-choice tests should not be the only method used to assess student learning. The course syllabus is important because it provides further suggestions about course development.

THE COURSE SYLLABUS: A TOOL TO ENHANCE STUDENT LEARNING

Courses are the building blocks of the curriculum that incorporate and integrate the organized subject matter and related activities, including laboratory and clinical experiences, that are planned to help students achieve specific learning objectives. Although competency-based education (Goudreau et al., 2009) and the concept of learning badges (Gibson, Ostashewski, Flintoff, Grant, & Knight, 2015) challenge traditional ideas about what a course is, courses typically are offered within a given time period and have specific start and end dates.

Courses are influenced by the school's philosophy, conceptual framework, program outcomes, and level outcomes/objectives, and they are placed strategically to simultaneously build on prior knowledge and provide a foundation on which future learning and practice will be built. The essence of each course is reflected in the syllabus, which serves as an implied contract between the school of nursing and student (Comer, 2016; Zucker, Baker-Schena, & Pak, 2010).

Often, the syllabus is filled with an extensive amount of "legalese" that outlines consequences of missing class or submitting late papers, options for make-up tests, and similar situations. Although it is important to be clear about how such situations will be managed, Wasley (2008) warned against such practices and challenged faculty to consider whether the purpose of such "legalese" is to prepare students for the demands of the course or to protect the teacher.

Whetten (2007) noted that one of the most important aspects of teaching is our careful choice of reading materials, assignments, activities, and learning objectives, all of which are included in the syllabus. We should remember, therefore, that the syllabus gives clues to our personality and priorities, and it should facilitate learning and a positive learning environment, not turn the teacher–learner relationship into an adversarial one.

The well-designed syllabus clarifies the overall purpose and specific goals of the course, requirements students will be expected to fulfill, and general operating principles of the course (Scheckel, 2016). These principles might take the form of group norms, as described by Clark (2017), who urges nurse educators to engage in open discussions with learners to establish group norms that will ensure civil behaviors. Group norms might relate to the use of phones or computers during class, lateness, acknowledgement of contributions to the discussion, words to be used or avoided, respect, valuing various perspectives, how to manage disagreements, and so on. Once they are established and agreed on by all participants, they can be incorporated into the syllabus to ensure that all agree to adhere to and respect the norms established by the group. When things go wrong in a course, unclear expectations are almost always to blame; therefore, clarifying norms of behavior as well as the core purpose and requirements for a course can be critical to the success of that course.

The components of a well-crafted syllabus include the following:

- Course title, which should clarify its unique focus
- Course credits; how those credits are allocated among theory, clinical, and laboratory components; and what the hours:credit ratio is
- Prerequisites, or specific courses on which this one is built
- Corequisites, or courses that must be taken concurrently with this one
- An informative but succinct description that provides an overview of the intent of the course and addresses both theory and clinical components but does not outline specific teaching strategies or evaluation methods used
- The course objectives, which should reflect the curriculum concepts, be appropriate for the level of the learners, and build on previous knowledge.
- An outline of the topics to be addressed in the course and the sequence of those discussions
- The teaching and learning strategies to be used
- The evaluation methods used, with the percentage of final course grade for each specified
- Due dates
- Textbooks and other key resources

When deciding on the topics to be addressed, it is important to remember that nurse educators need to select carefully from an enormous number of possibilities. Thus, faculty need to acknowledge that they cannot "cover it all" and to select carefully so that the topics, as well as the teaching strategies and evaluation methods, help students achieve the specified objectives. Zaretsky (2012) urged faculty to look at the syllabus "through new eyes," and Whetten (2007) addressed this concern when he called for a paradigm shift regarding the course syllabus, asserting that we must move from a teacher-focused approach to a learner-focused one, the latter of which helps set the tone for learning (Bart, 2015). Figure 16.5 summarizes the differences in these approaches in terms of the overall focus, the role of the teacher, how success is determined, and assumptions about teaching.

FIGURE 16.5 Teacher-focused versus learner-focused syllabus.

Teacher-Focused Syllabus	Learner-Focused Syllabus
Focus	
• What teacher wants to teach • How teacher can cover the designated material	• What learners need to learn • How teachers and students can collaborate to accomplish specific learning objectives
Role of the Teacher	
• Provide/deliver instruction • Transfer knowledge to learners • Classify and sort	• Produce learning • Elicit learner discovery and knowledge creation • Develop each learner's talents
Determinants of Success	
• Teacher's performance • Inputs/resources	• Students' performance • Learning • Development of students' understanding and skill and values
Assumptions About Teachers	
• Any expert can teach	• Teaching is complex and requires considerable preparation for the role

CONTEXT IN WHICH CURRICULUM EXISTS

The process of developing or revising/refining a curriculum calls for an awareness of the context in which the curriculum exists: the parent institution's mission and goals, the student population being served, requirements of external regulation and accreditation bodies, resources available, and faculty qualifications. This was examined in Chapter 15. To have a curriculum that is internally consistent, where each key component clearly connects with every other component (see Figure 16.6), faculty need to engage in extensive collaboration, extended discussions about values, and continuous environmental scanning. This is essential to ensure that the curriculum will be effective in preparing graduates to function effectively in the ever-changing, technology-infused, ambiguous, uncertain, regulated, stressful health care environment. The same is true for educators in health care settings who develop curricula for orientation and varied types of educational programs.

FIGURE 16.6 Integration among curriculum components.

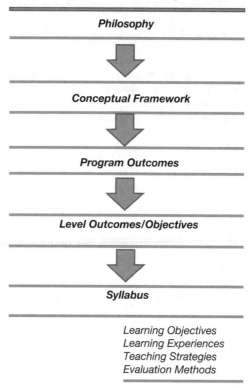

Philosophy

Conceptual Framework

Program Outcomes

Level Outcomes/Objectives

Syllabus

Learning Objectives
Learning Experiences
Teaching Strategies
Evaluation Methods

SUMMARY

The driving principle in curriculum development and revision is student learning, as faculty articulate values related to teaching and learning, select key concepts for the curriculum framework, formulate program outcomes and level outcomes/objectives, and design courses. Such attention was expressed by Whetten (2007) who, after careful reflection on the purpose of education, expressed the following: "I have come to understand that the most important things I can do to influence student learning involves carefully planning what my students—not their teacher—will do before, during, and after each class. In sum, I have learned that the most effective teachers focus their attention on course design" (p. 341).

It is the faculty who select the model for the curriculum, after a careful analysis of the advantages, disadvantages, and implications of each. It is the faculty who have responsibility for ensuring the interrelationship among all components of the curriculum. And it is the faculty who construct course syllabi to enhance student learning. These are challenging and time-consuming activities, but the benefit to students and, ultimately, to patient care and the strength of our profession makes them worthwhile.

REFERENCES

Bart, M. (2015). A learner-centered syllabus helps set the tone for learning. *Faculty Focus.* Retrieved from http://www.facultyfocus.com/articles/effective-classroom-management/a-learner-centered-syllabus-helps-set-the-tone-for-learning

Billings, D. M. (2012). Developing learner-centered courses. In D. M. Billings & J. A. Halstead (Eds.), *Teaching in nursing: A guide for faculty* (4th ed., pp. 160–169). St. Louis, MO: Elsevier Saunders.

Boland, D. L. (2012). Developing curriculum: Frameworks, outcomes, and competencies. In D. M. Billings & J. A. Halstead (Eds.), *Teaching nursing: A guide for faculty* (4th ed., pp. 138–159). St. Louis, MO: Elsevier Saunders.

Clark, C. M. (2017). *Creating and sustaining civility in nursing education* (2nd ed.). Indianapolis, IN: Sigma Theta Tau International.

Comer, A. R. (2016, July 27). The syllabus as a contract. *Chronicle of Higher Education.* Retrieved from http://www.chronicle.com/article/The-Syllabus-as-a-Contract/237251

Dickoff, J., & James, P. (1970). Beliefs and values: Bases for curriculum design. *Nursing Research, 19*(5), 415–427. doi:10.4103/0301-4738.195613

Duke University School of Nursing. (2017). Sample program and level outcomes. Durham, NC: Duke University School of Nursing.

Gibson, D., Ostashewski, N., Flintoff, K., Grant, S., & Knight, E. (2015). Digital badges in education. *Education and Information Technologies, 20*, 403–410. doi:10.1007/s10639-013-9291-7

Goudreau, J., Pepin, J., Dubois, S., Boyer, L., Larue, C., & Legault, A. (2009). A second generation of the competency-based approach to nursing education. *International Journal of Nursing Education Scholarship, 6*(1), Article 15. doi:10.2202/1548-923X.1685

Iwasiw, C. L., & Goldenberg, D. (2015). Establishing philosophical and educational approaches for an evidence-informed, context-relevant, unified curriculum. In C. L. Iwasiw & D. Goldenberg (Eds.), *Curriculum development in nursing education* (pp. 209–236). Burlington, MA: Jones & Bartlett.

Morin, K. H., & Bellack, J. P. (2015). Student learning outcomes. *Journal of Nursing Education, 54*(3), S3–S4. doi:10.3928/01484834-20150217-10

Payne, L. K., & Mullen, P. (2014). Outcome measures for traditional and accelerated nursing graduates: An integrative literature review. *Nursing Education Perspectives, 35*, 238–243. doi:10.5480/12-1008.1

Scheckel, M. (2016). Designing courses and learning experiences. In D. M. Billings & J. A. Halstead (Eds.). *Teaching in nursing: A guide for faculty* (5th ed., pp. 159–185). St. Louis, MO: Elsevier.

Valiga, T. M. (2012). Philosophical foundations of the curriculum. In D. M. Billings & J. A. Halstead (Eds.), *Teaching in nursing: A guide for faculty* (5th ed., pp. 118–129). St. Louis, MO: Elsevier.

Wasley, P. (2008, March 14). The syllabus becomes a repository of legalese. *Chronicle of Higher Education, 54*(27), A1, A8–A11. Retrieved from http://www.chronicle.com/article/The-Syllabus-Becomes-a/17723

Whetten, D. A. (2007). Principles of effective course design: What I wish I had known about learning-centered teaching 30 years ago. *Journal of Management Education, 31*(3), 339–357. doi:10.1177/1052562906298445

Zaretsky, R. (2012, August 14). Looking at an old syllabus with new eyes. *Chronicle of Higher Education.* Retrieved from http://www.chronicle.com/article/Looking-at-an-Old-Syllabus/133631

Zucker, K. D., Baker-Schena, L., & Pak, M. (2010, January). The course syllabus: Contract, culture, and compass. *The Teaching Professor, 3.*

17

Program Evaluation

DONNA L. BOLAND

OBJECTIVES

- Describe the evolution of the science of program evaluation
- Provide direction in designing a meaningful evaluation plan consistent with identified needs
- Identify the complexities of generating essential information that support program relevance and accountability to stakeholders

---

In today's world of increasing accountability, evaluation has moved to the forefront of importance, especially in the educational arena. At the most basic level of conceptual interpretation, evaluation is about making judgments regarding the value or worth of something. In this case it is about the value of an institution or educational program based on preconceived expectations and the worth of the institution or educational program to one or more entities. It is an expectation that judgments made about value and worth are based on information collected through a variety of qualitative and quantitative methods deemed appropriate by those charged with the responsibility of making the judgment calls. Evaluation provides decision makers with information about the institution or program's aims, purpose, and goals, and how well it is functioning in relation to these intentions.

This chapter focuses on various theories and theoretical frameworks that underpin evaluation efforts and discusses evaluation models and their use in approaching evaluation systematically. The chapter also examines research methodologies for generating useful evaluative information, especially within the context of nursing programs, connections between accountability and accreditation, and approaches to developing and implementing program evaluation meaningful to nursing programs.

THEORETICAL UNDERPINNINGS

The ability to understand the theory that drives evaluation is critical from a variety of perspectives. Theory provides an explanation as to why we do something: in this case, evaluate. It positions us to examine our practice and revise it as guided by the knowledge gained through the assessment of that practice. Theory also plays a valuable role in shaping our thinking about how to approach and carry out meaningful evaluation. There is continued discourse as to whether evaluation is grounded in science, or is a tool that allows us to implement the scientific method to achieve evaluation purpose and goals. Program evaluation has matured as both theory and method in response to societal needs and requirements for productivity and efficiency. Embedding evaluation into the need for accountability has pushed the science of evaluation into a publicly credible field, seeded by specific theories and nurtured by models.

Alkin and Christie (2004) discuss the roots of evaluation and the various contributions made by those recognized within this scientific field. Some of the most recognized leaders in evaluation research included in Alkin and Christie's classic discussion are highlighted in the following presentation on theoretical development of the field of evaluation. They conceptualized the evolution of theories into three distinct theoretical branches, based on their review, and they attached conceptual labels to each of these branches, based on their perceptions of theoretical similarities among the works. These labels were *use*, *methods*, and *valuing* (Alkin & Christie, 2004, p. 12). Although Christie and Alkin (2013) continue to refer to these three branches in their recent publication, the theorists and their branch categories are not mutually exclusive, based on characteristics identified. What are important to the development of evaluation science are the theoretical underpinnings evident in most of today's evaluation models. The following discussion highlights some of the notable theorists and their contributions to the evolution of the current state of evaluation science.

USE- OR UTILIZATION-ORIENTED EVALUATION THEORISTS

Theorists who fall into this category share the philosophy that evaluation should be used to generate information valuable to decision makers; they include such notables as Daniel Stufflebeam, Michael Patton, David Fetterman, and Marvin Alkin (Christie & Alkin, 2013). These theorists share the point of view that the main emphasis of evaluation efforts is concentrated on the collection of information that facilitates decision making. Using this theoretical orientation, the ultimate goal of evaluation is to facilitate decisions that support changes important to the institution or program.

The value placed on the contribution of evaluation was directly related to decision making. An example of this theoretical orientation was the Context, Input, Process, and Product (CIPP) Model developed by Daniel Stufflebeam and Egon Guba. CIPP includes the four essential components they believed to be critical in creating a useful evaluation (Stufflebeam, 2013). Stufflebeam advocated for an evaluation process that was both cyclic and sustainable, in that information should be continually available to support quality improvement efforts. According to Stufflebeam, evaluation designs should attend to such conceptual standards as utility, feasibility, propriety, and accuracy.

- The *utility* standard is intended to ensure that an evaluation will serve the information needs of intended users.
- The *feasibility* standards are intended to ensure that an evaluation will be realistic, prudent, diplomatic, and frugal.
- The *propriety* standards are intended to ensure that an evaluation will be conducted legally, ethically, and with respect for the welfare of those involved in the evaluation, as well as those affected by its results.

- The *accuracy* standards are intended to ensure that an evaluation will reveal and convey technically adequate information about the features that determine worth, or merit, of the program evaluated (Alkin & Christie, 2004, p. 45).

Michael Quinn Patton's Utilization-Focused Evaluation Theory was built on the foundation laid by Stufflebeam. Patton, however, argued that it was critical to identify and involve in the evaluation process those stakeholders who would be primarily users of evaluation findings, in an effort to increase utility of the evaluation process and resulting outcomes. Patton (2008, 2012) continues to refine his view of utilization-focused evaluation in a reality where we are able to generate more information than we can assimilate and apply to complex and often convoluted decisional issues.

Michael Scriven's early writings argued that evaluators needed to place a value on their findings in an effort to increase the usefulness of evaluation to decision makers. He suggested that the focus of evaluation efforts is to examine how causal associations relate directly to program quality. This thinking continues to be in vogue in today's reality. Scriven was a proponent of *goal-free* evaluation, determining which program outcomes to examine, rather than starting with the objectives of the program. He believed evaluation should determine the real accomplishments (and nonaccomplishments) of the program (Alkin & Christie, 2004, p. 33; Scriven, 1991, 2013). Few evaluation theorists have supported Scriven's sense of assigning a good or bad dichotomous approach in interpreting evaluation results. Egon Guba and Yvonna Lincoln also supported the notion of valuing as critical to evaluation. However, they placed the responsibility for making valuing interpretations on the shoulders of the stakeholders, based on the belief that "there are multiple realities based on the perceptions and interpretations of the individuals in the program to be evaluated" (Alkin & Christie, 2004, p. 42). Their approach to the role of evaluator was to navigate these various perceptions in facilitating stakeholders' ability to reach consensus on the issues and decisions to be made.

METHODS-FOCUSED EVALUATION THEORISTS

Other evaluation theorists directed their attention to methodological issues related to attainment of specified program goals and objectives. Ralph Tyler, known to many in the discipline of nursing, was an early leader in promoting the need to set behavioral objectives, identify situations in which the learners are able to demonstrate those behaviors, and find measures that generated the best information in determining how well the program or institution was meeting its goals. This information was used to support or reject assumptions regarding the effectiveness of a particular program (Madaus, 2013). Other theorists who expanded on Tyler's orientation to evaluation included Donald Campbell, who, joined by Stanley, wrote the 1966 classic text on experimental and quasi-experimental designs for research, which continues to serve as a valued resource for evaluation researchers when exploring methods and their contribution to evaluation efforts.

In the late 1960s, evaluation research gained in popularity as a legitimate science, thanks to the works of Edward Suchman, who argued that scientific methods were important to the legitimization and value of evaluation studies (Christie & Alkin, 2013). Suchman is credited with the creation of five criterion categories that provide a framework for evaluation research. They include:

1. Effort (quantity and quality of activity that takes place)
2. Performance (criteria that measure the results of effort)

3. Adequacy of performance (degree to which performance is adequate to the total amount of needs)
4. Efficiency (examination of alternative paths or methods in terms of human and monetary costs)
5. Process (how and why a program works or does not work; Christie & Alkin, 2013, p. 21)

These categories are still used today in designing evaluation research activities.

Also included in the methods branch was Thomas Cook, who explored the application of scientific designs for use in evaluation research. Additionally, he advanced the importance of the role of stakeholders within the design structure. He argued that the key to good evaluation was stakeholder involvement in the integration of the evaluation process. Stakeholders make valuable contributions to the identification of the problem to be examined, integral to the generation and interpretation of evaluation information. By including stakeholders early in the design of program evaluation efforts, the gap between expectations and outcomes of these efforts narrows, increasing the chances that evaluation findings are likely to be implemented (Bowman, 2015). Cook recognized that, although the identification of appropriate methodologies was critical to evaluation outcomes, there are variables that are difficult to control for, but that have a confounding effect on evaluation findings and interpretation of those findings. The concept growing out of this orientation was that program evaluation had to be studied within each program's unique context, and that study methods needed to match the contextual uniqueness surrounding each program (Christie & Alkin, 2013).

CONTEXTUALLY FOCUSED THEORISTS

Theory-driven evaluation came into vogue in the early 1980s, due to the contributions of Huey-Tsyh Chen and Peter Rossi, who believed that theory-driven evaluation is critical to the generation of meaningful evaluation outcomes (Christie & Alkin, 2013). Context is central in theory-driven evaluation, but Chen drew on social science theories to help inform the context surrounding program evaluation activities. From his perspective, theory informs context and improves the internal and external validity of evaluation outcomes (Chen, 2013).

In keeping with the context theme, Carol Weiss was among the first to reason that politics intrudes on program evaluation in three ways: "(a) programs are created and maintained by political forces; (b) higher echelons of government, which make decisions about programs, are embedded in politics; and (c) the very act of evaluation has political connotations" (Weiss, 1991, p. 213). Guided by her thinking, the scientific approach to evaluation activities is essential but not all-inclusive of factors. Certainly the focus on accountability is politically driven, which continues to support her supposition. Lee J. Cronbach incorporated the concept of policy into his orientation by suggesting that evaluation should inform conversations and decisions of those responsible for setting program policies. He believed that stakeholders were critical, both in shaping the questions that drive evaluation activities and in arriving at judgments based on the issues at hand (Alkin & Christie, 2004; Bowman, 2015).

CURRENT EVALUATION THEORISTS

Evaluation theories continue to emerge from the groundwork laid by these and others devoted to developing the science of evaluation. Over the past 15 years, the

Theory of Empowerment Evaluation has gained in popularity. Although empowerment evaluation incorporates the tenets of utilization and decision making, it distinguishes itself from other theories, including Utilization Evaluation Theory, by emphasizing the use of information to drive decisions that enable the decision makers to improve "their lives and the lives of those around [them, which] produces an extraordinary sense of well-being and positive growth" (Wandersman et al., 2012, p. 12). The principles that guide empowerment evaluation have historical roots and are guided by theoretical and philosophical tenets. These principles also resonate with both internal and external expectations to which higher education programs are being held.

Wandersman et al. (2012) identified nine principles associated with empowerment that educators should incorporate into their perspectives on evaluation (Exhibit 17.1). In nursing it is important that stakeholders understand that evaluation processes and resulting outcomes can be perceived as either good or not so good within the context of the desired aim or purpose of the evaluation process. There are various reasons that affect the perceived value or worth of the process. It is therefore important that cyclic evaluation processes be evaluated on a periodic basis. Evaluation of evaluation can employ both formative (process-oriented) and summative (outcome-oriented) methods. Formative evaluation considers how the evaluation process is conceived and implemented. At the center of summative evaluation are outcomes, judgments, and decisions made as a result of the information generated (Wandersman et al., 2012).

EXHIBIT 17.1 Perspectives on Evaluation: Nine Principles Associated With Empowerment

- *Principle one* argues the need to focus on program improvement as the end goal of evaluation activities. Improvement both provides a clear end goal and acts as a purposeful guide to evaluation designs.

- *Principles two and three* focus on the inclusion and engagement of stakeholders in the establishment of goals, design, collection, interpretation, and application of evaluation information. They argue that the more involved the community of interest is, the more meaningful and useful the results.

- *Principle four* highlights the need for democratic participation in the evaluation process. This principle is translated to mean that participation should be authentic, and every attempt should be made to leverage individual talent held among stakeholders in moving the evaluation process forward. Participatory equality leads to transparency of the evaluation process and a valued sense of control over the process.

- *Principle five* addresses the need for a social justice orientation. Although the concept of social justice grew out of a social-political theoretical framework, it can be easily applied to nurse educators, assuming that as a collective, program improvement anchored in quality and social relevance is their main goal.

- *Principle six* is critical to nursing education programs, as the need to partner with an appropriately defined community of interest is in the best interests of both the program and the community. Professional accreditation bodies recognize the value of engaging those within the community of interest in clarifying the problems and seeking workable solutions to real and evolving issues and challenges.

(continued)

EXHIBIT 17.1 Perspectives on Evaluation: Nine Principles Associated With Empowerment (*continued*)

- *Principle seven* underscores the value of the scientific approach to evaluation design and implementation. Evaluation activities should incorporate evidence-based practices that are appropriately aligned to the program being evaluated, the resources at hand, the decisions to be made, and the perceived value of the information being generated to finding answers/solutions to issues raised.
- *Principle eight* suggests that the more knowledgeable and skilled the evaluator(s) is/are, the greater the contribution to the utility of the evaluation process being conducted. The end result of this expertise is better outcomes. The underlying assumption is that the program environment supports the need for expertise and values both the evaluation process and outcomes generated. The value of learning generated from evaluation to programs and institutions is the focal point of principle nine. An established and supported culture of learning within an institution of higher education is not about sustaining what is, but rather about envisioning and reaching for what could and should be given—external and internal accountability and responsibility to society. If one defines learning as change, then evaluation is the vehicle driving change, hence the value and utility of evaluation.
- *The final principle (nine)* relates to accountability of all from inception to completion of the evaluation process. It is the responsibility of all involved in evaluation to be accountable for their actions and to hold others involved accountable.

Source: From Wandersman et al. (2012).

Historically, philosophically, and theoretically, evaluation is rooted in various divergent but often complementary ways of thinking. Few evaluation experts would argue against evaluation being a science grounded in theoretical properties. Evaluation has evolved into a broadly based applied science in which both applicability and utility are of value to various disciplines (McPherson, 2015). The versatility of evaluation allows stakeholders to respond to calls for accountability, especially in the areas of program productivity and quality, assessment of learning, impact of teaching on learning outcomes, and determination of best educational practices.

For nurse educators, evaluation practices provide answers to professional accreditation standards in the broad areas of effectiveness of program, efficiency of use of resources to promote program quality, and impact of program in meeting internal and external expectations (Astin & Antonio, 2012). It should be noted, however, that evaluation practices should not be limited to addressing accreditation expectations, as this narrow view of evaluation constrains the depth and breadth of the contributions of evaluation in developing and revising nursing programs on a continuous basis, as established by stakeholders and decision makers.

Given the evolution of evaluation, it is important that nurse educators focus on the following propositions when designing or constructing evaluation models that provide a framework for evaluation activities in their programs. Evaluation should:

- Be of use to those with decision-making authority
- Include an array of both primary (frontline) and secondary (interested parties) stakeholders to capture diverse needs and viewpoints
- Occur within a social-political environment, in that the context in which evaluation is carried out is known
- Incorporate methodological strategies that generate valid and meaningful results
- Be transparent and consistent with clearly stated goals

EVALUATION MODELS

The majority of evaluation models being employed today are a reflection of one or more theoretical or philosophical orientations noted earlier. Evaluation models are helpful in providing the framework in which evaluation activities occur. Prior to identifying an evaluation model, evaluators, along with stakeholders, must determine whether the outcomes of the evaluation will actually make a difference to program decisions needing to be made, agree that the evaluation process can be completed in a time frame for the results to be used in the decision process, and question whether the program and/ or the decisions needing to be made are of a scope that warrants the time and effort to carry out evaluation (Royce, Thyer, & Padgett, 2016). If the perceived need to conduct evaluation does not meet this broad litmus test, then the deliberations as to what evaluation model to use are irrelevant.

If the deliberations result in the need to conduct an evaluation of the program or of some aspects of the program critical to its viability, the next discussion needs to center on what one hopes to achieve from the evaluation process. It is important to ask what information is needed, by whom the information is needed, and what purpose the outcomes of evaluation are to serve. Evaluation is essential to determining the value of the program to stakeholders and to the broader community of interest. Decisions linked to program value or worth include the addition, revision, or deletion of the program. Evaluation models at this level of decision making should be comprehensive and inclusive to be effective in generating adequate information that informs decisions. Evaluation models should be part of any new program design, and not an afterthought once the program has been implemented. The chosen model should stand up to the test of time with modest tweaking. Evaluations with a focus on answering noncyclic questions or specific needs should be less elaborate in design and resource requirements.

Depending on the source you consult, you are likely to discover that there is no set nomenclature for evaluation models. Evaluation models used in higher education are relevant in guiding one's thinking as it relates to how to approach evaluation and what the outcome of the evaluation should achieve. Evaluation models should be chosen for their ability to generate findings that address desired goals. There are some consistencies in evaluation models in use today, as many of the evaluative processes are directed or guided by external expectations. Some of the more commonly used evaluation models and their focus are presented to give you a sense of the options that are available for the purpose of guiding your thinking.

GOAL-ORIENTED/FOCUS EVALUATION MODELS

Goal-oriented/focus evaluation models are utilitarian by nature, and are generally employed to examine change within or across institutions of higher education and their program offerings. This type of model is popular in determining the degree to which a course or program influences student learning. The key to this type of model is efficiency, as the model is most often employed to measure the impact on student learning or on educational outcomes. Decisions related to program impact are designed to compare predetermined goals, outcomes, or objectives to that which has been achieved. The key to goal-oriented thinking requires that the goals be clearly articulated and that consensus be reached prior to conducting an institutional and/or program evaluation (Patton, 2013).

A decision-making evaluation model emphasizes informed judgments as the end result of the evaluation process. Stufflebeam's CIPP Model is a good example of a decision-making model that continues to be used extensively (Stufflebeam, 2013). It is therefore important to understand how each element of the model can be interpreted for possible use by evaluators.

- *Context evaluations* assess needs, problems, assets, and opportunities to help decision makers define goals and priorities and to guide the broader group of users to judge goals, priorities, and outcomes.
- *Input evaluations* assess alternative approaches, competing action plans, staffing plans, and budgets for their feasibility and potential cost-effectiveness to meet targeted needs and achieve goals. Decision makers use input evaluations when they choose among competing plans, write grant proposals, allocate resources, assign staff, schedule work, and help others judge an effort's plans and budget.
- *Process evaluations* assess the implementation of plans to help staff carry out activities and later to help the broad group of users judge program performance and interpret outcomes.
- *Product evaluations* identify and assess outcomes—intended and unintended, short- and long-term—to help keep the organization focused on achieving important outcomes and help the broader group of users gauge the effort's success at meeting targeted needs (Stufflebeam, 2004, p. 246).

The CIPP Model is flexible in that it can be used to meet both formative and summative evaluation needs when the intent of evaluation is program improvement. Decision-driven models such as the CIPP Model tend to center on the effectiveness, quality, and/or impact of the program. In today's higher educational reality, in which scrutiny of program effectiveness is on everyone's mind, the ability to make informed decisions about program effectiveness is essential.

DISCREPANCY EVALUATION MODELING

Discrepancy evaluation modeling is close to decision-making models, as this type of modeling focuses on the ability of programs to meet internal and external standards. Currently, professional accreditation is built on the idea of compliance with standards. Nurse faculty are expected to provide data as to the program's ability to meet specified standards. Program evaluation plans have been designed around the need to collect, monitor, and interpret program data, based on the standards the accrediting body dictates for compliance purposes. When a discrepancy is noted, faculty need to determine the precipitating factors associated with the discrepancy and present a plan of action to address this discrepancy, along with a timetable for resolution. The challenge in using any type of decision-making approaches is in the identification of who can and should be making decisions related to program integrity. The path followed in making decisions is often convoluted and populated with unexpected or unanticipated hurdles.

GOAL-FREE EVALUATION MODELS

As noted earlier in the chapter, Scriven was the primary advocate for goal-free evaluation models. This approach focuses on measuring what *is* without the context of established goals or expected outcomes that could potentially bias the observations made and the interpretation of findings (Youker & Ingraham, 2013). The value of this type of evaluation model lies in determining the degree to which the information collected meets the needs of those using the information (Scriven, 2013). Scriven recognizes five dimensions that need to be included in a goal-free approach to evaluation: *"process, outcomes, cost, comparative advantage,* and *generalizability"* (Scriven, 2004, p. 188). Goal-free evaluation can be conducted either formatively or in a summative fashion, depending on the needs of the program. This model is closest to naturalistic inquiry philosophy. The strength of this approach is that data generated can highlight both intended and unintended consequences of the program. It also negates the need to compare the achievement of expected goals/outcomes to actual achievement of goals/outcomes (Cook, Scriven, Coryn, & Evergreen, 2010).

UTILIZATION-FOCUSED EVALUATION MODEL

The utilization-focused evaluation model is designed around the identification of the information needed, those needing the information (potential users), and the decisions needing to be made (Ramirez & Brodhead, 2013). The caveat in this thinking is that users can be fully known, and all information collected is useful to decision makers. It is also important to note that for evaluation findings to be useful to the decision makers, they must be accepting of the findings, and that the seeking of solutions might be beyond what they are willing to explore. Although institutions of higher education have been cautious in their approach to change, the social and political environment is ready for and demanding of organizational change to meet a dynamic, globally focused society. Critical elements identified by Patton (2012) include stakeholder engagement, an understanding of the context in which the program exists, planning, and open communication channels throughout the evaluation process. A utilization-oriented modeling approach can be used in both the formative and summative approaches to an evaluation project. The steps in using this type of model include the need to establish an evaluation committee, identify the purpose of the evaluation and the roles of the evaluators, develop guidelines for the evaluation process, identify the methods to be employed, implement the evaluation plan, analyze the information collected, and present logically the findings that resonate with the users (Patton, 2012).

OTHER CURRENT EVALUATION MODELS

Relying more on a contextual theoretical underpinning, four other current evaluation models used in education are *Success Case Studies, Systems-Focused, Transformative,* and *Logic* models. In the *Success Case Study Model,* the goal is to compare the successful programs with those that are less successful to identify the variables associated with success. This model tends to generate case-specific contextual information that might or might not be generalized beyond the scope of the programs under study. When one is using a case study model design, it is essential to determine the expressed purpose of the evaluation effort, questions that you wish to answer, the basic assumptions that affect the collection and interpretation of data, a clearly defined unit of analysis being used, and a set of criteria that will guide the interpretation of the study results.

System-Focused Evaluation Models are constructed on concepts related to systems thinking, which has been around since the early 1930s. However, system-focused evaluation resonates with nurse educators, as this model is inclusive rather than reductionistic in its approach. The context in which the program operates is important to the evaluation process. Mertens (2009) argued that evaluation models need to be genuine and respectful of the people and culture being evaluated. The ability to holistically examine the relationships between and among all aspects of a program can provide the evaluator with a realistic view of the functionality of a program under study. Critical pieces of a system-focused evaluation include the identification of the boundaries of the system's environment, input, output, process, state, hierarchy, goal-directedness, and information (Centers for Disease Control and Prevention, Program Performance and Evaluation Office, 2017).

Culturally responsive models that have incorporated Mertens's thinking must incorporate approaches that include appreciation for the cultural backgrounds of the stakeholders. Cultural orientation plays a key role both in determining the value or worth of the data being collected and in making decisions based on these data. To ensure a high level of visibility, there needs to be a collaborative effort among the evaluator and stakeholders, especially in relation to the culture and politics surrounding the entity being evaluated (Askew, Beverly, & Jay, 2012). For example, evaluation results generated from an evaluation of a nursing program designed to recruit from an educationally disadvantaged population needs to be interpreted within the context of variables such as characteristics of the learner population, community needs, institutional mission and goals, and uniqueness of the educational design.

Another type of contextual model is the *Transformative Model*, which is grounded in philosophical thinking that addresses social issues as well as building on a scholarly base. Core to a Transformative Evaluation Model is the incorporation of marginalized groups into the evaluation process (Mertens, 2009, 2016). The assumption of broadening the circle of participation is grounded in the argument of the value of diverse points of view, especially from the population groups served by the program and/or institution undergoing evaluation. The focus of a Transformative Model is on objectivity that balances the diversity of experiences with evaluation findings in a way that controls for bias as a result of a lack of understanding regarding the context in which the program lives (Mertens, 2010). Participatory involvement in decisions related to evaluation methods and interpretation of findings is critical to maintaining rigor, credibility, validity, and representative truth.

Mertens (2010, 2016) indicated that a Transformative Evaluation Model needs to focus on (a) determining which theoretical tenets best guide a program's approach to evaluating the program; (b) identifying stakeholders and approaches for meaningful engagement in the evaluation process, which in the case of a nursing program might include such characteristics as gender, age, ethnicities, races, languages, economic and family backgrounds, and educational backgrounds; and (c) developing data collection methods that measure findings that will be meaningful to the stakeholders and fuel potential future change. A transformative framework should be able to answer questions related to whether evaluation findings are either emerging or have been stable over a period of time. This type of model also needs to differentiate between evaluation outcomes and program practices, in that outcomes might or might not be the result of current practice expectations. As with any evaluation model, it is important to determine the significance of the outcomes to what is of value to stakeholders (Bowman, 2015).

A *Logic Model* also recognizes the importance of context, in that evaluation must consider the environment surrounding the program. This model focuses on input that includes human and institutional resources; processes that highlighted audience needs, collection and summarization of information, and information dissemination; and outputs that spoke to the usefulness of initial outcomes and the intermediate or actual use of evaluation outcomes and the long-term intended outcomes (Stame, 2014). The common steps in designing an evaluation using a Logic Model include the need to describe the program, fully explain how the program is delivered, determine a list of questions that need to be answered, determine how best to collect information to answer the questions posed, describe the existing program resources and the context in which they and the program exist, and implement the evaluation plan. Widely used in health care, these models provide a vehicle in managing the many aspects of program evaluation. (McLaughlin & Jordan, 2015).

Examples of more utility-oriented models are the Success-Focused, Meta-Analysis, and Appreciative Inquiry Models. *Success-Focused Evaluation Models* are grounded in Patton's (2013) outcome theoretical frame of reference. At the heart of the model's focus is the *so what?* question. The outcome of the evaluation process needs to be interpreted within the framework of impact and change from the perspectives of those who will be using the results. Fundamentals of this framework are inputs, outputs, and outcomes—elements that also define a systems approach. However, Patton is fairly clear on critical features that need to be examined within each of these elements. Inputs include information regarding program resources, findings of a needs assessment, available expertise within and outside the program, physical resources to support the program, and regulatory bodies that guide program implementation. The outputs comprise a determination of the extent of the evaluation to be undertaken, the products being delivered and the size of the population being served, the validity of the observations made, and the results of information collected. The *so what?* question is addressed by the third element of this modeling approach, and it looks at impact or benefit to those who will be using the information generated. It is also critical to evaluate the outcomes to determine whether the right kind of data has been generated to answer the *so what?* question. If not, then adjustments need to be made in the input and output core elements that will generate more useful information for end users (Patton, 2013).

Meta-analysis is most often considered a statistical approach. However, its application to evaluation provides us with a model that allows the synthesis of a variety of evaluation efforts that are directed toward well-defined questions, especially around outcomes targeting best methods. Meta-analysis as a model provides a mechanism that gives evaluation researchers the means to prepare, maintain, and disseminate evaluation outcomes that have been generated through meticulous, systematic collation of information that can be used to shape best practices (Stufflebeam, 2011). There are challenges in using a Meta-Analysis Model, which include the need to be clear about the question being asked, establish clear rules on what and how to identify and interpret data, and have guidelines for determining validity of data and reporting of results of the analysis. Meta-analysis requires time, talent, and access to a comprehensive and complex database.

Appreciative inquiry is a conceptual model that has limited use in higher education, but that does have conceptual utility, given its focus. This model attempts to ascertain what is working well within a program or organization and to explore how to align resources and functions that support a positive vision for a desired future. Critics of this type of approach to evaluation fear that problems and concerns might be glossed over. Proponents argue that problems are not necessarily ignored, but rather approached from a more positive perspective. Appreciative inquiry is constructed through the application of four process steps: discovery of or appreciation for what is working well; ability to dream or visualize what the future could be; design or construction of the desired future based on a vision; and achievement of this vision through action, monitoring, and revising as directed by the evaluation results (Stratton-Berkessel, 2015). Appreciative inquiry has continued to evolve and is used in organizations as a framework, especially in the context of quality improvement that focuses on strengthening best practices. Appreciative inquiry should be designed to be highly inclusive and supportive of the democratic engagement of a diverse group of stakeholders. As this framework emphasizes best practice, it can be a good choice in the early implementation of a new or newly revised program. Again, being able to focus on what is working allows for positively motivated corrections in direction. This type of approach also encourages consensus among primary stakeholders.

Although the approach to thinking about evaluation models is varied, there are some common themes to developing an evaluation model to fit diverse goals. The following checklist summarizes the themes that need to be considered when adopting or adapting an evaluation model:

1. Identify and engage stakeholders.
2. Clarify goals of the evaluation.
3. Assess resources needed for evaluation.
4. Design the evaluation.
5. Determine appropriate methods of measurement and procedures.
6. Develop a work plan, budget, and timeline for evaluation.
7. Collect the data using agreed-upon methods and procedures.
8. Process and analyze data.
9. Interpret and disseminate the results.
10. Take action.

This list corresponds to essential competencies that have been identified (Lee, Altschuld, & Lee, 2012). The critical competencies needed by effective evaluators include the ability to identify and understand the norms and values shaping the program being evaluated, the technical skills to conduct evaluation from a systematic inquiry approach, the analytical skills to understand the context in which the program exists from both a social and political perspective, expertise in managing all the evaluation project elements in a coordinated and timely fashion, communication/interpersonal skills required to keep information and interactions focused on the purpose of each evaluation effort undertaken, and the ability to package the findings in a way that is most meaningful to the primary decision makers (Patton, 2012).

The choice of evaluation models is primarily dependent on which model is believed to be the most useful, the most practical, and the most cost-effective from the perspective of benefits obtained (Alkin, 2011). As many of the models tend to share commonalities, an evaluator might use a combination of models to accomplish desired outcomes (Horne & Sandmann, 2012). Scriven (2013) argued that the discipline of evaluation has generated theory, models, and guidelines that have applicability to various disciplines. What evaluation science brings to the table is a sense of order and rigor for those engaging in evaluation. The main challenge in developing a one-size-fits-all approach to evaluation frameworks or models is the uncertainty of that which is to be evaluated. It is difficult to determine that all will be known about a program under investigation. Due to the increasing environmental complexities, it is impossible to identify specific direct cause-and-effect relationships that make the argument for a single model irrational. Lastly, it is challenging for evaluators to always identify what all stakeholders want as an outcome of evaluation efforts, given likely hidden agendas. Therefore, being able to measure for unknown variables is not feasible (Hermans, Naber, & Easerink, 2012; Centers for Disease Control and Prevention, Program Performance and Evaluation Office, 2012).

EVALUATION RESEARCH METHODOLOGIES

Methodologies differ widely, but there are some critical criteria that must be met for the findings of any evaluation research to be perceived as valid. Wholey (2013) indicated that "performance measurement systems and program evaluation studies can and should be mutually reinforcing," arguing that a single measure cannot meet the complex needs of all involved stakeholders (p. 262). The focus of an evaluation project must be clearly stated, as this provides the framework for the process, from developing the design through making conclusions. A clear focus also indicates whether the evaluation project will be formative, summative, or descriptive in nature. The level of analysis needed, as well as the precision in the collection of information, hinge on the focus or purpose of the evaluation to be undertaken (Scriven, 2013). Credibility of the evaluative findings is most reflective of the believability of those providing information. The level of believability relates to bias and relevance of the informant to the issues under study. Reporting of findings and conclusions should be concise and capable of being understood by stakeholders. All evaluation designs must be ethically and legally defensible and respect the rights, responsibilities, and diversity of those involved in the process. The last critical criterion in the design of any evaluation plan is ensuring that the cost of the project proposed is realistic and reflects existing resources (Scriven, 2013). Generalizability is not necessarily an issue in evaluation research unless the purpose of the project is to identify best practices that can be shared widely.

MIXED-METHOD APPROACH

Measurement instruments that complement evaluation are plentiful, but they need to be chosen with great skill because technology has the ability to generate an intense amount of information from complex measures (Zhanjun, Weifeng, & Jiangbo, 2016). Commonly, most evaluators use a mixed-method approach in the collection of information. Evaluators need to identify measures that are germane to the study purpose and that show an understanding of the culture and political environment surrounding the program. Measurement instruments must also generate the type of information that will be most meaningful to the stakeholders. To be of worth or value to those making decisions, the data generated have to "speak to them" both in the short- and more long-term decision discussions. One of the ideas that underpins program evaluation is the ability to identify outcomes that were intended from those outcomes that were not intended when making decisions (Jordan, Chazdon, & Alviz, 2016, p. 78). Higher education decision makers should focus on the impact of both internal and external environmental changes at the micro and macro levels. Evaluation data and outcomes often have to be interpreted within the context of the institution, its goals and achievements, and the regional, national, and international social policy arenas (Zhanjun et al., 2016, p. 90). Today, much of the evaluation data involve repeated observations that extend over a period of time, so measurements must be stable and perform consistently across data sets when making decisions related to the system. However, measurements are less stable when the focus is visionary.

   One of the main arguments that supports the notion that evaluation is not a true science is the assumption that all factors under study are known and can be controlled if the correct research design is chosen and implemented according to its standing protocols. It is an accepted premise that in evaluation research, it can be the case that not all factors are known, but they are often discovered within the process; a part of that premise is the concept that the ability to control factors within a human organization is impossible. Mixed methods are helpful in the collection of both existing and new or yet-to-be-discovered information. Stakeholders are essential in the identification of existing data sources and serve as informants in uncovering data that provide meaning and understanding in relation to the program function and outcomes.

USEFULNESS OF DATA COLLECTED

When collecting evaluation data, it is important to weigh the data against the usefulness of the information being collected. The evaluators need to ask such questions as, "Are the data helpful in better understanding the issues under study?" "Can the information be useful as the evaluation process progresses?" "Is the collection and analysis of the information worth the cost?" "Is the information presented from a biased perspective, and, if so, are there other sources of information that offset this bias?" If a program has had prior experiences with evaluations, then it is important to know what the process was like and what information was the most valuable. It is also critical to understand what programmatic changes have been made since the last evaluation and what changes are being contemplated for the future, as change will affect both the collection of information and the interpretation of that information. For example, if new educational programs have been implemented or are being considered, then the proposed evaluation must take into account the impact of those programs from such perspectives as meeting stakeholder needs; physical, fiscal, and human resources; outcomes; relevancy to practice and the job market; potential applicant pools; fit of new or proposed programs with institutional goals; value of programs to community of interest; and impact of graduates on the professional, educational, and social community.

PROCEDURAL STEPS IN PROGRAM EVALUATION

Once the first step (determining the purpose, goals, aims, and decisions to be made) of conducting a program evaluation is done, it is important to identify factors that might affect the ability to achieve evaluation goals. Possible constraints include a restricted budget or time frame; the availability of and access to information; expertise of the evaluator(s); stakeholder support for the evaluation being proposed; and potential, yet-to-be determined environmental challenges. It is also important to identify both short- and long-term goals and desired outcomes. Incorporated into your desired outcomes is a vision of potential impact outcomes may have on desired achievements (McLaughlin & Jordan, 2015).

The next procedural step is to identify the variables that are to be measured. Consistent with research practices, the variables under study need to be articulated in terms specific enough to be able to identify the appropriate collection method. It might be that one or more measures will need to be developed to facilitate data collection. If new data collection methods must be designed, then the time, talent, and energy should be calculated into the overall costs to justify these additional expenditures. One of the critical elements in program evaluation is the ability to measure the concept of "learning," which is essential to an institution's or program's documentation of effectiveness. When considering the culmination of the learning experiences, evaluators employ a summative thinking approach to their choices for measurement methodologies (Getha-Eby, Beery, O'Brien, & Xu, 2015). As most nurse educators will be involved with summative evaluation approaches, it is important to choose those measurements that provide useful summative information on learning as it relates to program effectiveness and ultimately to accountability of the program in meeting internal and external expectations.

QUALITATIVE AND QUANTITATIVE MEASUREMENT APPROACHES

Evaluators have a rich array of both qualitative and quantitative measurement approaches available. Common quantitative instruments employed by nurse educators in program evaluation include student performance and achievement tests, including teacher-made tests that are specific to coursework, nationally normed tests, high-stakes tests, document reviews, case logs, performance-focused observations (often employing simulation that incorporate scales or performance checklists), oral examinations, and surveys and questionnaires using a closed-ended question approach (Chen & Lo, 2015). More common qualitative measures employ participant and nonparticipant observations, case studies that focus more on open-ended, guided discussions, stories that highlight variables being studied, interviews (often with key informants), focus groups, and open-ended surveys or questionnaires.

PORTFOLIOS

Portfolios have become a popular assessment strategy over the past decade, particularly electronic or e-portfolios. Portfolios have a flexibility that is attractive in both program evaluation and assessment of learning, which is a key element in program evaluation. Portfolios can be constructed to meet the needs of the teacher and the learner. The traditional use of portfolios has been the assessment of the educational maturation of learners as they progress through a program of study. Portfolios are now being paired with outcomes assessment to appraise the learner's progression toward program goal attainment (Cosgrove, 2013). Determination of progression is based on products the learner has produced over her or his course of study. Other, more process-oriented documentation that can go into the construction of a portfolio includes artifacts of a learner's perception of growth and abilities, such as a diary or log. Incorporating metacognitive experiences into the portfolio not only enriches the learning experience but also adds another critical voice (the student's) to evaluation of program outcomes.

Portfolios have made inroads into program evaluation over the last few years. In this capacity, portfolios are more commonly used to judge achievements in relation to organizational mission and goals and to provide evidence associated with professional standards and public accountability. Portfolios provide a great deal of flexibility, depending on how they are constructed. Documentation can be in the form of visual, written, oral, and/or electronic information sources. The construction of a portfolio requires the identification of specific goals that must be addressed by the documentation gathered from various and diverse sources. It also requires a careful selection of evidence that obviously reflects the outcomes. If portfolios are to be used as summative evaluative tools, then there must be a standardization of the evidence included; the documentation must be clearly defined for all learners; assessment criteria must be articulated and applied consistently; evaluators should be trained in application of assessment criteria; and interrater reliability must be established (Rhodes, 2012; Senger & Kanthan, 2012).

HIGH-STAKES TESTING

As all nursing programs are embedded in institutions of higher learning, assessment of student learning is focused not only on discipline-specific outcomes, but also on college skill proficiency outcomes. In many cases, the focus of college proficiency outcome assessment has been based on nationally recognized *high-stakes* tests. In taking a value-added approach to learning, these tests tend to be administered at the beginning and end of a student's program of study (Simon, McGinnis, & Krauss, 2013). However, evaluators continue to raise questions related to validity of these high-stakes testing methods. A major caution in using high-stakes testing as a singular measure of college-level skill proficiency is that these measures do not address the difference in learner populations and institutions. The argument is that, for the purpose of evaluation, there needs to be a systematic approach to interpretation of this type of information, which must be done within a context of other performance variables (Stobart & Eggen, 2014). At present there is no one standardized test, or set of tests, that is in place for all institutions, but as the calls for improved student achievement increase, the need grows to develop and test reliable assessment methods that cross disciplines as well as meet discipline-specific outcomes. As these assessment methods are developed, they must address critical measurement issues that include conflicts related to the unit of analysis (student vs. institution) and myriad confounding variables that are difficult to control. There is concern that the use of national tests such as the Collegiate Assessment of Academic Proficiency will be used to make erroneous decisions regarding institutional quality as calls for accountability continue to increase (Banta, 2011). However, the Collegiate Assessment of Academic Proficiency is currently being used in some universities and colleges as a measure of student learning and an indicator of the value-added learning in the areas of reading, writing, mathematics, science, and critical thinking.

ALTERNATIVES TO USE OF HIGH-STAKES TESTS

With the need to continue to explore alternatives to the use of high-stakes tests, the Association of American Colleges and Universities (AACU) developed a Valid Assessment of Learning in Undergraduate Education rubric structure to incorporate knowledge beyond what most standardized tests measure. The knowledge elements included in this rubric are "creative writing, critical thinking, information literacy, inquiry and analysis, written and oral communication, problem-solving, quantitative literacy, reading, teamwork, civic knowledge and engagement, ethical reasoning, foundations and skills of lifelong learning, intercultural knowledge and competence, and integrative and applied learning" (AACU, 2010).

A number of universities and programs are incorporating these rubrics into their evaluation processes, especially if they use institutional portfolios as a measure of learning. The essence of each of these elements is woven into their institutional and program/discipline outcomes. The rubric framework is then constructed so that there is continuity from expected learning to actual or measurable learning. Although the portfolio provides a great deal of flexibility, there need to be strategies for dealing with potential reliability and flexibility issues. Interrater reliability is critical, and those asked to judge portfolios must agree not only on how to interpret the assessment values, but on the consistency in assigning these values. Portfolio evaluators need to be trained and monitored to be effective in the use of this type of methodology. Other alternatives to high-stakes testing revolve around the concept of marketability. The underlying premise of this type of approach assumes that program decision makers understand market demands and expectations and are able to prepare graduates who can perform accordingly. In an era where the health care industry expects graduates to have specific skills, there is growing emphasis on programs to design high-stakes testing. Students are being required to demonstrate their application of knowledge to various care scenarios throughout the program and at the end of it. These clinically oriented high-stake evaluation situations, supported by simulation, generate evaluative data but are not without their challenges in providing stakeholders with reliable quality information on which to base critical performance decisions (Kardong-Edgren, Oermann, Rizzolo, & Odom-Maryon, 2017).

EVALUATION AND ACCOUNTABILITY: ACCREDITATION

In the world of nursing education, accountability is synonymous with accreditation. Accreditation, though time-consuming, has enormous benefits. Accreditation is usually a voluntary process, although some states mandate that institutions and programs be accredited through established governmental rules and regulations. The accreditation process provides valuable information and data about the ability of a program to meet specified outcomes and standards. It requires faculty and students to be engaged in the process of evaluation, in generating information related to program quality and relevance.

TYPES OF ACCREDITATION

There are two general types of accreditation critical to education. These are institutional and program/specialized accreditation.

INSTITUTIONAL ACCREDITATION

All institutions of higher education hold some type of accreditation (focusing on the whole of the institution), depending on the type and focus of the institution. Currently there are 12 regional agencies recognized by the U.S. Department of Education and the Council for Higher Education Accreditation, with the authority to accredit public institutions of vocational and higher education. Although each regional agency has developed its own accreditation standards, there are common themes that run through those standards. These themes include having the ability to promote learning; an identified mission and goals; and the ability to demonstrate that the goals are being achieved, there are sufficient resources, and programs are sustainable. Accreditation provides a mechanism for institutions and programs to benchmark their performance against national, regional, and professional standards of expected practice. Accreditation engages faculty and administrators in generating and tracking evaluative information, not only about student performance, but also about graduates' relevance in the job market, the value of the program to the public, and the impact of achievements on the citizens and community the program serves.

Like all voluntary accreditation organizations, accreditation agencies are self-regulated, and their accreditation standards are periodically peer-reviewed and updated as appropriate to ensure that institutions are making decisions and changes consistent with their mission and goals. Accreditation processes encourage institutions and programs to look openly at strengths and weaknesses as part of continuous quality improvement.

NURSING PROGRAM ACCREDITATION

Although nurse educators participate in institutional accreditation activities based primarily on the contribution their programs and graduates make to the institution's mission and goals, programmatic accreditation requires faculty to focus their evaluation on the programs being offered through their educational unit. At present, there are three nursing professional accreditation agencies: the National League for Nursing's (NLN) Commission for Nursing Education Accreditation (CNEA), the Accreditation Commission for Education in Nursing (ACEN), and the Commission on Collegiate Nursing Education (CCNE). The accrediting agencies operate autonomously as voluntary self-regulatory agencies. They base their accreditation operations on accepted practices that include the establishment of accreditation standards, a process for the development of materials for those applying to the agency for accreditation status, a systematic system for peer review of nursing units seeking accreditation, a decision process for determination of accreditation status, an established communication route to publicize accreditation actions, and a procedure for systematic review of standards and processes. The NLN CNEA, established in 2013, accredits practical/vocational, diploma, associate, bachelor, master's, and clinical doctorate programs. The ACEN accredits all types of nursing programs, and is the only nursing program accreditor recognized by the U.S. Department of Education as a Title IV gatekeeper for nursing programs that require this function. The CCNE accredits baccalaureate and higher degree nursing programs (Halstead, 2017).

Accreditation is an external force for institutional and programmatic evaluation; however, it is seldom the singular vehicle guiding evaluation activities. The majority of institutions of higher education are accountable to state regulations, boards of governors, and other stakeholders. Higher education institutions establish internal systematic evaluation processes that require the participation of all existing programs as well as proposed programs. Depending on the nature of a program, the questions that need to be asked and answered differ. Evaluative questions asked of an established program usually focus on quality, impact, and achievement of outcomes. The focus of an evaluation of a new program is on examining what is working and what improvements need to be made to increase productivity. Information associated with a proposed program centers on program need, innovation, contribution, and potential value that is different from existing programs. Often the introduction of new programs influences existing resources and therefore requires a cost-benefit analysis evaluation approach to identify the gains made with the addition of a new program.

DEVELOPING AND IMPLEMENTING PROGRAM EVALUATION

Whether one is implementing an institutional or program evaluation, the development of a program plan is fundamental. A systematic evaluation plan guides the collection of essential documentation that provides programs and institutions with evidence of compliance with accreditation standards and publicly held expectations. As nursing units are attached to parent educational institutions, the nursing unit's evaluation plan should be designed to be integrated into a broader institutional evaluation plan. Many existing evaluation plans incorporate accreditation standards into their design. It is important to understand, when designing an evaluation plan, that accreditation standards are integral to the evaluation process, but that they should not be singularly driven by accreditation expectations. Program evaluation plans need to generate valuable information to meet the comprehensive needs of faculty and administrators.

SYSTEMATIC EVALUATION PLAN

The nursing professional accreditation standards assist in the identification of the major dimensions that should be a part of any nursing program evaluation design. These dimensions are mission, governance, faculty and staff, students, resources, curriculum, and evaluation. These evaluative features provide the broad structure on which to begin to shape your evaluation plan. In general, evaluation plans are at least two-dimensional in design. The dimensions serve as one facet, whereas the other part of the design includes expected outcomes, achievements made, and decisions or actions prompted by the differences. In today's reality of accountability, the focus must be on the rationale for existence and how programs work or do not work (Zhanjun et al., 2016, p. 89). Therefore, the evaluation plans need to not only identify the dimensions but also reflect how the different dimensions interact in determining the contributions and social value of these contributions to internal and external stakeholders.

STEPS IN PROGRAM EVALUATION

STEP 1

Conducting program evaluation requires that you have a systematic plan of attack. The first step in this plan should be to determine what you want to accomplish from evaluation activities. It is important that there be agreement on why you are conducting an evaluation and what you hope to gained from such activities, as noted earlier in this chapter. For nursing, one of the major reasons for conducting evaluation is accreditation. However, there is a potential for many other needs for program evaluation based on internal and external social and political factors. When determining what is to be accomplished from evaluation activities, it is important to understand the mission, goals, and outcomes of the parent institution as well as those of the nursing unit. By looking for congruency among these missions, goals, and outcomes across the layers of an organization, you are able to answer questions related to the fit of the nursing unit and program offerings with the parent's institutional mission and goals, and the contribution of the program in the context of societal needs and expectations of the health care system. During this clarification process, the engagement of community and institutional stakeholders is important to ensure that everyone understands the process and has the same outcome expectations. The establishment of goals or outcomes of evaluation might feel counterintuitive to a more grounded approach to theory, but logically it is critical if evaluation is to be meaningful. The major hesitation in establishing outcomes upfront is the concern that faculty and administrators will be held accountable for outcomes they cannot control. The goals and expected outcomes provide the foundation on which to build an evaluation model that is logically consistent with the identified intent of the goals and expected outcomes (Chyung, 2015, p. 84).

STEPS 2 AND 3

The next two steps in designing a program evaluation are the identification of documentation/evidence needed and the activities involved in gathering this information. Integral to these steps is identification of the type of evidence to be collected; location of the evidence, personnel, and stakeholders responsible for data retrieval; time frame in which the collection is to occur; and the frequency or cycle of repeated collection. Evidence and data can take many forms, including written, verbal, observational, and electronic. Data retrieved can be either qualitative or quantitative in nature, depending on what information exists. However, data should be able to be validated. Often this validation is accomplished through the use of mixed methodologies and cross-referencing/triangulation. One of the discovery outcomes of data retrieval is the ability to note nonexisting data, or data that do not exist in a format compatible to interpret accurately against established outcomes/goals. The measurements used in the collection of information should be valid, and the processes identified in the collection of information should be systematic and efficient.

STEP 4

The logical next step in evaluation planning is the incorporation of processes that will be used to interpret the information collected. These processes should reflect a systematic review and interpretation of information and a summation of findings. The summary of the findings should be presented to stakeholders in a way that supports goals and expected outcomes and is linked to program improvement, accountability, and contributions. If the main purpose of evaluation planning is summative in nature, then examining aggregated information over time is of the most value to stakeholders. When designing an evaluation plan for a proposed or newly implemented program, history would not exist or would be preliminary. This type of preliminary information needs to be interpreted with caution both by evaluators and decision makers. Some theorists describe the evaluation of new or proposed programs as formative as opposed to summative.

QUESTIONS TO GUIDE EVALUATION PLAN DESIGN

There are a number of decisions that faculty and administrators must address on a cyclic basis that guide thinking about designing the evaluation plan to ensure that these questions get answered. There is no one acceptable list of questions commonly used by program evaluators. In nursing, many of the questions that might be considered in program evaluation can be generated from the accreditation criteria. These questions often address the areas listed in Exhibit 17.2. Although the questions might seem overwhelming when taken as a collective, they can be distributed across the dimensions suggested earlier: mission, governance, faculty and staff, students, resources, curriculum, and evaluation. Table 17.1 displays these questions under each dimension, with potential decisions/answers to the questions posed as a clearer visualization for those designing a program evaluation plan. It is important to keep in

EXHIBIT 17.2 Areas That Guide Design of Evaluation Plan

- Expected and unexpected outcomes of the program and their impact on the program
- Balance between the cost of program delivery and the quality of the outcomes achieved
- Impact on mission and goals
- Adequacy of resources
- Appropriate qualifications and credentials for faculty, staff, and unit leader (dean, director, other)
- Existence of numbers and quality of physical and fiscal resources
- Appropriate allocation and use of resources to meet mission goals and needs of existing and potentially new programs
- Ability to implement program in a way that promotes achievement of program outcomes
- Quality and quantity of learning experiences to promote program outcomes
- Program barriers and enablers that positively or negatively affect program effectiveness
- Strategies to facilitate program improvement
- Quality and quantity of learning resources to promote student success
- Quality of graduates
- Alumni ability to perform to expectations
- Contributions of faculty, staff, students, and alumni to the professional and social community
- Value of the program in comparison to similar existing programs

Source: From Commission on Collegiate Nursing Education (2013).

TABLE 17.1 Evaluation Questions by Evaluative Dimensions

Dimensions	Potential Questions to Consider	Potential Decisions
Mission and goals	• Are the mission and goals of the nursing unit consistent with that of the parent institution? • Have professional standards and practice guidelines been incorporated into the goals and outcomes of the nursing unit? Are the standards consistent with community workforce needs and regional health care practices? • Is there an ongoing systematic review process in place to ensure continued accountability?	• Worth/contribution of the nursing unit to the mission and goals of the institution. • Program goals and outcomes are in alignment with professional practice expectations, which indicate program relevance. • Faculty are periodically reviewed for relevance and are accountable to practice for alumni performance.
Governance	• What is the process for faculty and student participation in setting goals, developing policies, and addressing issues related to quality of education and learning experiences? • Are educational policies and practices consistent with the learner population, consistently applied, equitable in interpretation and facilitating of student acceptance to and progress through to graduation? Do the policies in place protect individual rights and freedoms?	• Faculty and students take responsibility to provide meaningful input into the academic environment and learning culture that enhance their educational experiences. • The right policies for the right populations are administered at the right time in the right place by the right people. Individual freedoms are protected with appropriate due process mechanisms executed as written.
Faculty and staff	• Are the quantity and quality of the faculty and staff consistent with educational needs and abilities to promote achievement of program goals and student learning outcomes? • Do faculty and staff have the knowledge and skills to contribute to student learning, achievement of student goals, and attainment of nursing and institutional mission and goals through scholarship, practice, and service activities?	• Instructor-to-student ratios are within practice guidelines and consistent with best evidence for promoting learning. Faculty and staff hold professional and educational credentials consistent with role expectations, practice guidelines, community partner expectations, university expectations, and student and peer expectations.

(continued)

TABLE 17.1 Evaluation Questions by Evaluative Dimensions (*continued*)

Dimensions	Potential Questions to Consider	Potential Decisions
		• Faculty and staff contributions bring value and relevance to the institution, nursing, and professional self. Contributions are consistent with mission and unit goals and facilitate student achievement of outcomes.
Students	• Are student academic support systems in place, accessible, and of the quality needed to support student attainment of academic outcomes and personal goals? • Are support services able to meet the learning needs of students enrolled in programs relying on technology to deliver or enhance the learning experience for students?	• The quality, quantity, and accessibility of academic support facilitate student retention and achievement. • All students are able to meet program outcomes with appropriate leveraging of technological resources and services.
Resources	• Are physical resources and equipment of the quality and quantity to support student attainment of program and learning outcomes? • Are fiscal resources commensurate with program needs and of the quality to promote achievement of learning outcomes and program goals and mission? • Does a systematic process for review and modification exist to sustain the quality and quantity of resources required to meet mission and goals? Do faculty have a voice in the resource allocation process necessary to ensure resource sustainability?	• Physical resources meet program needs and provide the ability to implement learning experiences that promote achievement of learning outcomes and program goals/mission. • Fiscal resources are adequate to meet program mission and goals. They are aligned with institutional fiscal resources and based on goal achievement. • The nursing unit and its faculty and staff are able to acquire resources of the quantity and quality needed to meet the mission and goals of the nursing unit.
Curriculum	• Are the mission, goals, and expected learning outcomes consistent with stakeholders' expectations, professional standards, and best practice guidelines?	• Program outcomes are consistent with mission and goals. Program is relevant and provides the knowledge and skills consistent with evidence-based best practices.

(*continued*)

TABLE 17.1 Evaluation Questions by Evaluative Dimensions (*continued*)

Dimensions	Potential Questions to Consider	Potential Decisions
	• Has the curriculum been designed to promote attainment of knowledge and skills commensurate with established learning outcomes across programs? Are learning experiences consistent with and do they complement achievement of learning outcomes? • Are students able to acquire and use the knowledge from their liberal arts foundation in the acquisition of discipline-specific knowledge and skills needed to meet program and course outcomes?	• Students demonstrate the ability to meet course and program learning outcomes. • Demonstrated student behaviors are consistent with institutional and nursing program mission and goals.
Program effectiveness	• What is the overall contribution of value and impact of the program on the professional workforce and the social community? • What factors impede or enhance program effectiveness?	• The performance quality of the graduates meets or exceeds employer expectations. Program costs balance with the ability of graduates to achieve outcomes. Program is effective in meeting goals. • Barriers and enablers have been identified and decisions made to remove or reinforce to support efforts for continuous quality improvement of program.

TABLE 17.2 Matching Information Sources to Evaluation Questions

Dimensions	Question Elements	Information Sources/Documentation
Mission and goals	Consistency, contributions, reflect accepted standards of education and practice, and inform decisions	• Comparison of institutional mission and goals with nursing units • Comparison of professional standards with program outcomes • Committee documentation of systematic review and actions taken as part of the review process • Verification from practice partners that standards used to develop program outcomes reflect current practice expectations

(continued)

TABLE 17.2 Matching Information Sources to Evaluation Questions (*continued*)

Dimensions	Question Elements	Information Sources/Documentation
Governance	Faculty and student involvement in governance, contribution of involvement in promoting institutional and nursing mission and goals	• Listing of faculty and student involvement in governance structure • Determination of level of involvement • Contribution made to policy setting and alignment to implementation of polices • Committee minutes noting policy application to such activities as admission, progression, graduation
Faculty and staff	Qualifications, experience consistent with program needs	• Documentation of credentials, experience consistent with role • Professional contributions consistent with role expectations and educational outcomes that promote learning
Students	Student credentials consistent with academic success	• Admission credentials • Documentation of prior success • Identification of support services and impact on student success • Retention rates and progression to graduation data along with documentation of use of information by appropriate personnel
Resources	Commensurate with program needs to meet program goals	• Documentation of finances in relation to program needs, costs to administer program
Curriculum	Curriculum design facilitates learning	• Documentation of performance, achievement in relation to benchmark performance expectations • Performance evaluations using a 360-degree perspective
Program effectiveness	Meeting goals, impact of graduates as it relates to preparation for practice	• Percent graduating on time • Percent employed by specified time • Percent securing appropriate practice credentials • Results of employer surveys documenting ability to meet practice expectations

mind that this table is not an exhaustive list of questions to consider or decisional outcomes to achieve.

Once the questions and their expected outcomes have been built into the evaluation plan, it is important to identify what information is needed and how best to gather that information. As discussed earlier in the chapter, the most informative data should be collected in a timely and cost-effective way. Table 17.2 provides examples of possible data sources for answering some of the evaluation questions posed in Table 17.1.

REPOSITORY OF EVALUATION INFORMATION

A common repository should be created to ensure that information is collected and analyzed on a systematic and cyclic basis. The more complex the operations of the nursing unit and institution are, the more critical it is to establish and preserve evaluative information, especially summative data, to enhance retrieval and distribution to appropriate stakeholders in a timely fashion. As noted earlier in the discussion, evaluation that supports such formative activities as conducting a needs assessment about the possible development of a new program or other initiatives or assessing the implementation of a new program requires specific documentation directed "to implement or not," or "make corrective adjustments midstream." These types of evaluations tend to generate less information, and the need for future retrieval is limited.

The incorporation of electronic informational systems has facilitated not only data retrieval and storage, but also enhanced reporting and dissemination of information in a timely and meaningful fashion for stakeholders, especially for those stakeholders with authority and responsibility for decision making. The design of information systems ranges from fully designed to being customized for a specific institution or program. Start-up costs can be high, as is the time taken for customization and updating the system.

Within informational systems, there should be support tools that facilitate the ability to display information for specific audiences and needs. A couple of tools currently being used in institutions of higher education are the dashboard and report card display mechanisms. These tools allow institutions and programs to share summaries of performance, highlight key traits of performance or factors that are unique to the institution or program, and make comparisons with other national and regional performance indicators. Information shared using tools such as the dashboard or report card can be kept as an internal tracking mechanism or designed for more public use. Dashboards that display more strategic information about institutional operations focus more on decision makers' need to know. Other dashboards focus on performance indicators and are often embedded within the context of goals and outcomes. Often the designs focus on performance and are created for public informational purposes to highlight institutional or program mission and abilities. Measuring performance and goal attainment can be evidenced by the use of a numeric, alphabetic, or color scheme scale designed to quickly communicate the level of success.

ANALYSIS, REPORTING, AND USE OF EVALUATION INFORMATION

The last implementation steps in evaluation are the analysis, reporting, and use of the information collected. Evaluators are often challenged in distributing the information to the right stakeholders at the right time, as the information required by the stakeholders might need to be collected, or existing data might have to be analyzed differently to meet emerging needs. As an evaluator, you will most likely have to assist stakeholders in interpreting information in a way that is most useful in meeting individual needs.

In today's environment, many institutions and programs are being required to provide information associated with costs (Powell, Gilleland, & Pearson, 2012). Program evaluation plans often include processes that allow administrators to determine program costs in relation to program outcomes. Two types of approaches frequently used are cost-effectiveness and cost-benefit analysis. Cost-effectiveness analysis relates the costs of a program to the key outcomes or benefits of the program. In cost-benefit analysis, the process focuses on comparing costs with the dollar value of all (or most) of the program's benefits, which is a challenge when working with human factors. As funding continues to be closely tied to institutional and program outcomes, cost analysis will be integral to evaluation.

EXHIBIT 17.3 Elements to Support an Institution's Evaluation Activities

1. Clear goals
2. Commonly shared use of evaluation terminology across disciplines and campuses
3. Faculty ownership of evaluation and assessment activities
4. Continuous faculty development activities related to evaluation practices
5. Top-down support for evaluation activities that include budgeting and planning at the institutional and unit levels
6. Established goals and outcomes that can be measured
7. Evaluation plan that can be and is implemented and participated in by faculty, staff, administration, students, and other primary stakeholders
8. Systematic and cyclic institution plan for program reviews
9. Ongoing evaluation of institutional effectiveness in relation to its mission and goals
10. Support of initiatives that promote evaluation efforts
11. Means of recognizing and celebrating evaluation efforts and successes

Source: From Weiner (2009).

BUILDING A CULTURE OF EVALUATION

Building and sustaining a culture in which evaluation plays an important role is critical to sustain evaluation activities in the life of the institution and the various disciplines and programs housed within it. Institutions and programs need to build an environment in which decisions are based on valid information, collected using accepted research practices. Weiner (2009) identified elements that need to be in place to support evaluation in an institution (Exhibit 17.3).

Mayne (2010) suggested that a strong culture of evaluation is sustained by valuing self-reflection and self-examination. The information obtained through these processes facilitates the monitoring of organizations, as well as incorporating information into their decisional approach to dealing with challenges. A strong evaluative culture engages in learning from the evidence generated and encourages experimentation and innovation as ways to improve performance and strengthen a program. The greatest gain from self-examination is more internally focused.

Ndoye and Parker (2010) examined the challenges to the establishment of an assessment culture. Informants indicated that faculty involvement, resources, and the systematic use of information affected the ability to sustain such a culture. Another key to the establishment and sustainability of a culture of assessment and evaluation is having one or more people in the environment who have the skills needed to support evaluation practices. These skills include knowledge of evaluation and assessment, ability to ask the appropriate questions that will drive the process, management skills to coordinate and ensure that the evaluation plan is systematically and consistently implemented as designed, ability to know when and how to make adjustments to the plan, and skills to communicate findings to stakeholders by making connections between findings and expected outcomes (Bowman, 2015).

SUMMARY

Evaluation is critical to institutions and programs, given the pressures from accreditation requirements; state mandates; funding and allocation priorities within a continually shrinking budget; and pressures from students, families, and employers.

Evaluation science has grown in sophistication to keep abreast of these pressures. Program evaluation plans are more complex and consume more time and expense for nursing programs today than in the past, and this trend is likely to continue. However, with the aid of technology and experienced evaluators, evaluation activities can be more effective and efficient. As nurse educators, not only do we know what information is needed, but we are also learning how best to use evaluative information to maintain the quality and integrity of our programs. Making decisions based on valid evidence ensures that we continue to provide sustainable relevant educational programming through a continuous quality improvement process, program evaluation.

REFERENCES

Alkin, M. C. (2011). *Evaluation essentials: From A to Z.* New York, NY: Guilford Press.

Alkin, M. C., & Christie, C. A. (2004). An evaluation theory tree. In M. C. Alkin (Ed.), *Evaluation roots: Tracing theorists' views and influences* (pp. 12–65). Thousand Oaks, CA: Sage.

Askew, K., Beverly, M. G., & Jay, M. L. (2012). Aligning collaboration and culturally responsive evaluation approaches. *Evaluation and Program Planning, 35,* 552–557.

Association of American Colleges and Universities. (2010). *VALUE: Valid assessment of learning in undergraduate education.* Retrieved from http:/www.aacu.org/value/rubrics/pdf/All Rubrics.pdf

Astin, A. W., & Antonio, A. L. (2012). *Assessment for excellence: The philosophy and practice of assessment and evaluation in higher education* (2nd ed.). Lanham, MD: Littlefield.

Banta, T. W. (2011). Will we just stand by and watch this happen? *Assessment Update, 23.* Retrieved from http://www.assessmentupdate.com/sample-articles/will-we-just-stand-by.aspx

Bowman, S. F. (2015). *Evaluation in instructional design practice: A view from the stakeholders* (Doctoral dissertation, Capella University,. UMI: 3712122).

Centers for Disease Control and Prevention, Program Performance and Evaluation Office. (2012). Introduction to program evaluation for public health programs: A self-study guide. Step 1: Engage stakeholders. Retrieved from https://www.cdc.gov/eval/guide/step1/index.htm

Centers for Disease Control and Prevention, Program Performance and Evaluation Office. (2017). *Framework for program evaluation in public health* (No. RR-11). Retrieved from https://www.cdc.gov/mmwr/PDF/rr/rr4811.pdf

Chen, H. Y. (2013). The roots and growth of theory-driven evaluation: An integrated perspective for assessing viability, effectuality, and transferability. In M. C. Alkin (Ed.), *Evaluation roots: A wider perspective of theorists' views and influences* (pp. 113–129). Thousand Oaks, CA: Sage.

Christie, C. A., & Alkin, M. C. (2013). An evaluation theory tree. In M. C. Alkin (Ed.), *Evaluation roots: A wider perspective of theorists' views and influences* (pp. 11–58). Thousand Oaks, CA: Sage.

Chyung, S. Y. (2015). Foundational concepts for conducting program evaluations. *Performance Improvement Quarterly, 27*(4), 77–96. doi:10.1002/piq.21181

Commission on Collegiate Nursing Education. (2013). *Standards for accreditation of baccalaureate and graduate degree nursing programs.* Retrieved from http://www.aacn.nche.edu/ccne-accreditation/Standards-Amended-2013.pdf

Cook, T. D., Scriven, M., Coryn, C. L. S., & Evergreen, S. D. H. (2010). Contemporary thinking about causation in evaluation: A dialogue with Tom Cook and Michael Scriven. *American Journal of Education, 31,* 105–117. doi:10.1177/1098214009354918

Cosgrove, L. (2013). Portfolios: The next wave of student assessment? Retrieved from http://createquity.com

Getha-Eby, T., Beery, T., O'Brien B., & Xu, Y. (2015). Student learning outcomes in response to concept-based teaching. *Journal of Nursing Education, 54,* 193–200. doi:10.3928/014834-20150318-02

Halstead, J. A. (2017). The accreditation process in nursing education. In M. H. Oermann (Ed.), *A systematic approach to assessment and evaluation of nursing programs* (pp. 79–91). Philadelphia, PA: National League for Nursing/Wolters Kluwer.

Hermans, L. M., Naber, A. C., & Easerink, B. (2012). Theory-based evaluation: Challenges to this approach. *Evaluation and Program Planning, 35,* 427–438.

Horne, E. M., & Sandmann, L. R. (2012). Current trends in systematic program evaluation: An integrative literature review. *Journal of Nursing Education, 51,* 570–581. doi:10.3928/01484834-20120820-06

Jordan, C. M., Chazdon, S., & Alviz, K. (2016). Evaluating beyond the ivory tower: Lessons learned from the scholars program. *Journal of Community Engagement and Higher Education, 8,* 66–79.

Kardong-Edgren, S., Oermann, M. H., Rizzolo, M. A., & Odom-Maryon, T. (2017). Establishing inter- and intrarater reliability for high-stakes testing using simulation. *Nursing Education Perspectives, 38*, 63-68. doi:10.1097/01.NEP.0000000000000114

Lee, Y., Altschuld, J. W., & Lee, L. (2012). Essential competencies for program evaluators in a diverse cultural context. *Evaluation and Program Planning, 35*, 439–444.

Madaus, G. F. (2013). Ralph W. Tyler's contribution to program evaluation. In M. C. Alkin (Ed.), *Evaluation roots: A wider perspective of theorists' views and influences* (pp. 157–164). Thousand Oaks, CA: Sage.

Mayne, J. (2010). Building an evaluative culture: The key to effective evaluation and results management. *The Canadian Journal of Program Evaluation, 24*(2), 1–30.

McLaughlin, J. A., & Jordan, G. B. (2015). Using logic models. In K. E. Newcomer, H. P. Hatry, & J. S. Wholey (Eds.), *Handbook of practical program evaluation* (pp. 62–87). Hoboken, NJ: Wiley.

McPherson, C. L. (2015). *Implicit and explicit evaluation theories of expert evaluation practitioners* (Doctoral dissertation). Retrieved from ProQuest: 3737837)

Mertens, D. M. (2009). *Transformative research and evaluation.* New York, NY: Guilford Press.

Mertens, D. M. (2010). *Research and evaluation in education and psychology: Integrating diversity with quantitative, qualitative, and mixed methods.* Thousand Oaks, CA: Sage.

Mertens, D. M. (2016). Assumptions at the philosophical and programmatic levels in evaluation. *Evaluation and Program Planning, 59*, 102-108. doi:10.1016/j.evalprogplan.2016.05.010

Ndoye, A., & Parker, M. A. (2010). Creating and sustaining a culture of assessment. *Planning for Higher Education, 38*, 28–39.

Patton, M. Q. (2008). *Utilization-focused evaluation.* Thousand Oaks, CA: Sage.

Patton, M. Q. (2012). *Essentials of utilization-focused evaluation.* Thousand Oaks, CA: Sage.

Patton, M. Q. (2013). The roots of utilization-focused evaluation. In M. C. Alkin (Ed.), *Evaluation roots: A wider perspective of theorists' views and influences* (pp. 293–303). Thousand Oaks, CA: Sage.

Powell, B. A., Gilleland, D. S., & Pearson, L. C. (2012). Expenditures, efficiency, and effectiveness in U.S. undergraduate higher education: A national benchmark model. *Journal of Higher Education, 83*(1), 102–127. doi:10.1353/jhe.2012.0005

Ramirez, R., & Brodhead, D. (2013). *Utilization focused evaluation: A primer for evaluators.* Penang, Malaysia: Southbound Sdn. Bhd.

Rhodes, T. L. (2012). Show me the learning: Value, accreditation, and the quality of the degree. *Planning for Higher Education, 40*(3), 3–36.

Royce, D., Thyer, B. A., & Padgett, D. K. (2016). *Program evaluation: An introduction to an evidence-based approach* (6th ed., pp. 1–33). Boston, MA: Cengage.

Scriven, M. (1991). Pros and cons about goal-free evaluation. *American Journal of Evaluation, 12*(1), 55–62. doi:10.1177/109821409101200108

Scriven, M. (2004). Reflections. In M. C. Alkin (Ed.), *Evaluation roots: Tracing theorists' views and influences* (pp. 183–195). Thousand Oaks, CA: Sage.

Scriven, M. (2013). Conceptual revolution in evaluation: Past, present, and future. In M.C. Alkin (Ed.), *Evaluation roots: A wider perspective of theorists' views and influences* (pp. 167–179). Thousand Oaks, CA: Sage.

Senger, J., & Kanthan, R. (2012). Student evaluations: Synchronous tripod of learning portfolio assessment-self-assessment, peer-assessment, instructor assessment. *Creative Education, 3*(1), 155–163.

Simon, E. B., McGinnis, S. P., & Krauss, B. J. (2013). Predictor variables for NLCEX-RN readiness exam performance. *Nursing Education Perspectives, 34*, 18–24.

Stratton-Berkessel, R. (2015). *Appreciative inquiry: Overview of method, principles and applications.* Retrieved from http://www.positivitystrategist.com

Stame, N. (2014). Positive thinking approaches to evaluation and program perspectives. *Canadian Journal of Program Evaluation, 29*(2), 67–86. doi:10.3138/cjpe.29.2.67

Stobart, G., & Eggen, T. (2014). High-stakes testing - value, fairness and consequences. In T.J.H.M. Eggen & G. Stobart (Eds.), *High-stakes testing in education* (pp. 1-6). New York, NY: Routledge.

Stufflebeam, D. L. (2004). The 21st-century CIPP model: Origins, development, and use. In M. C Alkin (Ed.), *Evaluation roots: Tracing theorists' views and influences* (pp. 245–266). Thousand Oaks, CA: Sage.

Stufflebeam, D. L., (2011). Meta-evaluation. *Journal of MultiDisciplinary Evaluation, 7*(15), 99–158. Retrieved from http://www.jmde.com

Stufflebeam, D. L. (2013). The CIPP evaluation model: Status, origin, development, use and theory. In M. C. Alkin (Ed.), *Evaluation roots: A wider perspective of theorists' views and influences* (pp. 243–260). Thousand Oaks, CA: Sage.

Wandersman, A., Snell-Johns, J., Lentz, B. E., Fetterman, D. M., Keener, D. C., Livet, M., . . . Flaspoher, P. (2012). The principles of empowerment evaluation. In D. M. Fetterman, A. Wandersman, & R. A. Millett (Eds.), *Empowerment evaluation principles in practice* (pp. 27–41). New York, NY: Guilford Press.

Weiner, W. F. (2009). Establishing a culture of assessment. *Academe, 95*(4), 28–32.

Weiss, C. (1991). Evaluation research in the political context: Sixteen years and four administrators later. In M. W. McLaughlin & D. C. Phillips (Eds.), *Evaluation and education: At quarter century* (90th Yearbook of the National Society for the Study of Education; Part II, p. 213). Chicago, IL: University of Chicago Press.

Wholey, J. S. (2013). Using evaluation to improve program performance and results. In M. C. Alkin (Ed.), *Evaluation roots: A wider perspective of theorists' views and influences* (pp. 261–266). Thousand Oaks, CA: Sage.

Youker, B. W., & Ingraham, A. (2013). Goal-free evaluation: An orientation for foundation evaluators. *Foundation Review, 5*(4). doi:10.9707/1944-5660-1182

Zhanjun, W., Weifeng, Q., & Jiangbo, L. (2016). Data-intensive evaluation: The concept, methods, and prospects of higher education monitoring evaluation. *Chinese Education & Society, 49,* 86–98. doi:10.1080/10611932.2016.1192400

Scholarship and Nursing Education
Around the World

18

Evidence-Based Teaching in Nursing

MARILYN H. OERMANN AND JAMIE L. CONKLIN

OBJECTIVES

- Describe evidence-based teaching in nursing, including each of its phases
- Compare different types of evidence and the use of evidence in making educational decisions
- Search for evidence about a teaching method

Evidence-based teaching is the use of research findings and other evidence to guide educational decisions and practices. Available evidence should be used when developing the curriculum and courses, selecting teaching methods and approaches to use with students, planning clinical learning activities, and assessing students' learning and performance. Yet many nurse educators rarely search for evidence when they make educational decisions. They update their courses by incorporating new evidence about the content, but they might not seek evidence on how those courses are best designed, taught, and evaluated. How much practice do students need to retain their motor skills? What are best practices for debriefing? What characteristics of online courses are critical to learning and retention? These are the types of questions that every educator should be raising no matter what course or level of learner they are teaching.

Teachers can then search the literature for research studies and other evidence to answer these questions and guide their educational practices. By reviewing the literature, the teacher can also learn about the experiences of other educators, to build on those rather than to start anew. This chapter describes evidence-based teaching in nursing, the need for better research in nursing education, and a process for engaging in evidence-based teaching.

EVIDENCE-BASED TEACHING IN NURSING: WHAT IS IT?

Evidence-based teaching is the use of research findings and other knowledge to guide educational practices in nursing. Cannon and Boswell (2016) defined evidence-based teaching as a dynamic and holistic system using educational principles validated by evidence to promote learning in a variety of settings (p. 22). Nursing, medicine, education, and other fields have a body of knowledge that can be used to inform practice as a nurse, physician, or teacher: This knowledge provides the evidence to guide what we do. In evidence-based teaching, nurse educators use knowledge about how students learn, how best to promote their learning and performance, effective teaching and assessment methods, and other practices to guide what they do as educators.

Definitions of evidence-based nursing provide a framework for conceptualizing evidence-based teaching in nursing. Many of these definitions view evidence-based nursing as the integration of research evidence with clinical expertise and the values and preferences of the patient. The goal of evidence-based nursing is to integrate current knowledge into health care decisions to improve patient outcomes (Stevens, 2013). Scott and McSherry (2009) analyzed 83 articles to identify the key concepts associated with evidence-based nursing. Based on their analysis, they defined evidence-based nursing as an ongoing process by which evidence, nursing theory, and the nurse's clinical expertise are evaluated critically and considered in conjunction with patient involvement, with the goal of providing optimal nursing care to the patient (p. 1089). This analysis and resulting definition are useful for conceptualizing evidence-based teaching in nursing: it is the integration of the best research evidence with theories and concepts about learning, teaching, assessment, and other areas related to nursing education, the teacher's expertise, and the learner's preferences and goals.

In an online survey of 551 nurse educators, respondents had positive views of evidence-based teaching and believed it contributed to advancing the science of nursing education (Kalb, O'Conner-Von, Brockway, Rierson, & Sendelbach, 2015). They reported using academic, accreditation, and professional standards; their clinical knowledge; data from course evaluations; and findings from quantitative and qualitative research studies as evidence for their teaching. They used evidence for revising their courses, developing the curriculum, and teaching. Engaging in evidence-based teaching is promoted when there are colleagues who also seek evidence to guide their teaching, mentors, supportive administrators, and other resources available to faculty, such as librarians (Kalb et al., 2015).

NURSING EDUCATION RESEARCH AND EVIDENCE-BASED TEACHING

We need rigorous research in nursing education to generate evidence that can be used to guide teaching. Early on, many researchers explored nursing education topics, but over the years the focus of research has shifted to the study of clinical problems, with limited funding available for nursing education. Although the emphasis of nursing research is no longer on education, nursing education studies continue to be done with the aim of building an evidence base for understanding how nursing students learn and how to promote their learning, and to guide educational decisions in nursing. Many of these studies, though, are conducted with small samples of students in one setting only, with investigator-developed tools that have not been validated. Many are pilot studies, and, though valuable, they need to be followed up and replicated. One of the issues in nursing education is that few studies are replicated across schools of nursing and across students (Oermann, 2009). The lack of funding has made it difficult to conduct large, multisite educational studies in nursing (Beischel, Hart, & Turkelson, 2016; Oermann et al., 2012). Addressing these shortcomings is critical, though, to generalizing the findings and determining whether the educational practice can be used with different students and settings. Nursing education research is hampered by a lack of funding, protected time for nurse educators to conduct research, focus on programs of research about education, and expertise of faculty in educational research methods (Broome, Ironside, & McNelis, 2012).

Yucha, Schneider, Smyer, Kowalski, and Stowers (2011) found that most nursing education studies in their sample were done with a single group, either as cross-sectional or posttest only studies ($n = 74$, 55.6%). Less than 20% ($n = 25$, 18.8%) were single-group pre- and posttest. Studies in both nursing and medicine often compare the outcomes of a new educational approach using the learners' baseline as their own control. These studies are relatively easy to conduct as part of a typical teaching situation, and they can be done with minimal or no funding. The issue, however, is that these studies limit generalizability to other students and settings, and they do not contribute sufficient knowledge about the effectiveness of a teaching approach to guide future decisions. Too many studies in nursing education focus on student satisfaction with a new teaching method; though important, satisfaction should not be the only outcome examined.

Nurse educators develop many educational innovations and new initiatives, but without research to document their effectiveness and outcomes, it is not known whether the new approaches are better than the prior ones. Providing an evidence base for nursing education is not only important to advance the science of nursing education; faculty need evidence to make sound decisions about their teaching methods, considering the limited time available for student learning and extent of knowledge and skills they need to develop. Yucha et al. (2011) suggested that the methodological quality of nursing education studies could be improved if the researchers used objective measures of the outcomes, used instruments that were valid and reliable, employed more experimental designs, and included the impact of educational approaches on patient outcomes. Although the effects of education on patient outcomes are important to study, some researchers in medical education have cautioned that they should not be the main focus of medical education research (Cook & West, 2013). The same is true when evaluating the impact of educational interventions in nursing: the focus needs to remain on the students and their learning and development.

Levin (2004) developed a model of educational research that provides a framework for understanding the current state of nursing education research. *Stage 1* includes preliminary ideas, hypotheses, observations, and pilot studies. *Stage 2* involves controlled laboratory experiments and interventions tested in the classroom, as well as observational studies of master teachers. *Stage 3* studies are randomized controlled trials of educational interventions comparing a new approach to the standard one. Levin emphasized that in Stage 3 the interventions are assigned randomly to different groups of learners and educational situations, which are both realistic and controlled. With rigorous studies, effective interventions can be tested across settings (*Stage 4*). Most nursing education studies are at Stages 1 and 2. However, with rigorous studies at Stages 1 and 2 that are replicated in various schools of nursing and settings, research findings can be synthesized to create an evidence base for nursing education (Oermann, 2009).

PHASES OF EVIDENCE-BASED TEACHING

Evidence-based teaching includes four phases: (a) questioning educational practices and identifying the need for evidence to guide teaching, (b) searching for research studies and other evidence on educational practices, (c) evaluating the quality of the evidence, and (d) deciding whether the findings are applicable to one's own program, courses, students, and context in which one is teaching (Oermann, 2009). Similar to evidence-based practice in nursing and other fields, the teacher also considers theories and concepts about learning and teaching, and the teacher's own philosophy of nursing education and expertise as an educator. Students also need to have input as to their preferences for learning and their personal goals to be met in the course. The evidence alone does not dictate what methods and practices to use. It is up to the teacher to integrate the evidence with these other considerations, as the teacher understands the students and context in which the education takes place.

QUESTION EDUCATIONAL PRACTICES AND IDENTIFY NEED FOR EVIDENCE

The first phase in evidence-based teaching is for nurse educators to recognize that it is their responsibility to reflect on their educational practices and question whether there is a better way of teaching students (Oermann, 2009). Reflection and questioning our practices as teachers are defining characteristics of a professional, and they are critical to thinking about changes in education that could lead to improved learning and performance.

The questions can be general questions about an educational practice or intervention being considered. These are descriptive questions that guide a search of the literature for information about the practice, but not necessarily about whether it is superior to another practice in terms of outcomes. Examples of these general questions are: How can team-based learning be used for instruction in online nursing courses? What are strategies for incorporating audience response systems that allow the teacher to ask questions and gather students' responses in large group lectures? What are best practices in debriefing in simulation-based learning? These general questions are valuable too, because they allow the teacher to learn about the experiences of other nurse educators. With this type of question, the teacher can search the literature and other resources to learn more about the educational practice and build on those experiences.

Another type of question leads to a search for evidence to support an educational practice or intervention. With this type of question the teacher is searching for studies on the outcomes of various practices to make a decision as to the best approach to use. Examples of this type of question include the following: Is there a difference in knowledge retention between online courses that use team-based learning and traditional online courses with video recordings of lectures? What are the effects of audience response systems on learning outcomes in nursing education? Does scripted versus nonscripted debriefing and/or simulator realism affect performance of nurses in simulated cardiopulmonary arrests? In nursing education, this type of question is often more difficult to answer than it would be in other disciplines, as the research might not have been done, and the evidence is not available, or the studies are of such poor quality that the findings cannot be used for making educational decisions.

SEARCH FOR EVIDENCE ON EDUCATIONAL PRACTICES

In the second phase, teachers search the literature for studies on the topic and for other articles and resources to answer their questions. This research requires knowledge of bibliographic databases to search, search skills, and awareness of other resources, such as websites that report evidence on educational practices. Research also requires time, which can pose a barrier to completing a literature search (Patterson, 2009); however, seeking the assistance of librarians and accessing nursing and education literature readily made available through libraries can save time in evidence-based teaching as it has been shown to do in evidence-based practice in patient care (Marshall et al., 2013).

Although there are many bibliographic databases that contain reports of studies that might be relevant to teaching in nursing, three databases are recommended for a search in nursing education:

1. MEDLINE, which has more than 23 million references to biomedical and life sciences journal articles, including nursing education (United States National Library of Medicine, 2016). MEDLINE can be searched through PubMed, available at www.ncbi.nlm.nih.gov/pubmed.
2. Cumulative Index to Nursing and Allied Health Literature (CINAHL), the database covering nursing and allied health literature (EBSCO Industries, Inc., 2016).
3. Education Resources Information Center (ERIC) database, from the Institute of Education Sciences of the United States Department of Education (n.d.), which indexes education research and also conference proceedings and other reports that might provide evidence about a teaching practice.

For some questions, other bibliographic databases such as PsycINFO®, which covers studies and other peer-reviewed literature in the behavioral and social sciences (American Psychological Association, 2016), might be relevant, depending on the topic.

It is important to search multiple databases, because different journals are indexed in them, and thus a broad search of the literature provides a better evidence base. An example can be seen in a search for evidence on audience response systems. A search in PubMed using the phrase "audience response system" revealed more than twice as many articles as in the CINAHL database, and only some of these articles overlapped. If searching only one database, the nurse educator might miss some relevant studies.

The questions asked about the topic or educational practice guide the search for studies. Nurse educators need to be proficient in *searching the literature*. They should be knowledgeable about the databases and the literature in them, as well as about how they are organized. Educators also need skills in selecting keywords, using controlled vocabularies (for example, Medical Subject Headings [MeSH] terms in PubMed and subject headings in CINAHL), and combining search terms. Those skills are critical to locate relevant educational studies. Exhibit 18.1 lists strategies nurse educators can use to prepare themselves to conduct a search for evidence on teaching.

EXHIBIT 18.1 Strategies Nurse Educators Can Use to Prepare Themselves to Conduct a Search

Ask the Question

Learn how to ask clear questions to guide a search.

Develop a PICO(TS) as applicable.

Write a focused question based on the PICO(TS).

Identify the main concepts from the focused question.

Plan search strategies in advance.

Locate the thesaurus, if one is available, in each of the databases to be used in the search.

Identify subject headings and text word terms for your topic or to answer your question.

Find a few sample articles and confirm or alter the search terms.

(continued)

EXHIBIT 18.1 Strategies Nurse Educators Can Use to Prepare Themselves to Conduct a Search (*continued*)

Select and Search Appropriate Databases

Select relevant databases to search and use multiple databases.

Become familiar with different bibliographic databases, including MEDLINE, CINAHL, Education Resources Information Center (ERIC), PsycINFO, and others, depending on the subject.

Review the types of literature indexed in each of the databases.

Learn how each database is organized.

Learn to use the databases through tutorials, help guides, and practice.

Learn how to broaden and narrow a search, use filters, combine searches, conduct advanced searches, and use other search strategies in each database.

Review sample records and different views of each record to become familiar with them.

Critically Evaluate the Search Terms and Process Based on Citations Returned

Be prepared to adjust or change search terms or strategies and/or databases used to match needs.

Refer to Exhibit 18.2 for specifics on evaluating the nursing education studies retrieved in the search.

Organize Citations and Information Returned

Learn how to save searches, create collections, and manage citations as appropriate.

Learn how to save and manage references in bibliographic management software.

Develop a system for recording results of references; review available resources such as PRISMA (Preferred Reporting Items for Systematic Reviews and Meta-Analyses) flow diagram (www.prisma-statement.org).

Use PRISMA checklist and flow diagram if conducting systematic review or meta-analysis.

PICO(TS), population or problem, intervention, comparison, outcomes, timing (if applicable), and setting (if applicable).

Teachers also should be aware of other resources, such as websites that report evidence on educational practices. For example, the Best Evidence Medical and Health Professional Education (BEME) Collaboration is an international group with the aim of developing evidence-based education in medicine and other health professions. Researchers conduct systematic reviews to provide the best available evidence for teaching in the health fields and to disseminate the findings of their reviews at their website and in journals (BEME, 2016b). Nurse educators can search for evidence reviews related to their topic or question at the BEME website (www.BEMEcollaboration.org/Published+Reviews). Although these reviews are not specific to nursing education, they include nursing education studies, and most of the reviews are applicable to teaching in nursing. Teachers can also search websites of nursing education organizations for summaries of evidence and reports of relevant studies.

SYSTEMATIC REVIEWS

For areas of education that have been well studied, the teacher should begin by searching for a systematic review in which experts critically appraise and synthesize the findings of multiple studies on a particular educational topic to identify best practices. These reviews include an assessment of the original studies; in evidence-based practice, such studies are referred to as *appraised resources*.

One type of systematic review is a meta-analysis, which uses quantitative methods to synthesize the findings from individual research studies. Meta-analyses typically calculate effect sizes, which determine whether the differences between groups are significant and the magnitude of these differences, when considering the studies as a whole (Oermann, 2009). Shin, Park, and Kim (2015) conducted a meta-analysis on the effectiveness of patient simulation in nursing education. Of 2,503 potentially relevant studies, 20 were included in the final analysis. Studies indicated that simulation improved learning outcomes with medium to large effect sizes when compared to traditional education or no intervention. In another meta-analysis, they examined outcomes based on the fidelity of the simulation (Kim, Park, & Shin, 2016). Of 2,279 possible studies, 40 were included in the meta-analysis. The effect sizes were larger for high-fidelity simulation (0.86), medium-fidelity simulation (1.03), and standardized patients (0.86) compared to low-fidelity and hybrid simulations (Kim et al., 2016). Simulation was particularly valuable for learning in the psychomotor domain.

Often when multiple individual studies are synthesized, it becomes clear that more research is needed to arrive at a sound conclusion about an educational approach. For example, Cheng et al. (2014) conducted a meta-analysis of research on debriefing with technology-enhanced simulation. From a review of 10,903 potentially eligible studies, they identified 177 studies that used debriefing. Key aspects of debriefing, however, such as educator presence, method used, timing, and others, were inadequately reported, so it was impossible to draw conclusions. There also were varied results when comparing concurrent debriefing to debriefing held at the end of the simulation. While an individual study may suggest an approach to use, that same approach may not be supported when multiple studies are considered as a whole.

With a systematic review, the researchers use an organized method of searching for studies; decide which studies to include in the review, based on specific criteria; appraise the quality of each study; and synthesize the findings. The protocol for conducting the review ensures that each study in the review is critiqued similarly, and a standardized process is used. For example, reviews done by BEME follow a protocol that includes the description of the background of the topic, review questions and objectives, search sources and strategies, selection criteria for studies to review, procedures for extracting data, and synthesis of the evidence, among other areas (BEME, 2016a). While systematic review methods in education are mostly similar to those in evidence-based practice, Patricio and vaz Carneiro (2012) point out a few differences in degree, in that educational reviews typically have more confounding variables, more complexity in both the question formation and appraisal of individual studies, and explanatory syntheses of what makes interventions work, for whom, and when rather than numerical syntheses of results (e.g., point estimates, relative confidence intervals).

LITERATURE REVIEWS

With a literature review, the author selects studies to review based on specific criteria, evaluates the studies, and integrates the findings. A literature review is an examination of the literature from the author's perspective. The benefit of systematic reviews and meta-analyses is that only studies that meet certain criteria are included, and the reviews follow an established protocol (Oermann, 2009). An issue with literature reviews is that they are frequently summaries of the findings of studies, with little analysis of their quality and the impact of that quality on the results.

When a systematic review has not been done, however, other more rigorous types of reviews can be valuable in a search for evidence. Grant and Booth (2009) identified 14 types of reviews, including mixed methods, rapid, and state-of-the-art reviews, which include more comprehensive literature searching, critical appraisal, synthesis, or analysis. For example, De Gagne, Choi, Ledbetter, Kang, and Clark (2016) conducted a review of the literature on cyberincivility in health professions education. They reviewed 11 articles published in English from November 2007 to May–June 2015. There were three main themes: (a) online postings of unprofessional content by health professions students, (b) both student and faculty incivility in online courses, and (c) strategies to promote a culture of online professionalism.

INDIVIDUAL STUDIES

When systematic and literature reviews are not available, the teacher needs to review individual studies and critique their quality. With systematic reviews, the researchers assess the methodological quality of studies included in the review. However, when teachers are reviewing the literature themselves, they need to critically appraise each study to determine whether the findings are valid, whether they answer the educational questions raised earlier in the process, and whether they will be useful to the teacher considering his or her own students and context. The study validity depends on whether the research methods are rigorous enough for the findings to be as "close to the truth as possible" (Melnyk, Fineout-Overholt, Stillwell, & Williamson, 2010, p. 52). For example, were students randomly assigned to the teaching intervention and control groups, and were valid and reliable tools used to measure outcomes? Flaws in the study design, the lack of a control or comparison group, use of measurement tools without established validity and reliability, issues with the procedures used for data collection (e.g., the teacher distributing surveys to own students), errors in the statistical analysis, and so forth weaken the findings and limit their use.

The teacher also evaluates whether the results answer the questions identified for the review, support the educational practice or intervention, and are applicable to his or her own students and setting. The study might have been well-designed, but a small sample size in one school of nursing limits generalizing the findings to other groups of learners and settings. Exhibit 18.2 provides a general guide for analyzing nursing education research literature. Table 18.1 provides a form for recording a review of studies with a sample excerpt from a review.

EXHIBIT 18.2 Guide for Analyzing Nursing Education Research Literature

Title

Does it clearly describe the educational study reported in the paper? Is it informative?

Abstract

Does it emphasize the study's purpose, method, major findings, and conclusions?
Is this a quantitative, qualitative, or mixed-methods study in nursing education?

Introduction

Does it state the problem in nursing education and why it is important to learn more about it?
Does the introduction provide the background and rationale for the study?

(continued)

EXHIBIT 18.2 Guide for Analyzing Nursing Education Research Literature (*continued*)

What is the purpose of the study, and is it clear and understandable?

If a conceptual or theoretical framework is presented, does it relate to the purpose and describe the concepts underlying the study and their relationships?

Literature Review

Is the literature critically reviewed?

Are strengths and weaknesses of prior studies included in the review?

Does the review support the reason for conducting the study and identify gaps in our understanding of how best to promote student learning, teach students, develop nursing programs, and so forth?

Is the literature review up to date, that is, most articles in the past 5 years?

Are primary sources used?

Research Questions

Are the research questions clear, specific, and stated appropriately?

Are variables defined if appropriate?

Design

Is the design consistent with the questions?

What type of design is used?

What are strengths and weaknesses of the design?

Sample

What criteria were used to select the sample?

Is the sample size adequate?

Is the sample representative of learners, teachers, nursing programs, and so forth?

Instruments

Are the instruments and other measures described, and are they appropriate?

Are they valid and reliable?

Data Collection Procedure

Is the procedure clearly described?

Are methods for collecting and analyzing qualitative data appropriate for the type of study?

Findings

Are the findings interpreted correctly, including any statistical analyses?

Are the statistics appropriate for analyzing the data?

Are the findings presented clearly and in relation to the study questions or hypotheses?

Are the findings presented logically?

Are tables and figures easy to read, and do they support the text?

Are the statistics in the tables and figures and the statistics in the text consistent?

(continued)

EXHIBIT 18.2 Guide for Analyzing Nursing Education Research Literature (*continued*)

Discussion

Is the discussion related to the literature, and does it include how the study builds on earlier research in nursing education (and higher education if relevant)?

Are the limitations identified, and could they have been resolved?

Can the findings be generalized and, if so, to what populations?

Are there implications for teaching, assessment, program development, and so forth, and are they relevant?

Are the conclusions based on the study results and accurate?

Strengths and Weaknesses

Overall, what are the study's major strengths and weaknesses?

Source: Adapted from Oermann and Hays (2016). Copyright 2016. Reproduced with the permission of Springer Publishing.

TABLE 18.1 Form for Recording Evidence Review of Nursing Education Studies

Components of Review	Evidence Summary
Question to be answered	What are the effects of high-fidelity simulation on nursing students' knowledge and confidence in providing end-of-life care?
Search terms	simulation AND nursing students AND (end-of-life care OR terminal care) (limits: English language, 2011–2016)
Databases searched	PubMed (MEDLINE), CINAHL, ERIC
Number of relevant citations	22
Research study and level of evidence[a]	Dame and Hoebeke (2016).The aim was to evaluate the outcomes of an end-of-life simulation on nursing students' attitudes toward caring for dying patients. A convenience sample of 57 sophomore nursing students participated in an end-of-life care simulation. Students' attitudes were measured using the Frommelt Attitudes Toward Care of the Dying Scale-Form B. After participating in the simulation, students had a significant increase in positive attitudes toward caring for dying patients ($p<.001$). Level 2a

[a]Kirkpatrick's Four-Level Evaluation Model.

EVALUATE THE QUALITY OF THE EVIDENCE

There are many systems for rating the quality of the evidence that can be applied to nursing education. In traditional rating systems, evidence from systematic reviews and meta-analyses is at the highest level. These are followed by randomized controlled trials (of which there are few in nursing education); then cohort studies (e.g., two groups or cohorts of students, one of which receives the educational intervention, whereas the other does not); case control and descriptive studies; and last, expert opinion, the lowest level. The stronger the evidence, the more likely that it is valid and relevant for a particular educational situation.

As an example, a meta-analysis explored the effectiveness of feedback, information on performance from an instructor, a peer, or a computer, either during or after a simulation activity, in facilitating procedural skills learning (Hatala, Cook, Zendejas, Hamstra, & Brydges, 2014). There were 31 articles included in the review. The results suggested that there was a moderate benefit of feedback; feedback at the end of the simulation activity appeared to be more effective than concurrent feedback for novice learners; and multiple sources of feedback, including instructor feedback, were superior to any single source of feedback. In another study skills laboratory, faculty developed a creative strategy to reduce nursing students' stress during assessment of skills and improve first-round pass rates for skills competency assessments (Payne, Ziegler, Baughman, & Jones, 2015). Mock competencies were structured to allow students to practice their skills with feedback from peers. During the mock assessments, students rotated through multiple stations performing skills that might be required in the actual graded competency assessment, with peer evaluation. At the end of the mock assessments, faculty conducted a debriefing session in which they answered students' questions and provided feedback on any performance errors they observed. With the mock competency intervention, students had higher pass rates on first-time skill assessments and a reduction in stress-related behaviors. The results from the meta-analysis provide stronger evidence on feedback during skill learning and sources of feedback than the single study.

Other models have been developed for evaluating evidence from educational studies that are appropriate for use in nursing education. Levin's Model of Educational Research, described earlier, can be used for this purpose (Levin, 2004). With this model, the lowest level of evidence would be pilot and observational studies. These are followed by controlled experiments in the classroom, laboratory, and clinical setting, and observational studies of master teachers, and then randomized controlled trials of educational interventions, the highest level.

Kirkpatrick's Four-Level Evaluation Model has also been used to appraise educational evidence (Kirkpatrick, 1998). The levels of this evaluation model consist of the following:

1. Learners' reaction: How well did the students like the learning process?
2. Learning: What did they learn (i.e., the extent to which the learners gained knowledge and skills)?
3. Changes in behavior: What changes in behavior resulted from the learning process (i.e., changes in the learner's capability to perform newly learned skills)?
4. Results: What are the tangible results of the learning process in terms of reduced cost, improved quality, efficiency, and so forth?

Kirkpatrick's Model can be used for assessing the level of outcomes of an educational study, and it is appropriate for nursing education research. Studies that examine learners' perceptions of and satisfaction with an educational practice or intervention, curriculum, course, teaching or assessment method, learning activity, and so forth, are at the lowest level. At the next level are studies that measure changes in learner attitudes; knowledge (e.g., acquisition of concepts, principles, and cognitive skills); and psychomotor skills, as a result of the education. The next two levels of studies have outcomes relating to changes in behaviors, such as ability to transfer learning to the clinical setting, followed by changes in the organization and patient outcomes as a result of the educational practice or intervention (Exhibit 18.3).

EXHIBIT 18.3 Appraisal of Educational Evidence Using Kirkpatrick's Four-Level Evaluation Model

- Level 1 Participation in educational experiences: outcomes of the study include learners' views on the learning experience, teaching method, aspects of the instruction, quality of the teaching
- Level 2a Change in learners' attitudes or perceptions: outcomes of the study relate to changes in the attitudes or perceptions of learners or between groups of learners about the educational practice or intervention
- Level 2b Change in learners' knowledge and/or skills: outcomes of the study relate to the acquisition of concepts, principles, cognitive skills, problem-solving ability, psychomotor skills
- Level 3 Change in behaviors: outcomes of the study document the transfer of learning to the clinical setting, workplace, and other settings, or the willingness of learners to apply new knowledge and skills to clinical practice
- Level 4a Change in professional practice: outcomes of the study include changes in the organization or delivery of care related to the educational practice or intervention
- Level 4b Benefits to patients: outcomes of the study include improvement in patient outcomes as a direct result of the educational practice or intervention

Source: Adapted from Issenberg, McGaghie, Petrusa, Gordon, and Scalese (2005); and Yardley and Dornan (2012).

Although Kirkpatrick's Model is used for appraising educational evidence, including reviews by the BEME Collaboration, Yardley and Dornan (2012) suggested that this model was appropriate for relatively simple educational interventions and programs with short-term endpoints, but noted that the levels were not suitable for complex educational interventions with long-term outcomes, in which process evaluation was as important as the learning outcomes. Concerns they have with using these levels for appraising educational evidence are that teachers are not included, and the model does not allow for the rich variety of outcomes with both qualitative and quantitative educational studies (Yardley & Dornan, 2012). This is important, as many nursing education studies use qualitative methods and explore educational practices that are complex with many variables.

Yardley and Dornan (2012) suggested that, for experimental studies, the critical appraisal tools of evidence-based practice can be applied to education evidence. For other studies, evaluation of the quality of the evidence can be based on global judgments of trustworthiness, such as with the following BEME scale:

1. No clear conclusions can be drawn; not significant.
2. Results ambiguous, but there appears to be a trend.

3. Conclusions can probably be based on the results.
4. Results are clear and very likely to be true.
5. Results are unequivocal (Hammick, Dornan, & Steinert, 2010; Yardley & Dornan, 2012).

This scale of 1 to 5 could be used for rating the strength of the findings of a nursing education study.

DECIDE WHETHER FINDINGS ARE APPLICABLE TO OWN PROGRAM, COURSES, STUDENTS, AND CONTEXT

The fourth phase of evidence-based teaching is as important as the earlier phases: deciding whether the findings are ready for implementation based on the evidence and, if so, whether they are applicable to one's own teaching situation. Teachers should assess if the findings are relevant to their students, program, courses, and the context in which they teach. The key in making this decision is whether the characteristics of the students, nurse educators, and other aspects of the nursing program are similar to the research that has been done. The findings from a systematic review of studies with students in prelicensure nursing programs might not be applicable for teaching nurses and other staff. Studies done in a small school of nursing might not be transferable to a large school with a diverse student population.

As a next step, if a new educational practice is used, studies should be planned to evaluate its effectiveness. Is the new practice better than the previous approach? Did it improve learning and performance? What outcomes changed as a result of this new practice or educational intervention? The goal is to design studies that measure outcomes other than satisfaction with the new teaching approach and that provide strong evidence that can be used to guide future decisions about teaching in nursing.

SUMMARY

Evidence-based teaching is the use of research findings and other evidence to guide educational decisions and practices. Available evidence should be used when developing the curriculum and courses, selecting teaching methods and approaches to use with students, planning clinical learning activities, and assessing students' learning and performance. This evidence is generated from rigorous pedagogical research; for findings to be useful to nurse educators, they must be valid and the result of well-designed studies. Most of the studies in nursing education are done with small samples in one setting only. These need to be replicated and include diverse samples of learners, teachers, and programs to determine whether the educational practice is applicable across settings and with varied student groups.

Evidence-based teaching includes four phases: (a) questioning educational practices and identifying the need for evidence to guide teaching; (b) searching for research studies and other evidence on educational practices; (c) evaluating the quality of the evidence; and (d) deciding whether the findings are applicable to one's own program, courses, students, and the context in which one is teaching. Teachers also consider theories and concepts about learning and teaching, their own philosophy of nursing education, and their expertise as educators. The learner needs to have input and consideration as to preferences for learning and personal goals to be met in the course. The evidence alone does not dictate the educational practices to use. It is up to the teacher to integrate the evidence with these other considerations.

The first phase in evidence-based teaching is for nurse educators to reflect on their educational practices and to question whether there is a better way of teaching students. In the second phase, teachers search the literature for studies done on the topic and other articles and resources to answer their questions. This phase requires knowledge of databases to search, ability to conduct a search, and knowledge of other resources, such as websites that report evidence on educational practices. Although there are many databases that contain reports of studies that might be relevant to teaching in nursing, three databases are recommended for a search in nursing education: (a) MEDLINE (via PubMed), (b) CINAHL, and (c) ERIC.

For areas of education that have been well studied, the teacher should begin by searching for a systematic review in which experts evaluate and synthesize the findings of multiple studies on a particular educational topic to arrive at conclusions about best practices. When systematic reviews are not available, the teacher should search for literature reviews. If reviews have not been done, the next step is to locate individual studies and critique their quality. Typically, a few studies on an educational practice will not be sufficient to make a major educational change.

There are many systems for rating the quality of the evidence that can be applied to nursing education, such as Levin's Model of Educational Research, Kirkpatrick's Four-Level Evaluation Model, and a scale for making a global judgment, such as the BEME scale of 1 to 5. The review provided evidence about the educational practice or intervention, but the fourth phase is equally important: deciding whether the findings are ready for implementation based on the evidence and, if so, whether they are relevant for the teacher's own students, program, courses, and context.

REFERENCES

American Psychological Association. (2016). *PsycINFO®*. Retrieved from http://www.apa.org/pubs/databases/psycinfo/index.aspx

Beischel, K. P., Hart, J., & Turkelson, S. L. (2016). Conducting a multisite education research project: Strategies to overcome the barriers to achieve the benefits. *Nurse Educator, 41,* 204–207. doi:10.1097/NNE.0000000000000246

Best Evidence Medical and Health Professional Education. (2016a). *A guide to writing and submitting a BEME review protocol.* Retrieved from https://www.bemecollaboration.org/Step+4+Protocol+Preparation

Best Evidence Medical and Health Professional Education. (2016b). *The BEME collaboration.* Retrieved from https://www.bemecollaboration.org

Broome, M. E., Ironside, P. M., & McNelis, A. M. (2012). Research in nursing education: State of the science. *Journal of Nursing Education, 51,* 521–524. doi:10.3928/01484834-20120820-10

Cannon, S., & Boswell, C. (2016). *Evidence-based teaching in nursing: A foundation for educators* (2nd ed.). Burlington, MA: Jones & Bartlett.

Cheng, A., Eppich, W., Grant, V., Sherbino, J., Zendejas, B., & Cook, D. A. (2014). Debriefing for technology-enhanced simulation: A systematic review and meta-analysis. *Medical Education, 48,* 657–666. doi:10.1111/medu.12432

Cook, D. A., & West, C. P. (2013). Perspective: Reconsidering the focus on "outcomes research" in medical education: A cautionary note. *Academic Medicine, 88,* 162–167. doi:10.1097/ACM.0b013e31827c3d78

Dame, L., & Hoebeke, R. (2016). Effects of a simulation exercise on nursing students' end-of-life care attitudes. *Journal of Nursing Education, 55,* 701–705. doi:10.3928/01484834-20161114-07

De Gagne, J. C., Choi, M., Ledbetter, L., Kang, H. S., & Clark, C. M. (2016). An integrative review of cybercivility in health professions education. *Nurse Educator, 41,* 239–245. doi:10.1097/NNE.0000000000000264

EBSCO Industries, Inc. (2016). *The cumulative index to nursing and allied health literature.* Retrieved from https://www.ebscohost.com/biomedical-libraries/the-CINAHL-database

Grant, M. J., & Booth, A. (2009). A typology of reviews: An analysis of 14 review types and associated methodologies. *Health Information & Libraries Journal, 26*(2), 91–108. doi:10.1111/j.1471-1842.2009.00848.x

Hammick, M., Dornan, T., & Steinert, Y. (2010). Conducting a best evidence systematic review. Part 1: From idea to data coding. BEME Guide No. 13. *Medical Teacher, 32*(1), 3–15. doi:10.3109/01421590903414245

Hatala, R., Cook, D. A., Zendejas, B., Hamstra, S. J., & Brydges, R. (2014). Feedback for simulation-based procedural skills training: A meta-analysis and critical narrative synthesis. *Advances in Health Sciences Education: Theory and Practice, 19*(2), 251–272. doi:10.1007/s10459-013-9462-8

Institute of Education Sciences, U.S. Department of Education. (n.d.). *What is ERIC?* Retrieved from https://ies.ed.gov/ncee/projects/ERIC.asp

Issenberg, S. B., McGaghie, W. C., Petrusa, E. R., Gordon, D. L., & Scalese, R. J. (2005). Features and uses of high-fidelity medical simulations that lead to effective learning: A BEME systematic review. *Medical Teacher, 27*(1), 10–28.

Kalb, K. A., O'Conner-Von, S. K., Brockway, C., Rierson, C. L., & Sendelbach, S. (2015). Evidence-based teaching practice in nursing education: Faculty perspectives and practices. *Nursing Education Perspectives, 36*, 212–219. doi:10.5480/14-1472

Kim, J., Park, J. H., & Shin, S. (2016). Effectiveness of simulation-based nursing education depending on fidelity: A meta-analysis. *BMC Medical Education, 16*, 152. doi:10.1186/s12909-016-0672-7

Kirkpatrick, D. L. (1998). *Evaluating training programs: The four levels* (2nd ed.). San Francisco, CA: Berrett-Koehler.

Levin, J. R. (2004). Random thoughts on the (in)credibility of educational psychology intervention research. *Educational Psychologist, 39*, 173–184

Marshall, J. G., Sollenberger, J., Easterby-Gannett, S., Morgan, L.K., Cavanaugh, S. K., Klem, M. L., . . . Hunter, S. (2013). The value of library and information services in patient care: Results of a multisite study. *Journal of the Medical Library Association, 101*(1), 38–46. doi:10.3163/1536-5050.101.1.007

Melnyk, B. M., Fineout-Overholt, E., Stillwell, S. B., & Williamson, K. M. (2010). The seven steps of evidence-based practice. *American Journal of Nursing, 110*(1), 51–53. doi:10.1097/01.NAJ.0000366056.06605.d2

Oermann, M. H. (2009). Evidence-based programs and teaching/evaluation methods: Needed to achieve excellence in nursing education. In M. Adams & T. Valiga (Eds.), *Achieving excellence in nursing education* (pp. 63–76). New York, NY: National League for Nursing.

Oermann, M. H., Hallmark, B. F., Haus, C., Kardong-Edgren, S. E., McColgan, J. K., & Rogers, N. (2012). Conducting multisite research studies in nursing education: Brief practice of CPR skills as exemplar. *Journal of Nursing Education, 51*, 23–28. doi:10.3928/01484834-20111130-05

Oermann, M. H., & Hays, J. (2016). *Writing for publication in nursing* (3rd ed.). New York, NY: Springer Publishing.

Patricio, M., & vaz Carneiro, A. (2012). Systematic reviews of evidence in medical education and clinical medicine: Is the nature of evidence similar? *Medical Teacher, 34*, 474–482. doi:10.3109/0142159x.2012.682186

Patterson, B. (2009). The nature of evidence in teaching practice. *Journal of Nursing Education, 48*, 327–333.

Payne, C., Ziegler, M. P., Baughman, D. M., & Jones, J. (2015). Implementation of mock competency skill assessments to improve student outcomes. *Nurse Educator, 40*, 281–284. doi:10.1097/NNE.0000000000000173

Scott, K., & McSherry, R. (2009). Evidence-based nursing: Clarifying the concepts for nurses in practice. *Journal of Clinical Nursing, 18*, 1085–1095. doi:10.1111/j.1365-2702.2008.02588.x

Shin, S., Park, J. H., & Kim, J. H. (2015). Effectiveness of patient simulation in nursing education: Meta-analysis. *Nurse Education Today, 35*, 176–182. doi:10.1016/j.nedt.2014.09.009

Stevens, K. (2013). The impact of evidence-based practice in nursing and the next big ideas. *The Online Journal of Issues in Nursing, 18*(2), Manuscript 4. doi:10.3912/OJIN.Vol18No02Man04

United States National Library of Medicine. (2016). *Fact sheet: MEDLINE®*. Retrieved from https://www.nlm.nih.gov/pubs/factsheets/medline.html

Yardley, S., & Dornan, T. (2012). Kirkpatrick's levels and education "evidence". *Medical Education, 46*(1), 97–106. doi:10.1111/j.1365-2923.2011.04076.x

Yucha, C. B., Schneider, B. S. P., Smyer, T., Kowalski, S., & Stowers, E. (2011). Methodological quality and scientific impact of quantitative nursing education research over 18 months. *Nursing Education Perspectives, 32*, 362–368. doi:10.5480/1536-5026-32.6.362

19

Becoming a Scholar in Nursing Education

MARILYN H. OERMANN

OBJECTIVES

- Discuss scholarship of teaching in nursing and various forms of scholarship
- Examine the process of becoming a scholar in nursing education
- Identify phases in writing for publication

The role of the nurse educator includes more than teaching, assessing learning, and developing courses: it also includes scholarship and contributing to the development of nursing education as a science. Research in nursing education is essential, but scholarship is more than studies about students, teachers, and programs: scholarship can be conceptualized broadly as inquiry about learning and teaching. Scholars in nursing education question and search for new ideas; they debate and think beyond how it has "always been done." For the teacher's work to be considered as scholarship, it needs to be public, peer-reviewed and critiqued, and shared with others so they can build on that work. This chapter examines scholarship in nursing education and developing one's role as a scholar. Because of the importance of dissemination to scholarship, the chapter includes a description of the process of writing for publication and other strategies for dissemination. Assessment of teaching, by students and peers, and the scholarship of teaching are also discussed, including development of a teaching portfolio to document teaching excellence and scholarship. This chapter builds on Chapter 1, which examined career development as a nurse educator.

SCHOLARSHIP OF TEACHING IN NURSING

Scholarship is essential to nursing education because without it our educational practices cannot develop further. It is through research and other forms of scholarship that teachers make contributions to the science, the body of knowledge, of nursing education. There are many different views about the scholarship of teaching. Scholarship in nursing education can be conceptualized broadly as inquiry about learning and teaching. That inquiry can involve developing new concepts about learning, systematic reflection on learning and teaching that becomes public, the discovery of new knowledge and evidence on educational practices, and translating and using research findings to guide teaching. Through scholarship about teaching and learning, teachers provide evidence to guide educational practices and disseminate that evidence widely through various methods such as articles in peer-reviewed journals.

Nurse educators engage in a wide range of teaching activities. These activities include developing the curriculum and courses, teaching innovations, learning activities for students, and assessment methods and implementing them: these are the practices of teaching in nursing. Sharing these practices with other educators, in the literature, at conferences, and through informal sessions in one's own setting, provides ideas for teaching, builds community, and may lead to other educators reflecting on their own teaching experiences (Kern, Mettetal, Dixson, & Morgan, 2015, p. 6). Activities in which nurse educators engage when teaching others, however, may not reflect scholarly teaching. Scholarly teaching requires using research findings and evidence to guide teaching and assessment. In scholarly teaching, educators base their teaching on the scholarly literature (Kern et al., 2015; Zakrajsek, 2013). The scholarship of teaching and learning is the systematic study of teaching practices and includes disseminating those findings. Kern et al. (2015) emphasized that this scholarship builds the knowledge and theory base of teaching and learning in a field of study (p. 6).

BOYER'S FORMS OF SCHOLARSHIP

Views about the scholarship of teaching in nursing education have been influenced significantly by Boyer (1990) and Glassick, Huber, and Maeroff (1997), who provided a broader view of scholarship than only formal research. Boyer believed that scholarship also involves searching for connections, building bridges between theory and practice, and communicating one's knowledge to learners. He identified four separate but overlapping forms of scholarship:

1. Scholarship of discovery: conducting original research that expands current knowledge and understanding in a field
2. Scholarship of integration: developing connections across disciplines and synthesizing research done by others; essential for evidence-based teaching
3. Scholarship of application: applying knowledge to practice and translating research findings into practical interventions that solve problems
4. Scholarship of teaching: inquiry that focuses on student learning that results from our educational practices (Boyer, 1990)

CONCEPTUALIZATIONS OF SCHOLARSHIP OF TEACHING IN NURSING

Conceptualizations of the scholarship of teaching in nursing are not well developed. Some nurse educators view the scholarship of teaching as parallel to the scholarship of discovery, that is, research (Glanville & Houde, 2004). However, that view negates the creative work of nurse educators in developing innovations and new approaches to teaching. For example, the development of an interactive, virtual environment for learning community health nursing concepts is scholarship, but it is not traditional research with the aim of discovering new knowledge.

A second perspective is that the scholarship of teaching in nursing is excellence in teaching, but being an outstanding teacher does not mean the nurse educator is a scholar. Glanville and Houde (2004) suggested that expert teachers may not reflect on their teaching or view teaching and learning as "matters for inquiry and communication" (p. 9). The scholarship of teaching is more than excellence as a teacher.

Another perspective is that scholarship of teaching in nursing is applying theory and research to one's own educational practices (Glanville & Houde, 2004). Although this may lead to evidence-based teaching, there need to be products of one's scholarship, such as an article in a peer-reviewed journal, a presentation at a professional conference, or a description of an educational innovation.

Thoun (2009) expressed concerns that Boyer's framework did not reflect the richness and breadth of contributions of scholarship in nursing. She proposed three patterns of scholarship for nursing. The first is emergent scholarship that involves generating research and new knowledge. The second pattern of scholarship is educational and administrative scholarship: the inquiry of teaching, learning, and administrative processes (Thoun, 2009). That type also includes evaluation of teaching methods and educational technologies, curriculum development, and leadership in teaching and administration of nursing education programs. The third type, professional scholarship, is the inquiry of practice, resulting in new insights and understanding about clinical practice.

The scholarship of teaching in nursing needs to embrace the many forms that scholarship can take. This includes:

1. Conducting original research about teaching, with a focus on students and their learning
2. Evaluation studies of educational practices and teaching methods
3. Systematic and other types of reviews that synthesize knowledge and provide evidence for educational practices and decisions
4. Development and application of concepts and theories to guide teaching and assessment, which lead to dissemination
5. Development of educational innovations and new initiatives with outcomes evaluated
6. Development of new programs, courses, teaching methods, instructional materials, and assessment methods, among others, that are systematically evaluated (Oermann, 2014)

The scholarship of teaching in nursing can take any of these forms, but it is not the same as excellence in teaching, evidenced by outstanding student evaluations. It also is not the same as scholarly teaching, which is teaching grounded in sound principles and reflecting well-designed strategies of course design, transmission, interaction with learners, and assessment (Shulman, 2000). Scholarship involves inquiry and reflection, the development of products as a result of the scholarly work, and their dissemination. By disseminating one's scholarship, peers can critique its quality and use the information in their own teaching if relevant. The most common product of the teacher's scholarship is a journal article about education, but examples of other products are book chapters; books; essays on teaching; editorials; descriptions of teaching methods and materials, learning activities of students, educational innovations, a program or course, assessment strategies, and tools; a simulation scenario; and media and technology for teaching (McGaghie & Webster, 2009; Oermann, 2014).

SCHOLARSHIP OF TEACHING: CRITERIA TO BE MET

Shulman (2000) proposed that all forms of scholarship have to meet three criteria. First, the work needs to be public for others to consider and review it. Second, all forms of scholarship must be subject to peer review and critique. Third, the scholarly work must be shared with other nurse educators, so they, in turn, can build on that work. Educational studies disseminated beyond a school of nursing can be replicated, and findings can be accumulated. Innovations and new initiatives shared with others can be used to spread ideas throughout the nursing education community. Dissemination is critical to build evidence for teaching in nursing.

BECOMING A SCHOLAR IN NURSING EDUCATION

Meeting these three criteria transforms the teacher's work as an educator into scholarship. Teachers can begin this process by reflecting on their educational practices and experiences, discussing their ideas and reflections on teaching with other educators in their schools of nursing or other settings, and sharing their work with colleagues for critique. This process of reflection and critique can lead to new practices, which are then evaluated and disseminated.

Weston and McAlpine (2001) described a continuum of growth of teachers toward the scholarship of teaching. In phase 1, teachers develop personal knowledge about their own educational practices and their impact on students' learning. In phase 2, teachers dialogue with colleagues about learning and teaching and engage in conversations that demonstrate their knowledge. Phase 3 is growth in the scholarship of teaching, in which teachers develop knowledge about education that has significance for and impact on the field (Weston & McAlpine, 2001). Table 19.1 applies these phases to nurse educators.

TABLE 19.1 Progression Toward Scholarship of Teaching

Phase 1: Develop Personal Knowledge About Own Teaching	Phase 2: Share Ideas and Practices About Teaching and Learning With Colleagues	Phase 3: Develop Scholarship of Teaching
Reflect on own teaching	Engage in conversations about teaching and learning with others	Integrate nursing education research and evidence in teaching
Learn about own educational practices and impact on student learning	Develop expertise in an area of nursing education and be recognized for that in your school or other setting	Conduct studies, evaluate teaching innovations and practices, and develop products of own scholarship of teaching
Read nursing education literature	Attend nursing education conferences and discuss ideas about learning and teaching with colleagues	Publish papers in peer-reviewed journals, present scholarly work at conferences, and disseminate work through other venues

(continued)

TABLE 19.1 Progression Toward Scholarship of Teaching (*continued*)

Phase 1: Develop Personal Knowledge About Own Teaching	Phase 2: Share Ideas and Practices About Teaching and Learning With Colleagues	Phase 3: Develop Scholarship of Teaching
Learn about theories to guide teaching	Expand understanding of concepts and theories to guide teaching	Become an expert in an area of nursing education and know the research done on that topic
Conduct self-assessments of the quality of teaching and seek peer evaluations	Provide leadership in teaching at the course or program level, serve on educational committees	Provide leadership at the national level in advancing knowledge in an area of nursing education
	Mentor novice teachers	Mentor others on research and developing their scholarship of teaching

Source: From Weston and McAlpine (2001).

Nurse educators as scholars are creative and open to new ideas. They reflect on their educational practices, develop new approaches, and study their outcomes. They engage in conversations and debates with colleagues about learning and teaching. Scholars critically question ideas that are taken for granted, are brave enough to suggest unpopular ideas, and are resilient (Stockhausen & Turale, 2011). Strategies nurse educators can use to develop as scholars are presented in Exhibit 19.1.

EXHIBIT 19.1 Strategies to Become a Scholar in Nursing Education

1. Complete a self-assessment. Do you have attributes of a scholar: creativity, an inquiring mind, openness to new ideas, integrity, willingness to critically question and reflect on own educational practices, confidence in being questioned about own ideas and products of scholarly work, collegial, resilient, respectful of the scholarly process, and prepared to develop scholarship and grow as a scholar?[a] Set a goal to develop attributes you do not currently possess.

2. Identify an area of nursing education to learn more about and on which to focus your scholarship. Ask yourself what you are curious about in terms of teaching and learning. What problems and issues have you encountered with student learning? What do you want to know more about in terms of learning and teaching?

3. Discuss your questions and ideas for an area of scholarship with colleagues, and use their critique and feedback to refine them.

4. Do a quick search of the literature to answer your questions and learn more about your potential area of scholarship. What do we know about the topic, and what questions remain unanswered? Discuss your findings and continued thinking with colleagues. Consult with experts in the area of scholarship you are considering and confirm the gaps in knowledge that you identified from your literature review.

5. Select your area of scholarship and be open to modifying it as you engage in your scholarly work.

(continued)

EXHIBIT 19.1 Strategies to Become a Scholar in Nursing Education (*continued*)

6. Become known as an expert in that area of nursing education and share your expertise with colleagues.

7. Identify your products of scholarship and strategies for disseminating them; for example, writing an abstract for submission to a nursing education conference about a clinical evaluation tool you developed, or preparing a manuscript on the use of multiple patient simulations in your leadership course. In planning dissemination strategies, consider your time and resources.

8. Search for funding if planning a pilot study or evaluation.

9. Disseminate widely, including presentations and publications.

10. Attend nursing education conferences and interact with other nursing education scholars there. Share your work and ideas with them.

11. Be realistic in terms of the time you have available for your scholarly work. Set goals with dates for completion that are attainable.

[a] Stockhausen and Turale (2011).

DISSEMINATING YOUR SCHOLARSHIP

One of the issues related to the scholarship of teaching in nursing is that too few nurse educators share their work. There are many lost opportunities to spread new ideas and innovations: nurse educators in one setting develop an educational innovation and evaluate its effectiveness, but they never share that work with others. The reality is that the contributions of nurse educators are limited if they do not share their innovations with others (Clark & Webster, 2012). There are many venues for teachers to disseminate the products of their scholarship to make them public and accessible for critique and use by others. They can present their scholarship at conferences, both nursing education and others; describe their work in newsletters; post summaries of their studies, projects, and innovations on relevant websites and the school of nursing intranet; report at faculty meetings, which provide an opportunity for critique; and disseminate their scholarly work through publications. Articles published in peer-reviewed journals provide the widest dissemination, spreading the ideas to other educators for consideration and use in their own teaching. When research findings are published, these results can be synthesized to generate evidence for teaching, as discussed in Chapter 18.

Publications in peer-reviewed journals are a requirement for promotion and tenure in many schools of nursing; this is another reason for teachers to disseminate their scholarship through publications. Nurse educators need to be aware of the criteria for contract renewal, promotion, and tenure in their school of nursing and the importance given to journal publications. In some settings, databased articles (papers that report the findings of research studies) published in peer-reviewed journals, also called refereed, are considered more important in these decisions than descriptive articles, chapters, and books about teaching and other educational topics. Peer-reviewed journals—for example, *Nurse Educator, Journal of Nursing Education, Journal of Continuing Education in Nursing, Nursing Education Perspectives, Nurse Education Today,* and *International Journal of Nursing Education Scholarship,* among others—have experts (peers) who critically evaluate manuscripts submitted to the journal, ensuring their quality.

PLANNING PHASE OF WRITING FOR PUBLICATION

In planning the dissemination of the teacher's scholarship, the first step is to identify the purpose of the manuscript (Oermann & Hays, 2016). The term *manuscript* is the unpublished paper; once published, it is referred to as an article. The purpose of the manuscript might be to share new ideas and concepts about learning and teaching in nursing; describe a nursing program or course; present a research study and findings, or the results of an evaluation of an educational innovation; or report other educational topics. The purpose guides the development of the manuscript, and it should be stated early in the paper.

As part of the planning phase, the teacher reviews the literature to build on what has already been published. The two databases most valuable for this purpose are MEDLINE, searched through PubMed, and the Cumulative Index to Nursing and Allied Health Literature (CINAHL). Similar to searching for evidence for teaching, if those databases provide limited citations, then the teacher should also search the Education Resources Information Center (ERIC) database. A review of the literature might reveal that the teacher's ideas and topic for dissemination have been reported by others. Then the key is identifying how the scholarly work builds on those ideas and provides new knowledge for readers.

Typically, reviewing the literature for the prior 5-year period is sufficient, unless few citations are located; in that case the teacher should extend the time period for the search. Citations can be saved by using bibliographic management software, which allows the teacher to create citations and reference lists formatted in the appropriate style. Many nurse educators are familiar with the reference style of the American Psychological Association (APA, 2010), but not all journals use APA style. Some journals use a numbered citation format, such as the *AMA Manual of Style* (American Medical Association [AMA], 2007). The journal's author guidelines specify the style to use when preparing references.

Prior to beginning to write the paper, the teacher selects possible journals for submission of the manuscript. One consideration is whether readers of the journal would be interested in the topic. For example, if the manuscript reports the findings of a study on concept maps, potential readers would be nursing faculty members, and a journal intended for academic nurse educators would be more appropriate than one for nurse educators in professional development. In contrast, a manuscript on a simulation to improve interprofessional collaboration would be of interest to nurse educators in schools of nursing and clinical settings, expanding the number of possible journals. It is also important to determine whether the journal publishes the type of manuscript being planned. Some journals publish mainly research in nursing education, whereas others do not.

There are hundreds of possible journals in which nurse educators can publish their scholarship. To search for appropriate journals, nurses can use directories of journals available on the web such as the Directory of Nursing Journals, a joint service of *Nurse Author & Editor* and INANE, the International Academy of Nursing Editors (https://nursingeditors.com/journals-directory). Another way to locate possible journals is to search MEDLINE (via PubMed) and CINAHL for journals that publish similar types of papers. Using one of these directories or searching for journals indexed in MEDLINE (PubMed) or CINAHL avoids submitting a manuscript to a predatory journal.

Predatory journals are not reputable journals. Consistent with other open-access journals, they charge a fee for publishing the paper, but predatory journals have questionable publishing practices (Beall, 2016). They advertise a fast peer review process, but it is frequently of low quality (Oermann et al., 2016). Articles in predatory journals are not indexed in bibliographic databases such as MEDLINE and CINAHL, and as such, readers will not find the nurse educator's article in a search. Predatory journals typically seek authors through spam e-mails (Oermann et al., 2016).

Teachers should select about five possible journals for submission, rank-order them, and prepare their papers to be consistent with the journal format and author guidelines, available at the journal's website, which provide details about how to prepare the paper. The teacher can send a short query e-mail to the editors of the potential journals to determine their interest, although doing so is not essential. Though a manuscript can be sent to only one journal at a time, query e-mails can be sent to multiple editors. If the manuscript is rejected by a journal, the teacher at that point can revise the paper and submit it to the next journal on the rank-order list.

WRITING PHASE OF WRITING FOR PUBLICATION

The second phase is focused on writing the manuscript. This begins with an outline to guide writing the first draft and to ensure including the essential content to reflect the purpose of the paper. The outline also allows the teacher to plan the approximate number of pages to write for each content area and to avoid preparing a manuscript that is too short or too long. Although journals have different limits on the number of pages for a manuscript, the desired length is often between 15 and 18 double-spaced pages.

Using the outline, the teacher then writes the first draft. The goal of the first draft is to write quickly and without concern about grammar and writing style (Oermann & Hays, 2016). It is critical in this phase to include the citations as the content is developed. When the content is drafted sufficiently, the teacher revises the grammar, punctuation, writing style, and format. In preparing the final version of the paper, the teacher should explicitly follow the author guidelines in terms of format.

PEER REVIEW PHASE OF WRITING FOR PUBLICATION

Peer review of the manuscript is conducted by content experts who serve as reviewers for the journal. These experts evaluate the manuscript, identifying its strengths and weaknesses, and may suggest revisions. The peer-review process ensures that papers published in the journal are of high quality and have accurate and up-to-date content; peers also critique the research methods if the paper reports a nursing education study (Oermann, 2010; Oermann & Hays, 2016). In most nursing journals, peer review is a double-blind review: the author does not know who reviewed the paper, and the reviewers are unaware of the author's identity, removing potential bias. Some journals also use *single-blind review,* in which the author is not aware of the reviewers' identities, but the reviewers know the authors (Ali & Watson, 2016). Peer review also can be open, where the authors and reviewers are both known to each other (Ali & Watson, 2016). The type of peer review used by a journal will be described in the author guidelines or on the journal website. Typically, reviewers rate the quality of the manuscript on a web-based form and provide a narrative summary of their critique of the paper. An example of a review form is in Table 19.2. The narrative summary is usually provided to the author with the editor's comments and decision about acceptance. Authors submit their manuscript at the journal website, and communication with the author, including the results of the peer review comments, are done electronically.

The editor may accept the manuscript without or with revision, ask the teacher to revise and resubmit the paper for another review, or reject it. In revising the manuscript, the teacher should make the suggested revisions or provide a rationale for not making them (Oermann & Hays, 2016). A summary of the revisions proposed and made in

TABLE 19.2 Example of Form for Peer Review of Manuscript

Yes	No	Comments
—	—	Does the paper present new findings or ideas about nursing education?
		Is the content:
—	—	timely/relevant?
—	—	logically and clearly developed?
—	—	sophisticated enough for our readers?
—	—	innovative?
—	—	Introduction: Is the purpose of the paper clear?
—	—	Methods (*research paper*)
—	—	Are the sample and sampling method adequate?
—	—	Are the instruments reliable and valid?
—	—	Are statistical tests appropriate?
—	—	Methods (*other types of papers*)
—	—	Were the objectives clearly identified?
—	—	Were the outcomes evaluated adequately?
—	—	Do conclusions and implications go beyond what findings support?
—	—	Are the references current (the majority within the past 3–5 years)?
—	—	Does the content include implications for teaching in nursing? Other implications for nursing education?
—	—	Was the paper interesting to read?

Recommendation:

( ) **Accept for publication without revision**

( ) **Accept for publication after satisfactory revision**

( ) **Review again after major revision**

( ) **Reject**

Select the number that best indicates the overall quality of this manuscript:

1	2	3	4	5	6
Outstanding	Excellent	Good	Acceptable	Uncertain of acceptability	Unacceptable

Comments/Suggestions:

the manuscript needs to submitted with the revised paper (Exhibit 19.2). For rejected manuscripts, the teacher should consider the feedback from the reviewers, modify the paper as appropriate, and submit it to the next journal on the list established earlier.

PRESENTATIONS AT CONFERENCES AND OTHER DISSEMINATION METHODS

For scholarship not ready for dissemination in peer-reviewed journals, the teacher should plan to disseminate her or his scholarly work via other venues, such as presenting it at nursing education and other conferences. The teacher can begin by presenting a paper

EXHIBIT 19.2 Sample Summary of Manuscript Revisions

Ms. Ref. No.: 1034

Original Title: Differences in Performance of Nursing Students Trained With Computer-Based CPR Course With Voice Advisory Manikin and Instructor-Led Course With Traditional Manikin

Revisions Proposed and Made

REVIEWER 1:

Was there a conceptual framework for this study?

> Ericsson's Deliberate Practice Model. See lines 42–43 and 219 and citation 26

Please make sure you have more than two sentences in a paragraph.

> Revised throughout paper

Shorten the title. Need to be concise.

> We have shortened the title to: Comparison of Two Instructional Modalities for Nursing Student CPR Skill Acquisition.

Literature Review: describe outcomes in your Aims . . . what are you measuring?

> We added the outcomes in the aims statement: see abstract lines 3–4; text lines 37–41. The outcomes also are identified in lines 111–117.

Line 34: define beginning nursing students.

> Revised line 6 in the abstract to omit "beginning" because these details about the students are not essential in the abstract. In the Methods we added information about the schools: "Twelve schools of nursing from across the United States, including six associate degree programs and six bachelor of science programs . . ." (see lines 48–50).

Line 57: what is meant by the "quality of CPR"?

> We added an explanation. See lines 4–6.

Line 62: need reference for psychomotor and technical skills lost.

> We removed the sentence in original line 62 because we have this finding with a citation earlier in the paper (see line 19).

Line 64: what is the feedback received?

> We added examples of the feedback: "Use of a voice advisory manikin (VAM) can improve CPR skills by providing continuous verbal feedback, for example, 'do not compress so fast' and 'ventilate more slowly,' during training." See lines 11–13.

Line 71: delete the word "Some"

> Done

Line 75: what are their evaluations? define, otherwise appears like bias statement.

> Deleted this statement: it was not essential to our paper.

Line 86–88: Provide reference for statements in this paragraph.

> Added (lines 33–34): "The researchers speculated that their findings indicated a lack of initial skill acquisition rather than retention."

Line 90: What are the measurable outcomes? Include in the aim.

> We added the outcomes in the aims statement. See Abstract lines 3–4.
> See also text lines 37–41.

(continued)

EXHIBIT 19.2 Sample Summary of Manuscript Revisions (*continued*)

> **REVIEWER 2:**
>
> Title—too long.
>> Title revised to Comparison of Two Instructional Modalities for Nursing Student CPR Skill Acquisition
>
> 34 Define "beginning" nurse
>> Revised line 6 in the abstract to omit "beginning" because these details about the students are not essential in the abstract. In the Methods we added information about the schools. See lines 48–50.
>
> 41 Results: were they significant? Include in abstract
>> The results were significant, and we added this to the abstract.
>
> 92 Year group of nurses?
>> We removed the term "prelicensure nursing students" for clarity among readers who are nonnurses. See lines 48–50.
>
> 116 How was sport defined?
>> Removed sport reference from manuscript and tables.
>
> 150 How did you adjust for this in the data analysis?
>> See revised data analysis section to explain this (see lines 127–137).
>
> 255 Needs some evidence to support these points, for example, reference to self-directed learning.
>> Sentences (lines 219–220) were revised; two references were added.
>
> 266 Or was it their preferred learning style?
>> Paragraph removed for clarity.

CPR, cardiopulmonary resuscitation.

at local, state, and regional conferences and then progress to national and international ones. Organizations such as the National League for Nursing (NLN), Sigma Theta Tau International, and the regional nursing research societies (for example, Midwest Nursing Research Society) sponsor education summits and conferences at which teachers can present their work. These venues also provide an opportunity to engage in discussions about teaching and scholarship, critical to developing as a scholar in nursing education. Many of the organizations listed in Appendix D.4 sponsor conferences where teachers can present their educational research and other types of scholarly work.

Other dissemination strategies include writing about scholarly work in newsletters, in other non–peer-reviewed publications such as nursing magazines, and as letters to the editor, among others. Reports at faculty and committee meetings and sharing ideas through informal discussions provide other strategies for making scholarship public for review and critique by peers.

ASSESSMENT OF TEACHING AND SCHOLARSHIP OF TEACHING

The NLN's core competencies of nurse educators (NLN Academic Nurse Educator Certification Program, 2016), which were discussed in Chapter 1, describe the essential knowledge, skills, and attitudes of a teacher in nursing. Appendix D.3 presents sample activities of the teacher for each of the core competencies. These competencies are consistent with research findings on qualities of effective teaching in nursing and higher education. For effective teaching, the nurse educator needs to

1. Be an expert in the content area
2. Be clinically competent if teaching in the laboratory, simulation, and the practice setting

3. Have expert teaching skills
4. Develop positive interpersonal relationships with learners as a group and individually
5. Possess attributes such as enthusiasm, patience, friendliness, integrity, perseverance, and willingness to admit mistakes, among others (Oermann, Shellenbarger, & Gaberson, 2018)

In most settings in which nurse educators work, the quality of their teaching; scholarship; service to the nursing program, college or university, community, and profession; and clinical practice, if relevant, are assessed to provide feedback to the teacher (formative evaluation) and for annual performance reviews and personnel decisions such as contract renewal, promotion, and tenure (summative evaluation). This assessment is done by students during and at the end of a course; by peers; by formal committees such as the appointment, promotion, and review committee; and by administrators to whom the teacher reports. In health care settings, though there are differences in the formal committees responsible for evaluation, the quality of the teaching is evaluated by learners, peers, and administrators. Most important is that teachers periodically reflect on and assess the quality of their own teaching and scholarship.

STUDENT RATINGS

Student evaluations of teaching are one source of information about the teacher's effectiveness, but not the only one. Evidence suggests that students can make valid and reliable interpretations about the quality of teaching from their perspectives. Students can assess the teacher's effectiveness, teaching methods used in the course, whether the evaluation by the teacher was fair, the degree of interest the teacher exhibited in students and their learning, and the teacher's enthusiasm. It is unlikely, however, that students can assess the quality of the content of a course (for example, accuracy and depth of the teacher's knowledge), because they are not experts in the subject matter to assess this.

In a systematic review of the research on student evaluations of teaching in nursing, Annan, Tratnack, Rubenstein, Metzler-Sawin, and Hulton (2013) identified six themes of relevance to interpreting student ratings: faculty characteristics, student characteristics, course characteristics, online versus paper student evaluations, reliability and validity, and development of new instruments. They emphasized the need for nurse educators to understand these factors and how they might influence student ratings of their teaching. Student ratings and comments provide feedback to the teacher on improving teaching. Research suggests that discussing ratings with a peer or consultant, combined with students' feedback, is more useful for improving teaching than feedback alone (Benton & Cashin, 2012).

Most nursing programs have standard forms for the evaluation of teaching by students. There may be one form for assessing the quality of teaching in courses, a separate form for student rating of clinical teaching effectiveness, or a general tool that is used for all courses in the nursing program. Annan et al. (2013), based on their systematic review of student evaluations of teaching in nursing, concluded that tools used for student ratings should be specific to nursing and not generic tools. Exhibit 19.3 lists typical areas assessed by students when evaluating teaching effectiveness.

PEER REVIEW

Because student evaluations provide only one view of teaching effectiveness, it is important for any evaluation system for faculty to also include other sources of information about teaching effectiveness. This might include peer review and a teaching portfolio

EXHIBIT 19.3 Typical Areas Assessed on Student Evaluation of Teaching Forms

Teaching Skills
- Organized course well
- Gave clear explanations
- Used examples, illustrations, and other methods to promote understanding of content
- Was well prepared for class
- Was enthusiastic about content and teaching
- Stimulated students' interest in subject
- Motivated students to do best work
- Used learning activities, readings, and assignments that facilitated understanding of course content

Interactions With Students Individually and in Groups
- Encouraged student participation and discussion
- Showed respect for students' views and opinions
- Was readily available to students

Coverage of Subject Matter
- Presented different views and perspectives as appropriate

Assessment and Grading Practices
- Communicated student responsibilities clearly
- Explained course assignments, assessment methods, and grading procedures
- Was fair in assessment and grading
- Provided prompt and valuable feedback

Overall Course Evaluation
- Course difficulty (e.g., rated on scale of *too difficult* to *too elementary*)
- Workload in course (e.g., rated on scale of *too heavy* to *too light*)
- Course pace (e.g., rated on scale of *too fast* to *too slow*)
- Extent of learning in course (e.g., rated on scale of *a great deal* to *nothing new*)
- Overall course rating (e.g., rated on scale of *excellent* to *poor*)

Overall Teacher Evaluation
- Overall quality of the teaching (e.g., rated on scale of *excellent* to *poor*)

Clinical Teaching Items
Did the teacher
1. Encourage students to ask questions and express diverse views in the clinical setting?
2. Encourage application of theoretical knowledge to clinical practice?
3. Provide feedback on student strengths and weaknesses related to clinical performance?
4. Develop positive relationships with students in the clinical setting?
5. Inform students of their professional responsibilities?

(continued)

EXHIBIT 19.3 Typical Areas Assessed on Student Evaluation of Teaching Forms (*continued*)

6. Facilitate student collaboration with members of health care teams?
7. Facilitate learning in the clinical setting?
8. Strive to be available in the clinical setting to assist students?
9. Was the instructor an effective clinical teacher?

Source: Adapted from Oermann and Gaberson (2017). Copyright 2017. Reproduced with the permission of Springer Publishing.

in which faculty members display innovative teaching materials they developed that demonstrate their creativity and expertise (Annan et al., 2013). Peers can observe teaching performance and provide feedback to the nurse educator about areas to be improved; these observations are intended for formative evaluation, because there are many variables that can influence the reliability of observing teaching in the classroom or clinical setting (Oermann & Gaberson, 2017). Peers can review course and instructional materials, teaching methods and strategies developed for learners, online learning activities, tests, and other documents developed for teaching. That type of review can be done for formative evaluation, to provide feedback to the teacher, or for summative evaluation as part of an annual performance review and reviews for reappointment, promotion, and tenure.

In terms of the scholarship of teaching, peers can discuss the teacher's scholarly works, review products of scholarship, critique educational grants, review manuscripts, and assess the teacher's overall scholarly performance. This assessment can be used for formative purposes, to give feedback for continued development of the teacher's scholarship, or for summative purposes, such as in annual reviews and for making decisions about promotion (Oermann & Gaberson, 2017).

TEACHING PORTFOLIO

A teaching portfolio or dossier is a collection of materials selected by nurse educators to document the quality of their teaching, illustrate their creativity in teaching, present innovative teaching and assessment methods they have developed for their courses, and provide documentation of their overall teaching effectiveness. Teaching portfolios can be used to improve teaching (formative evaluation), providing an organized collection of documents for review and critique by others. Or, they may be submitted to the administrator to whom the faculty member reports and to committees such as the appointment, promotion, and review committee for formal peer review (summative evaluation). Types of documents typically included in the portfolio are listed in Exhibit 19.4. These provide a source of data for assessment by others of the nurse educator's expertise in teaching.

Glanville and Houde (2004) suggested that teaching portfolios can also be used to document the scholarship of teaching. Faculty members can include in their portfolios descriptions of their innovations in teaching and how they improved student learning; can explain creative strategies they developed for teaching and assessment; can describe their contributions on committees, on teams, and in organizations related to nursing education; and can summarize their dissemination of their scholarship beyond what is listed on the curriculum vitae. Portfolios allow educators to make their scholarship public and share it with others for peer review.

EXHIBIT 19.4 Types of Documents Included in Teaching Portfolio

- Philosophy of teaching and goals for teaching
- Syllabi
- Sample teaching methods and materials, student learning activities and assignments, assessment methods, evaluation tools, others
- Innovations in teaching and descriptions of their success
- Descriptions of technologies developed for teaching and their successful application
- Descriptions of and documents related to new courses and programs developed in school of nursing (with individual contributions described if work was done by a team)
- Accreditation and comprehensive program reports
- Publications of educational studies, teaching and assessment methods, innovations, new initiatives, and others on teaching and learning
- Presentations related to teaching and learning
- Educational grants
- Teaching awards and other recognition of teaching effectiveness
- Peer evaluations of teaching

CAREER DEVELOPMENT

Chapter 1 explored the nurse educator role and career development in that role. As teachers gain experience and develop their expertise, they can be recognized through the NLN's Academic Nurse Educator Certification Program. To be certified, nurse educators need to successfully pass an examination that assesses their knowledge about learning, methods for facilitating learning and development of the learner, assessment and evaluation, curriculum development and evaluation, quality improvement in the nurse educator role, and the scholarship of teaching, service, and leadership (NLN Academic Nurse Educator Certification Program, 2016). Further information about the NLN Certification Program and examination is provided in Appendices D.1 and D.2.

The importance of faculty development in nursing education was discussed in Chapter 1. In developing as a scholar, however, the teacher might need additional preparation and mentoring. Teachers need to set short- and long-term career goals for their scholarship and identify areas in which they need further learning and skills development. For some nurse educators, additional course work might be required; for others, continuing education programs and workshops such as those offered by the NLN, the American Association of Colleges of Nursing, other organizations, and schools of nursing will be adequate to meet their learning needs. Some of the organizations listed in Appendix D.4 provide educational programs that would enable teachers to gain skills essential to advance their scholarship. It is also valuable to bookmark websites that could serve as resources for teaching and scholarship.

SUMMARY

Scholarship in nursing education can be conceptualized broadly as inquiry about learning and teaching. That inquiry can involve the discovery of new knowledge and evidence on educational practices, translating and using research findings to guide teaching, and developing new concepts about teaching and learning in nursing.

The scholarship of teaching in nursing needs to embrace the many forms that scholarship can take. These include conducting original research about teaching and learning; evaluation studies; reviews that synthesize knowledge and provide evidence for teaching; development and application of concepts and theories to guide teaching; development of educational innovations and new initiatives; and development of new programs, courses, teaching methods, instructional materials, and others, that are systematically evaluated and disseminated.

To transform the teacher's work as an educator into scholarship, all forms of scholarship need to be public, peer-reviewed and critiqued, and shared with other educators so they, in turn, can build on that work. There are many venues for teachers to disseminate the products of their scholarship to make them public and accessible for critique and use by others. They can present their scholarship at conferences, at faculty meetings, and through other venues. Articles published in peer-reviewed journals, however, provide the widest dissemination. A section in the chapter presented the phases of writing for publication and important principles for disseminating scholarship through publications.

In most settings in which nurse educators work, the quality of their teaching, scholarship, service, and clinical practice, if relevant, is assessed by students, peers, administrators, and formal committees. This evaluation, including the use of teaching portfolios, was discussed in the chapter. However, the most important evaluation is that done by teachers themselves: nurse educators need to periodically reflect on and assess the quality of their own teaching and scholarship. With this self-assessment, combined with feedback from others, teachers can identify areas in which they need further development and mentoring, set short- and long-term career goals, find resources to help them with their career development, expand their teaching competencies, and advance their scholarship of teaching.

REFERENCES

Ali, P. A., & Watson, R. (2016). Peer review and the publication process. *Nursing Open, 3*(4), 193–202. doi:10.1002/nop2.51

American Medical Association. (2007). *AMA manual of style: A guide for authors and editors* (10th ed.). New York, NY: Oxford University Press.

American Psychological Association. (2010). *Publication manual of the American Psychological Association* (6th ed.). Washington, DC: Author.

Annan, S. L., Tratnack, S., Rubenstein, C., Metzler-Sawin, E., & Hulton, L. (2013). An integrative review of student evaluations of teaching: Implications for evaluation of nursing faculty. *Journal of Professional Nursing, 29*, e10–e24. doi:10.1016/j.profnurs.2013.06.004

Beall, J. (2016). Open-access and web publications. In M. H. Oermann & J. C. Hays (Eds.), *Writing for publication in nursing* (3rd ed., pp. 379–393). New York, NY: Springer Publishing.

Benton, S. L., & Cashin, W. E. (2012). *Student ratings of teaching: A summary of research and literature. Idea paper #50*. Manhattan, KS: The IDEA Center. Retrieved from http://www.theideacenter.org/sites/default/files/idea-paper_50.pdf

Boyer, E. (1990). *Scholarship reconsidered: Priorities of the professoriate.* San Francisco, CA: Jossey-Bass.

Clark, E., & Webster, B. (2012). Innovation and its contribution to the scholarship of learning and teaching. *Nurse Education Today, 32*, 729–731. doi:10.1016/j.nedt.2012.06.001

Glanville, I., & Houde, S. (2004). The scholarship of teaching: Implications for nursing faculty. *Journal of Professional Nursing, 20*, 7–14.

Glassick, C. E., Huber, M. T., & Maeroff, G. I. (1997). *Scholarship assessed: Evaluation of the professoriate.* San Francisco, CA: Jossey-Bass.

Kern B., Mettetal, G., Dixson, M.D., & Morgan, R. K. (2015). The role of SoTL in the academy: Upon the 25th anniversary of Boyer's *Scholarship Reconsidered. Journal of the Scholarship for Teaching and Learning, 15*(3), 1–14. doi:10.14434/josotl.v15i3.13623

McGaghie, W. C., & Webster, A. (2009). Scholarship, publication, and career advancement in health professions education: AMEE Guide No. 43. *Medical Teacher, 31*, 574–590.

National League for Nursing Academic Nurse Educator Certification Program. (2016). *Certified nurse educator (CNE) 2016 candidate handbook.* New York, NY: Author.

Oermann, M. H. (2010). Writing for publication in nursing: What every nurse educator needs to know. In L. Caputi (Ed.), *Teaching nursing: The art and science* (2nd ed., pp. 146–166). Glen Ellyn, IL: College of DuPage.

Oermann, M. H. (2014). Defining and assessing the scholarship of teaching in nursing. *Journal of Professional Nursing, 30*, 370–375. doi:10.1016/j.profnurs.2014.03.001

Oermann, M. H., Conklin, J. L., Nicoll, L. H., Chinn, P. L., Ashton, K. S., Edie, A. H., . . . Budinger, S. C. (2016). Study of predatory open access nursing journals. *Journal of Nursing Scholarship, 48*, 624–632. doi:10.1111/jnu.12248

Oermann, M. H., & Gaberson, K. B. (2017). *Evaluation and testing in nursing education* (5th ed.). New York, NY: Springer Publishing.

Oermann, M. H., & Hays, J. (2016). *Writing for publication in nursing* (3rd ed.). New York, NY: Springer.

Oermann, M. H., Shellenbarger, T., & Gaberson, K. B. (2018). *Clinical teaching strategies in nursing* (5th ed.). New York, NY: Springer Publishing.

Shulman, L. S. (2000). From Minsk to Pinsk: Why a scholarship of teaching and learning? *Journal of Scholarship in Teaching and Learning, 1*(1), 48–53.

Stockhausen, L., & Turale, S. (2011). An explorative study of Australian nursing scholars and contemporary scholarship. *Journal of Nursing Scholarship, 43*, 89–96. doi:10.1111/j.1547-5069.2010.01378.x

Thoun, D. S. (2009). Toward an appreciation of nursing scholarship: Recognizing our traditions, contributions, and presence. *Journal of Nursing Education, 48*, 552–556. doi:10.3928/01484834-20090716-01

Weston, C. B., & McAlpine, L. (2001). Making explicit the development toward the scholarship of teaching. *New Directions for Teaching & Learning, 2001*(86), 89–97.

Zakrajsek, T. D. (2013). Scholarly teaching: Suggestions for a road more traveled. *International Journal for the Scholarship of Teaching and Learning, 7*(1), Article 2. doi:10.20429/ijsotl.2013.070102

20

Preparing Students for Interprofessional Work in the Global Village: The Role of Nurse Educators

LYNDA WILSON, C. ANN GAKUMO, AND MARTHA A. DAWSON

OBJECTIVES

- Describe major global health challenges and the impact of globalization on nursing practice and on higher education
- Define global health and global nursing
- Review recommendations for incorporating global health and interprofessional educational competencies in nursing education programs
- Examine research to identify global health competencies for students in nursing, public health, and medicine
- Identify strategies to integrate global health competencies in nursing education programs

In today's increasingly globalized and complex world, health issues transcend national borders and social, political, and economic events in one part of the world have impacts in other world regions. In September 2015, members of the United Nations approved a set of 17 Sustainable Development Goals designed to "end all forms of poverty, fight inequalities and tackle climate change" by the year 2030 (United Nations, 2016). The goals build on the Millennium Development Goals that guided global development between 2000 and 2015. Although only one goal deals specifically with promoting health and well-being, all of the goals have a potential impact on individual and population health around the globe. Nurses and midwives comprise more than 50% of the global health workforce, although they also account for more than 50% of the global shortage of health workers (World Health Organization [WHO], 2016c).

Although there is general consensus among nurse educators about the need for nurses to be culturally competent, there is growing recognition that the current concept of cultural competence should be expanded to incorporate global cultural competence (Currier, Lucas, & Saint Arnault, 2009; Riner, 2011). Riner proposed a model of globally engaged nursing education and suggested that global cultural competence refers to "development of knowledge, attitudes, and skills about cultural differences, but also about the cultural, social, political, and economic systems that shape individuals' lives on a global scale, the complex interactions among people, the moral and ethical obligations people have to one another, and how these influence health and health care" (p. 312). The focus of this chapter is the role of nurse educators in preparing nurses for interprofessional work in the globalized world of the 21st century.

MAJOR GLOBAL HEALTH CHALLENGES

Although there have been significant improvements in global health indicators over the past 25 years, there continue to be significant disparities in the global burden of disease. Many of these disparities are related to effects of poverty and inequitable distribution of global resources (WHO, 2011). In 2005, the member states of the WHO made a commitment to promote Universal Health Coverage (UHC) to address these disparities. UHC refers to "the provision of, and access to, high-quality health services; and financial risk protection for people who need to use these services. . . . The term includes ways of taking action on social and environmental determinants both within and beyond the health sector" (WHO, 2013, p. xi). Current major global health challenges are reflected in the health-related targets of the Sustainable Development Goals and include reducing maternal, neonatal, and child mortality; noncommunicable and communicable diseases; mental health and substance abuse problems; road traffic accidents; mortality due to environmental pollution; child malnutrition; and violence. These goals also focus on improving access to sexual and reproductive health services, essential medicines, safe drinking water and safe environments, and an adequate health workforce (WHO, 2016b).

Climate change represents a significant global health challenge for the 21st century and beyond. Kjellstrom and McMichael (2013) summarized the direct and indirect health effects of climate change, including increased incidence of heat stroke, infectious and vector-borne diseases, stress-related illnesses, injuries due to extreme weather events, and poor nutrition related to decreased food availability. These authors stressed the urgency of global initiatives to mitigate these effects, including reducing greenhouse gas emissions, shifting to renewable energy sources, and promoting energy conservation.

In 2015, the Lancet Commission on Planetary Health (funded by the Rockefeller Foundation), published a landmark report, noting the paradox between improvements in global health that have occurred while global ecosystems are deteriorating at unprecedented rates (Whitmee et al., 2015). Members of this commission defined the concept of "planetary health" as "the achievement of the highest attainable standard of health, wellbeing, and equity worldwide through judicious attention to the human systems—political, economic, and social—that shape the future of humanity and the Earth's natural systems that define the safe environmental limits within which humanity can flourish. Put simply, planetary health is the health of human civilization and the state of the natural systems on which it depends" (p. 1978). The Sustainable Development Goals provide an opportunity to address the major challenges to global and planetary health in an integrated manner (Whitmee et al., 2015).

IMPACT OF GLOBALIZATION ON NURSING PRACTICE

Globalization has both direct and indirect effects on nursing practice related to increased opportunities for travel, communication, and migration of the global nursing workforce. Increased travel opportunities have positive effects, including promotion of greater cross-cultural and global understanding and awareness, and allowing nurses to learn first-hand about challenges as well as solutions to global health problems. However, increased travel opportunities can also promote the spread of disease, as seen in the recent outbreaks of Ebola and Zika virus infections. Nurses and all health professionals must be prepared to recognize the potential health effects of travel and also be prepared to advise those who plan to travel abroad about measures to promote health and prevent illness, including immunizations and safe practices related to eating, sanitation, and personal safety. Recognizing the potential for the global spread of disease means that public health agencies and associations in the United States and other countries, such as the Quad Council for Public Health Nursing, will have to shift their focus from individual, families, and population to planetary wellness, prevention, and health intervention (Swider, Krothe, Reyes, & Cravetz, 2013). The practice of geographical health boundaries is no longer effective in a globalized world. In addition, nurses must be leaders in addressing the impacts of environmental and climate changes on health (Kirk, 2002).

Hunter et al. (2013) presented a review of the growing field of global health diplomacy, and argued that because nurses play key roles as global health diplomats, they should be aware of implications of global health diplomacy on nursing and health care. Global health diplomacy (GHD) "refers to international diplomatic activities that (directly or indirectly) address issues of global health importance, and is concerned with how and why global health issues play out in a foreign policy context. GHD can encompass a broad set of activities and actors, such as formal country delegations holding bilateral and multilateral negotiations on health issues, a combination of governmental and nongovernmental actors negotiating on health-related issues, and, although often not considered 'diplomacy' in the traditional sense, official or semi-official representatives of one country acting in a health capacity in another" (Michaud & Kates, 2013, p. 24). Although GHD has many potential benefits in promoting global health, there may be ethical concerns when health priorities are determined by political goals, leading local communities to mistrust humanitarian motives of global health practitioners. Nurses should be aware of these challenges and of their roles as global health diplomats.

Nurses have increased opportunities to communicate with colleagues from around the globe thanks to the growing availability of open-access online journals as well as online communities of practice such as the Global Alliance for Nursing and Midwifery (GANM, 2016), and the Global Health Nursing Online & Midwifery (2016). Collaboration and sharing of best practices is also enhanced by numerous nursing networks such as the International Council of Nurses (ICN) Nursing Networks (ICN, 2016), the Global Network of WHO Collaborating Centers for Nursing and Midwifery Development (2016), and the International Nursing Networks of the Pan American Health Organization (2016). In addition, professional nursing organizations that represent different racial and ethnic groups in the United States are increasingly expanding their relationships and sharing best practices with other countries. For example, the strategic focus of the National Black Nurses Association (NBNA) Inc. includes global health and diversity (NBNA, 2016). The NBNA Diversity and Inclusivity Committee goal is to ensure that the nursing workforce increasingly represents the global patient population. NBNA's global health strategic direction focuses on achieving social justice, building nursing capacity, strengthening nursing education and eliminating health disparities globally. The NBNA has formed key partnerships with schools of nursing at home and aboard and strives to share educational resources and best practices at the local, state, regional, national and international levels. For example, the organization has a partner with the Haiti Nursing Foundation, and NBNA members provide education and service support to many areas around the globe (NBNA, 2016).

Globalization also has resulted in increased opportunities for migration of nurses and other health professionals. Although such migration can have positive impacts, particularly on individual nurses seeking greater economic and professional opportunities, migration of nurses from low-resource countries can also strain health systems with serious nursing shortages (All Party Parliamentary Group on Global Health, 2016). Nurse migration is also having a profound effect on workforce planning for both the sending and receiving countries. When nurses leave a country, the sending country may not have the replacement resources needed for safe practice. Therefore, it is important for all nurses to be aware of ethical issues and challenges associated with nurse migration and with recruitment of nurses from low-resource countries to work in higher resource settings. In 2010, the World Health Assembly approved the Global Code of Practice on the International Recruitment of Health Personnel, which provides guidelines for the ethical recruitment of health personnel (WHO, 2010b). All nurses should be familiar with these guidelines and ensure that they are followed in their respective work settings. The 2010 Institute of Medicine (IOM) Report (Committee on the Robert Wood Johnson Foundation Initiative on the Future of Nursing at the IOM, 2011) noted that receiving countries must be aware of variation in licensure, clinical and practicum preparation, and practices of migrating nurses. This report also addressed specific practice transition strategies that should be employed when integrating foreign-educated nurses (FENs) into a health care setting.

IMPACT OF GLOBALIZATION ON HIGHER EDUCATION

As early as 1997, Jarvis described the impact of globalization on nursing in higher education (Jarvis, 1997). Merson (2014) described growing student interest in addressing global health disparities, and suggested that universities can contribute to advancing global health in many ways, including education, research, innovation, capacity building, technical support, and service delivery. If universities and schools of nursing are to influence global health, they must be open to new admission and exit strategies, curriculum changes, and new pedagogical methods that support the diversification of their student population (American Association of Colleges of Nursing [AACN], 2016; Childs, Jonew, Nugent, & Cook, 2004). Students from different cultural backgrounds learn differently; therefore, teaching and instructional methods must vary to engage and support the learning style of all students. It is not enough to recruit and admit a diverse student population; schools of nursing must embrace the institution of policies and practices that help these students matriculate and graduate. The end goal should be an increase in the percentage of nurses from diverse cultural, racial, and ethnic backgrounds, not merely an increase in enrollment numbers.

The international faculty shortage is also having an impact on how nurses are educated across the globe. Many schools of nursing in the United States have partnerships with nursing programs in other countries and recruit international students. In addition, students who could not be admitted to U.S. nursing programs due to limitations on enrollment related to the faculty shortage are being educated abroad. Offshore nursing education is an emerging trend that could have profound impact on the nursing workforce. The IOM report

(Committee on the Robert Wood Johnson Foundation Initiative on the Future of Nursing at the Institute of Medicine, 2011) discussed offshore nursing schools and the possibility that many nursing students born in the United States are being educated abroad. After these students graduate, they are treated as FENs upon returning to the United States to practice. The dual licensure and practice of nurses who are educated offshore could strengthen the globalization of nursing education and practice environments.

Influences of globalization on higher education include the increasing availability of online courses and programs that transcend national borders, and also the "massification" of higher education through the growth of Massive Online Open Access Courses (MOOCs). For example, in 2014 Facebook announced that it was creating a pilot project in Rwanda, along with the MOOC platform edX (Biemiller, 2014; edX, 2017), the Government of Rwanda, Nokia, and Airtel Africa to create SocialEDU, promoting access to free courses by providing free content, data, and affordable smartphones to students in Rwanda (Biemiller, 2014). Other MOOC platforms, such as NextGenU (2017) and Coursera (2017), offer thousands of high-quality courses that are leading to the democratization of higher education. Shishani et al. (2012) described the development of a free online nursing "supercourse" to develop and share global health content for nurses.

DEFINING GLOBAL HEALTH AND GLOBAL NURSING

The concept of global health has evolved from an initial focus on "international health" that emerged in the 19th century, with a focus on control of global epidemics and programs to address health problems in low-resource countries or of indigenous groups in higher resource countries (Rowson et al., 2012). In 2014, Horton et al. (2014) published a manifesto in the journal *Lancet*, proposing that the concept of global health be expanded to incorporate the concept of planetary health. The authors urged that "an urgent transformation is required in our values and our practices based on recognition of our interdependence and the interconnectedness of the risks we face. We need a new vision of cooperative and democratic action at all levels of society and a new principle of planetism and wellbeing for every person on this Earth—a principle that asserts that we must conserve, sustain, and make resilient the planetary and human systems on which health depends by giving priority to the wellbeing of all" (p. 847).

In 2013, the Sigma Theta Tau International, the Honor Society of Nursing, convened a 17-member Global Advisory Panel for the Future of Nursing and Global Health (GAPFON) to establish a vision for the future of nursing that would advance global health (Klopper & Hill, 2015). To provide a framework for their work, seven GAPFON members conducted an extensive literature review and extracted major themes to reach a consensus definition of global health and global nursing (Wilson, Mendes, et al., 2016). Their proposed definitions, in Exhibit 20.1, can provide a useful framework for nurse educators as they develop ways to integrate these concepts into nursing curricula.

EXHIBIT 20.1 Definitions of Global Health and Global Nursing

*"**Global health** refers to an area for practice, study and research that places a priority on improving health, achieving equity in health for all people (Koplan et al., 2009) and ensuring health-promoting and sustainable sociocultural, political and economic systems (Janes & Corbett, 2009). Global health implies planetary health, which equals human, animal, environmental and ecosystem health (Kahn, Kaplan, Monath, Woodall, & Conti, 2014). It also emphasizes transnational health issues, determinants, and solutions; involves many disciplines within and beyond the health sciences;*

(continued)

EXHIBIT 20.1 Definitions of Global Health and Global Nursing (*continued*)

> promotes interdependence and interdisciplinary collaboration; and is a synthesis of population-based prevention with individual holistic care (Koplan et al., 2009, p. 1136)." (Wilson, Mendes, et al., 2016, p. 1536)
>
> "*Global nursing* is the use of evidence-based nursing process to promote sustainable planetary health and equity for all people (Grootjans & Newman, 2013). Global nursing considers social determinants of health, and includes individual and population-level care, research, education, leadership, advocacy and policy initiatives (Upvall, Leffers, & Mitchell, 2014). Global nurses engage in ethical practice and demonstrate respect for human dignity, human rights and cultural diversity (Baumann, 2013). Global nurses engage in a spirit of deliberation and reflection in interdependent partnership with communities and other health care providers (Upvall et al., 2014, p. 1137)." (Wilson, Mendes, et al., 2016, p. 1537)

Source: From Wilson, Mendes, et al. (2016).

INCORPORATING GLOBAL HEALTH AND INTERPROFESSIONAL EDUCATIONAL COMPETENCIES IN NURSING PROGRAMS

A key component in most definitions of global health is the focus on interprofessional and intersectoral collaboration. The need for greater emphasis on interprofessional education (IPE) and interprofessional collaboration (IPC) has resulted from factors including the global shortage of health workers and concerns about quality and safety. As early as 1972, the Institute of Medicine called for more team-based education for students in the health professions (Institute of Medicine, 1972). In 2010, the WHO published a Framework for Action on Interprofessional Education and Collaborative Practice (WHO, 2010a). In 2011, the Interprofessional Education Collaborative (IEC) proposed competencies for interprofessional collaborative practice (Interprofessional Education Collaborative Expert Panel, 2011). The IEC was sponsored by the AACN, American Association of Colleges of Osteopathic Medicine, American Association of Colleges of Pharmacy, American Dental Education Association, Association of American Medical Colleges, and the Association of Schools of Public Health. The proposed competencies address values/ethics for interprofessional practice, roles and responsibilities, communication, and interprofessional teamwork. In 2016, the IEC published a follow-up report, which documented the progress since the original publication, including the addition of nine other professional associations to the Collaborative, representing disciplines such as psychology, social work, physical therapy, and optometry (Interprofessional Education Collaborative, 2016).

Rodger and Hoffman (2010) conducted a study that was commissioned by the WHO to assess the extent of IPE integration globally. This study included 41 countries from six WHO regions, with the majority (91%) representing high-income countries. Rodger and Hoffman (2010) reported that respondents perceived that IPE had a positive impact on interprofessional consultations, understanding the role of other professionals, incorporation of diverse patient care data, improved work environment, and quality of care relative to access and patient outcomes. The findings were similar for both high-income and low-income countries. The authors suggested that there is a need for all countries to provide faculty education related to IPE, ensure that students receive clear objectives to support IPE learning activities, and conduct formal evaluations of IPE initiatives.

Concomitant with calls for IPE, there also have been calls to incorporate global health into curricula of health professional students. In 2010, Frenk et al. published the report of an independent commission of 20 academic and health professionals from different countries proposing reforms to prepare health professionals for the 21st century (Frenk et al., 2010). Commission members highlighted opportunities for education reform associated with increased global exchange of knowledge and technology as well as migration of health professionals and patients. The report proposed a vision that "all health professionals in all countries should be educated to mobilize knowledge and to engage in critical reasoning and ethical conduct so that they are competent to participate in patient and population-centered health systems as members of *locally responsive and globally connected teams*. The ultimate purpose is to assure universal coverage of the high quality comprehensive services that are essential to advance opportunity for health equity within and between countries" (p. 6).

RESEARCH TO IDENTIFY GLOBAL HEALTH COMPETENCIES

Over the past 10 years there have been a number of studies aimed at identifying global health competencies for students in the health professions, including medicine (American Academy of Family Physicians, 2012; Arthur, Battat, & Brewer, 2011; Battat et al., 2010; Drain et al., 2007; C. R. Howard, Gladding, Kiguli, Andrews, & John, 2011); dentistry (Donaldson et al., 2008; Giannobile, 2013); public health (Association of Schools of Public Health, 2011); and physical therapy (Cassady et al., 2014). The One Health paradigm promotes increased collaboration among the disciplines of human medicine, public health, and veterinary medicine (Fisman & Laupland, 2010), and core One Health competencies have been proposed (Global One Health Core Competency Working Group, 2013). Members of the Global Health Competency Subcommittee of the Consortium of Universities for Global Health have also proposed four levels of interprofessional global health competencies (Jogerst et al., 2015; Wilson et al., 2014).

Archambault (2010) recommended global health content that should be incorporated in nursing curricula, although she did not identify specific global health competencies. Similarly, the *Essentials of Baccalaureate Education for Professional Nursing Practice* document (AACN, 2008) lists global health as an example of content to be incorporated under one of the Essentials related to population health, but does not identify specific global health competencies. Clark, Raffray, Hendricks, and Gagnon (2016) conducted a literature review and identified 14 common competencies related to global and public health competencies for nurses that were described in 25 articles that were reviewed. The competencies were related to global burden of disease, travel and migration, determinants of health, environmental factors, cultural competency, communications, health systems/delivery, professionalism/ethics, social justice/human rights, partnership/collaboration, management skills, and key players.

Wilson and colleagues have conducted a series of studies to begin to identify essential global health competencies for undergraduate nursing students. The first study was conducted in collaboration with nurses in the United States, Brazil, and Mexico. The research team adapted a list of competencies that had been developed for medical students by the Association of Faculties of Medicine in Canada Resource Group on Global Health and the Global Health Education Consortium. The adapted list included 30 competencies divided into six categories (Exhibit 20.2). The list was translated into Spanish and Portuguese, and after receiving institutional review board approval, it was distributed via email survey to a convenience sample of nursing faculty members in the United States, Canada, Caribbean, and Latin American countries. Respondents were

EXHIBIT 20.2 List of Global Health Competencies for Undergraduate Nursing Students[a]

---

1. **GLOBAL BURDEN OF DISEASE**

   A basic understanding of the global burden of disease is an essential part of a modern nursing education. This knowledge is crucial for participating in discussions of priority setting, healthcare rationing and funding for health and health-related research. A nursing graduate should be able to demonstrate:

   Competency

   I a. Describe the major causes of morbidity and mortality around the world, and how the risk of disease varies with regions

   I b. Describe major public health efforts to reduce disparities in global health (such as Millennium Development Goals and Global Fund to Fight AIDS, TB, and malaria)

   I c. Discuss priority setting, healthcare rationing and funding for health and health-related research

2. **HEALTH IMPLICATIONS of MIGRATION, TRAVEL and DISPLACEMENT**

   The appropriate management of patients necessitates taking into consideration perspectives and risks posed by international travel or foreign birth. A nursing graduate should be able to:

   Competency

   II a. Demonstrate an understanding [of] the health risks posed by international travel or foreign birth

   II b. Recognize when travel or foreign birth places at patient at risk for unusual diseases or unusual presentation of common diseases and make an appropriate assessment or referral

   II c. Describe how cultural context influences perceptions of health and disease

   II d. Elicit individual health concerns in a culturally sensitive manner

   II e. Communicate effectively with patients and families using a translator

   II f. Identify world regions and/or travel activities associated with increased risk for life-threatening diseases including HIV/AIDS, malaria and multi-drug resistant tuberculosis

3. **SOCIAL and ENVIRONMENTAL DETERMINANTS of HEALTH**

   Social, economic and environmental factors are important determinants of health; furthermore, health is more than simply the absence of disease. Nurses should understand how social, economic and environmental conditions affect health, both to recognize disease risk factors in their patients and to contribute to improving public health. A nursing graduate should be able to:

   Competency

   III a. Describe how social and economic conditions such as poverty, education and life styles affect health and access to health care

   III b. List major social determinants of health and their impact on differences in life expectancy between and within countries

   III c. Describe the impact of low income, education and communication factors on access to and quality of health care

---

(continued)

EXHIBIT 20.2 List of Global Health Competencies for Undergraduate Nursing Students[a] (*continued*)

III d. Describe the relationship between access to clean water, sanitation, food and air quality on individual and population health

III e. Describe the relationship between environmental degradation and human health

4. **GLOBALIZATION of HEALTH and HEALTH CARE**

Globalization is profoundly changing disease patterns and the availability of healthcare workers worldwide. Besides the direct effects of diseases, healthcare workers and patients moving around the world, global agreements and institutions affect governments' and health care systems' ability to meet populations' health needs. A nursing graduate should be able to:

Competency

IV a. Analyze how global trends in healthcare practice, commerce and culture, multinational agreements and multinational organizations contribute to the quality and availability of health and healthcare locally and internationally

IV b. Describe different national models or health systems for provision of healthcare and their respective effects on health and healthcare expenditure

IV c. Analyze how travel and trade contribute to the spread of communicable and chronic diseases

IV d. Analyze general trends and influences in the global availability and movement of healthcare workers

IV e. Describe national and global healthcare worker availability and shortages

IV f. Describe the most common patterns of healthcare worker migration and its impact on healthcare availability in the country that the healthcare worker leaves and the country to which he/she migrates

5. **HEALTH CARE in LOW-RESOURCE SETTINGS**

Health care needs and resources markedly differ between high- and low-resource settings, yet much medical training occurs in high-resource settings. To effectively care for patients across a range of settings, a nursing graduate should be able to:

Competency

V a. Articulate barriers to health and healthcare in low-resource settings locally and internationally

V b. Demonstrate an understanding of cultural and ethical issues in working with disadvantaged populations

V c. Demonstrate the ability to adapt clinical skills and practice in a resource-constrained setting

V d. Identify signs and symptoms for common major diseases that facilitate nursing assessment in the absence of advanced testing often unavailable in low-resource settings (cardiovascular disease, cancer, and diabetes)

V e. Describe the role of syndromic management and clinical algorithms for treatment of common illnesses

V f. Identify clinical interventions and integrated strategies that have been demonstrated to substantially improve individual and/or population health in low-resource settings (e.g. immunizations, essential drugs, maternal child health programs)

(continued)

EXHIBIT 20.2 List of Global Health Competencies for Undergraduate Nursing Students[a] (*continued*)

> V g. For students who participate in electives in low-resource settings outside their home situations, a demonstration that they have participated in training to prepare for this elective
>
> 6. **HEALTH as a HUMAN RIGHT and DEVELOPMENT RESOURCE**
>
>   Human rights impact both individual and population health. Health also is an essential element of economic and social development. To effectively advocate for patients' and communities' health based on an understanding of the relationship between human rights, social and economic development and health, a nursing graduate should be able to:
>
>   Competency
>
>   VI a. Demonstrate a basic understanding of the relationship between health and human rights
>
>   VI b. Demonstrate familiarity with organizations and agreements that address human rights in healthcare and medical research
>
>   VI c. Describe role of WHO in linking health and human rights, the Universal Declaration of Human Rights, International Ethical Guidelines for Biomedical Research Involving Human Subjects (2002), Declaration of Helsinki (2008)

---

[a]Included in the original survey.

Source: From Wilson et al. (2012). Copyright Elsevier, 2012. Reprinted by permission of Elsevier.

asked to rate the extent to which they agreed that each competency was essential for an undergraduate nursing student using a 4-point Likert scale (1=strongly disagree; 2=disagree; 3=agree; 4=strongly agree). The final sample included 542 responses to the English survey and 51 responses to the Spanish survey (Wilson et al., 2012), and 212 responses to the Portuguese survey (Ventura et al., 2014). Because of the low number of responses to the Spanish survey, the survey was replicated by the Association of Latin American Nursing Schools in collaboration with the University of Mexico National Autonomous University School of Nursing, and an additional 111 responses were received (Wilson, Moran, et al., 2016).

In a subsequent study, Warren, Breman, Budhathoki, Farely, and Wilson (2015) received 63 responses to the survey from nursing educators in Africa. Mean responses to all 30 competencies were above 3.0 in all of these studies, suggesting a high level of agreement that these competencies are essential for undergraduate nursing students. However, respondents provided a number of qualitative comments, suggesting the need to revise the competency list to incorporate a more holistic nursing (as opposed to medical) focus (Wilson, Moran, et al., 2016). Qualitative content analysis of these comments suggested that competencies related to the following themes should be added to the original list:

1. Culturally competent, humanistic, and holistic care
2. Prevention, health promotion, and primary care
3. Multidisciplinary work and teamwork
4. Communication
5. Professional nursing issues in diverse settings
6. Policy/politics and historical context

7. War, disaster, pandemics, terrorism, and displacement
8. Program development, planning, and evaluation
9. Leadership, management, and advocacy
10. Vulnerable populations (Wilson, Moran, et al., 2016)

Further research is currently underway to seek consensus on a revised list of competencies that incorporates these themes, using a Delphi survey of nursing faculty in the United States with expertise in global health (Torres, Harper, & Wilson, 2016).

STRATEGIES TO INTEGRATE GLOBAL HEALTH COMPETENCIES IN NURSING PROGRAMS

The framework of educator, infrastructure, and curriculum strategies identified by the WHO to incorporate interprofessional competencies into higher educational programs might be used to integrate global health competencies into nursing educational programs (WHO, 2010a). Gilchrist and Rector (2007) conducted a literature review of best practices for recruiting, retaining, and graduating students from diverse backgrounds. Their findings supported the need for faculty development and diversification of the curriculum. Some of the approaches mentioned in this article are applicable to the improvement of global education in schools of nursing, including development of supportive environments to promote transformative learning approaches. Educator strategies include nurturing faculty who are global health champions, providing faculty development about global health priorities, and enhancing and embracing faculty and student diversity.

Schools of nursing should provide workload readjustment for faculty to integrate global learning into teaching, practice, research, and leadership initiatives. Faculty who mentor international students or scholars, offer study-abroad programs, and host international conferences should have released time to support these initiatives. When providing students with global health learning activities (at both local and international sites), faculty need the time to develop, implement, and evaluate student learning outcomes. Global learning supports the scholarship of teaching, practice, and research. Therefore, integration of global work should be considered for promotion and tenure by academic chairs and administrators.

Infrastructure strategies include providing administrative support for global initiatives and priorities, removing structural barriers that prohibit interprofessional and global learning initiatives, and ensuring that students and faculty have access to technology that facilitates global collaborations (e.g., videoconferencing or web-based communication platforms). Mill, Astle, Ogilvie, and Gastaldo (2010) argued that nursing faculty must move beyond providing international electives or citing isolated global examples within courses, and instead embed learning opportunities throughout the curriculum to help students become engaged global citizens. There are numerous curricular strategies that can facilitate integration of global health competencies: mapping existing curricula to identify how global health competencies are being integrated, offering separate global health elective courses, co-listing global health courses with other schools, including global health initiatives in the school's strategic plan, incorporating global perspectives and content into existing courses, promoting service learning opportunities both locally and at international sites, developing global health interest groups, sponsoring or hosting cultural events, offering global health case competitions, using technology to facilitate sharing and collaboration between students and faculty, and conducting research with a global focus. The remainder of this chapter expands on each of these curricular strategies.

MAPPING GLOBAL HEALTH COMPETENCIES ACROSS THE CURRICULUM

As an initial step in identifying strategies to enhance the integration of global health competencies in the nursing curriculum, Dawson, Gakumo, Phillips, and Wilson (2016) mapped courses in the bachelor of science in nursing (BSN), master of science in nursing (MSN), and doctor of nursing practice (DNP) programs of the University of Alabama at Birmingham School of Nursing, using the list of 30 competencies that had been developed by Wilson and colleagues (Wilson et al., 2012). These were presented in Exhibit 20.2. After reviewing course syllabi and online course materials, course faculty were interviewed to gather additional information about their integration of global health content into courses via classroom activities, online activities, readings, and/or student assessments. Findings from the mapping exercise were shared with individual faculty members and with faculty in each of the programs (BSN, MSN, and DNP), so that they might consider ways to address competencies that were not included, or were only minimally addressed across the curriculum.

In addition, a toolkit of resources was developed and made available through the School of Nursing shared server to help faculty members incorporate additional global health content in their courses. The Consortium of Universities for Global Health (Consortium of Universities for Global Health, 2014) and the World Federation of Academic Institutions for Global Health (World Federation of Academic Institutions for Global Health, 2016) have also developed toolkits of resources that are excellent resources for faculty.

OFFERING SEPARATE GLOBAL HEALTH ELECTIVE COURSES

Offering interdisciplinary global health elective courses provides an excellent interprofessional learning opportunity (Anders, Briggs, Hai-Jew, Caby, & Werick, 2011; Hanson, 2010; Lencucha, 2014; Moore, Sorensen, Cooper, & Daussat, 2012). Many such courses are available online through open-access platforms such as Coursera (Coursera, 2016), although these courses do not usually provide academic credit. Table 20.1 includes a sample of free online courses or modules related to global health. These courses can provide helpful resources for faculty who are developing their own elective courses for academic credit.

INTEGRATING GLOBAL HEALTH CONTENT WITHIN INDIVIDUAL COURSES

Because many nursing curricula are already overloaded with content, integrating global health competencies and concepts within existing courses may be a more effective strategy than offering separate elective courses. Faculty can assign readings, case studies, and/or review of websites that provide students with an exposure to global perspectives within each required nursing course. For example, in the introductory nursing course, when learning about basic nursing procedures, students could be encouraged to think about how they might adapt these procedures in a resource-

TABLE 20.1 Sample Listing of Free Online Global Health Courses or Modules

Online Global Health Courses or Modules	Description	URL
Coursera Courses on Global Health	Includes 17 pages listing many free open-access global health–related courses	www.coursera.org/courses/?query=global%20health&languages=en
EdX	Founded by Harvard University and the Massachusetts Institute of Technology, offers many open-access courses from universities around the world	www.edx.org/course
Global Health Gateway	Global Health Gateway is Australia and New Zealand's hub for global health careers. Site has links to many free online courses and podcasts related to global health	www.globalhealthgateway.org.au/index.php/education-and-training/free-online-courses
Global Health University—Unite for Sight	Offers courses and certificates related to global health	www.uniteforsight.org/global-health-university
Institute for International Medicine (INMED)	Offers on-site, hybrid, and self-paced courses in various topics	www.inmed.us/courses-info
Johns Hopkins Bloomberg School of Public Health	Has links to many online learning modules and courses	www.jhsph.edu/academics/online-learning-and-courses
Open Education Consortium, Global Health Courses	A global network of educational institutions, individuals, and organizations that support an approach to education based on openness	www.oeconsortium.org/courses/search/?search=Global+health
World Bank Open Learning Campus	An open and interactive learning environment	https://olc.worldbank.org
World Health Organization Management and Health Systems Delivery	Provides information about variety of online courses and programs	www.who.int/management/newitems/en/index1.html

limited setting. Students in pediatric or maternal–child health courses could be encouraged to review and compare data about maternal and child morbidity and mortality in several countries. Courses that address professional nursing issues might address issues such as international nurse migration and brain drain. Faculty members could share creative strategies used to incorporate global health through brown-bag lunches or online blogs and discussions. Exhibit 20.3 provides a sample listing of nonfiction readings, case studies, and websites that faculty could use to identify resources to integrate into their teaching. Table 20.2 provides a sample listing of organizations that might provide resources to support integration of global health concepts into nursing education programs.

EXHIBIT 20.3 Sample Listing of Nonfiction Readings, Case Studies, and Websites as Global Health Teaching Resources

Nonfiction Books About Global Health (Sample Listing)

Fadiman, A. (1997). *The spirit catches you and you fall down: A Hmong child, her American doctors, and the collision of two cultures.* New York, NY: Farrar, Straus and Giroux.

Farmer, P., Kim, J. Y., Kleinman, A., & Basilico, M. (2013). *Reimagining global health: An introduction.* Oakland: University of California Press.

Kidder, T. (2003). *Mountains beyond mountains: The quest of Dr. Paul Farmer, a man who would cure the world.* New York, NY: Random House.

Kristof, N., & WuDunn, S. (2009). *Half the sky: Turning oppression into opportunity for women worldwide.* New York, NY: Knopf.

Orbinski, J. (2008). *An imperfect offering: Humanitarian aid in the twenty-first century.* Toronto, ON: Doubleday Canada.

Global Health Case Studies

Blas, E., Sommerfeld, J., & Sivasankara, K. A. (Eds.). (2011). *Social determinants approaches to public health: From concept to practice, a collection of 13 case studies addressing social determinants of health.* Geneva, Switzerland: World Health Organization. http://www.who.int/social_determinants/tools/SD_Publichealth_eng.pdf?ua=1

BMC *International Health and Human Rights Journal*—Published an issue in 2011 focused on global health research case studies: lessons from partnerships addressing health inequities. http://www.biomedcentral.com/bmcinthealthhumrights/supplements/11/s2

Case Studies for Global Health—http://www.casestudiesforglobalhealth.org

Denton, M., Prus, S., & Walters, V. (2004). Gender differences in health: A Canadian study of the psychosocial, structural and behavioural determinants of health. *Social Science and Medicine, 58*(12), 2585–2600. (Case study on gender differences in health in Canada.)

Global Health Delivery Case Studies. http://www.ghdonline.org/cases

Standing, H. (1997). Gender and equity in health sector reform programmes: A review. *Health Policy and Planning, 12*(1), 1–18.

White, M., & Evert, J. (2014). Developing ethical awareness in global health: Four cases for medical educators. *Developing World Bioethics, 14*(3), 111–116.

Websites With General Global Health Resources

Child Family Health International: Global Health Programs. https://www.cfhi.org/global-health-programs-resources

Consortium of Universities for Global Health. www.cugh.org. *The resources section of this website has many global health education resources, including videos, modules, case studies, and discussion forums.*

Education Portal. International Health. http://education-portal.com/directory/category/Medical_and_Health_Professions/Public_Health_and_Safety/International_Health.html

(continued)

EXHIBIT 20.3 Sample Listing of Nonfiction Readings, Case Studies, and Websites as Global Health Teaching Resources (*continued*)

Global Health Delivery and GHD Online. http://www.ghdonline.org
Global Health Training Center. https://globalhealthtrainingcentre.tghn.org
International Training and Education Center for Health (ITECH). http://www.go2itech.org/what-we-do/heath-systems-strengthening
Nightingale Initiative for Global Health. http://www.nighvision.net/our-work.html
United States National Institutes of Health Fogarty International Center. E-learning Resources for Global Health Researchers. http://www.fic.nih.gov/Global/Pages/training-resources.aspx
United States Agency for International Development Global Health eLearning Center. https://www.globalhealthlearning.org/about

TABLE 20.2 Selected Organizations That Provide Resources Relevant to Global Health or Global Nursing

Organization	URL
Asian American/Pacific Islander Nurses Association	www.aapina.org
Centers for Disease Control and Prevention – Global Health	www.cdc.gov/globalhealth/index.html
Consortium of Universities for Global Health	http://cugh.org
Fogarty International Center	www.fic.nih.gov
Global Alliance for Nursing and Midwifery	https://knowledge-gateway.org/ganm
EDUCAUSE Library—Globalization	https://library.educause.edu/topics/information-technology-management-and-leadership/globalization
Global Nursing Caucus	www.globalnursingcaucus.org
International Council of Nurses	www.icn.ch
National Alaska Native American Indian Nurses Association	www.nanainanurses.org
National Association of Hispanic Nurses	www.nahnnet.org
National Black Nurses Association	www.nbna.org
National Coalition of Ethnic and Minority Nurses	http://ncemna.org
Nightingale Initiative for Global Health	www.nighcommunities.org
Pan American Health Organization	www.paho.org
Philippine Nurses Association of America	http://mypnaa.org/m
Sigma Theta Tau, International	www.nursingsociety.org/connect-engage/our-global-impact/stti's-global-initiatives
World Federation of Academic Institutions in Global Health	www.wfaigh.org
World Health Organization	www.who.int/en
World Health Organization Nursing & Midwifery Collaborating Centers	www.who.int/collaboratingcentres/networks/networksdetails/en/inIdex1.html

Faculty teaching at the graduate level could incorporate learning about international health systems into core courses that focus on role development, care delivery systems, and the use of evidence-based practice/research (AACN, 2011). Faculty members can develop cases in the form of debates and media presentations that focus on nurse migration, global workforce planning, and the impact of global diseases such as Ebola and Zika virus. These nonclinical cases provide an environment to engage students in learning and discussing multiple global issues relating to resource allocations, challenges to health maintenance and disease prevention, control of health care costs, access to care, and health outcomes. Using creative teaching strategies, faculty can avoid addressing global issues as single lecture topics and provide more stimulating, interactive learning environments. Exhibits 20.4 and 20.5 provide examples of learning activities that can be used to integrate global health content into a nursing course.

EXHIBIT 20.4 Example: Media Simulation Assignment

Students prepare a 5-minute live media interview on an assigned team topic, which addresses various current or historical global health issues. Preparation for the simulation includes researching the topic, reviewing media interviewing guidelines, attending an online media class, and posting a brief written overview of the topic prior to the simulation. Faculty members serve as the news anchors and evaluators. Faculty and students conduct postinterview debriefings using the "Gather-Analyze-Summarize" and "Plus Delta" debriefing methods. Examples of media topics include:

- Global Health: Ebola Arrives in America
- Ethical Issues in Research: Henrietta Lacks
- World Health: The Zika Virus

EXHIBIT 20.5 Example: Debate

Simulated debates allow students to engage in evidence-based learning to develop skills in influencing practice and policy at the institutional, local, state, national, and international levels. The debate is based on a case study that describes the nursing shortage (compounded by decreasing enrollment in area nursing schools and regional migration of nurses to states that pay higher wages), and the increased staffing needs due to addition of new intensive care unit beds. The debate focuses on whether the institution should employ foreign-educated nurses to supplement nurse staffing. The debate includes an opening argument and a rebuttal. After the opening argument, each team has 1 week to prepare a rebuttal. During this week, students and faculty engage in an online discussion forum to explore issues and share information related to the topic. The team is evaluated based on level of participation, incorporation of evidence in the response, demonstration of critical thinking, and reflection. The activity helps students learn about a variety of issues including workforce planning, impact of nurse migration, quality and safety, personnel management, legal issues, advocacy, and public policy.

The use of reflection as a teaching strategy can help students to think deeply about their learning experiences, including readings, films, clinical or service learning, and classroom experiences (Martinez, Artze-Vega, Wells, Mora, & Gillis, 2015; Martins de Oliveira & Tuohy, 2015). Buy et al. (2016) published a collection of 63 reflective essays written by students about their global health experiences. This resource could provide students with an example of how to use reflection as a tool to facilitate their global health learning.

Faculty also can incorporate the use of arts (literature, movies, films, photographs, or other art forms) to enhance students' global health learning (Frei, Alvarez, & Alexander, 2010; Rieger & Chernomas, 2013). Information about films with global health relevance can be found on websites of many global health centers and the WHO (University of Southern California Institute for Global Health, 2016; WHO, 2016a). Websites with photos that depict global health issues can also be a rich resource to encourage student reflection and learning (Global Health Council, 2016; The Guardian Global Development, 2016).

PROMOTING SERVICE LEARNING OPPORTUNITIES

Although there are differences in the specific definitions of service learning, most authors agree that service learning involves both service to the community and academic learning tied to specific curricular objectives, and most service-learning programs involve collaboration between the communities being served and those providing the service (Amerson, 2014; Dalmida et al., 2016; J. Howard, 2012). Underwood has provided a conceptual model to guide development of collaborative partnerships (Underwood, Gleeson, Konnert, Wong, & Valerio, 2016). Although there is a need for further research to document outcomes of service learning on students, findings from both qualitative and quantitative studies suggest that such learning activities include increased cultural and global competence, ability to work with diverse populations, empathy, civic awareness, and social responsibility (Amerson, 2014; Caldwell & Purtzer, 2015; Dalmida et al., 2016; J. Howard, 2012). Ideally, service-learning programs also benefit the communities served (Amerson, 2014; Dalmida et al., 2016; J. Howard, 2012). Riner (2011) proposed a model that provides a useful framework for designing, implementing, and evaluating local and international global experiential learning experiences.

The Sigma Theta Tau International (STTI) Service Learning Task Force recently conducted an extensive literature review and survey of 500 STTI chapters to make recommendations that could guide development of collaborative partnerships and local/global service-learning initiatives (Dalmida et al., 2016). The members of the Task Force concluded that service learning and volunteer initiatives involving nurses or nursing students should be based on principles of collaboration, sustainability, bidirectionality, equitable partnerships, and the Sustainable Development Goals. The authors emphasized the importance of avoiding North American–centric approaches, and basing volunteer and service initiatives in principles of nursing ethics and social justice. It is essential to ensure that nurses comply with the licensure requirements of the host country if they are providing direct nursing care (Dalmida et al., 2016).

Others have emphasized the importance of ensuring ethical practice during service learning and study-away experiences, and avoiding unintentional harm to the communities that such experiences are intended to serve (Caldwell & Purtzer, 2015; Crigger & Holcomb, 2007; Melby et al., 2016). Caldwell and Purtzer (2015) noted that service learning can be a transformative educational strategy when it incorporates reflection and "critical pedagogy," a concept derived from the work of Freire (1974), which encourages students to "question authority and its effects, struggle with ongoing relations of power, and prepare . . . to be critical, active citizens in . . . local, national, and global public spheres" (Freire, 1974, p. 28).

The National League for Nursing has developed toolkits that faculty could use to enhance diversity and to develop study-away opportunities for students (Adams, 2016). Other authors have also provided guidelines for development of service learning and study-away initiatives (Palmer, Wing, Miles, Heaston, & de la Cruz, 2013; Saenz & Holcomb, 2009; Wright, 2010). It is critical to ensure that any service-learning program adheres to ethical guidelines, including guidelines for licensure if the program is conducted outside of the United States (Crump & Sugarman, 2008; Dalmida et al., 2016).

DEVELOPING GLOBAL HEALTH INTEREST GROUPS

An excellent strategy for helping students and faculty learn about global health issues is the development of interdisciplinary (or discipline-specific) global health interest groups. These groups are often led by students, providing opportunities for development of skills in leadership and in interprofessional collaboration. One such group is Nursing Students Without Borders (2016). At the University of Alabama at Birmingham, students in the School of Public Health organized a global health interest group that sponsors monthly meetings open to all students and faculty in which speakers discuss current global health topics (University of Alabama at Birmingham Global Health Interest Group, 2016).

OFFERING GLOBAL HEALTH CASE COMPETITIONS

In 2009, the Emory University Global Health Institute initiated a global health case competition (Ali, Grund, & Koplan, 2011; Baggett, 2009; Emory University Global Health Institute, 2016). Students formed teams of five members representing at least three different disciplines, and the teams worked together to propose a solution for a global health case focused on child malnutrition in Ethiopia. The winning team at Emory then competed with winning teams from other universities to address a different case. This competition has grown each year since it was initiated, and in 2016, 24 universities sent teams to compete in the international competition at Emory. Participating universities develop their own procedures for the preliminary competitions.

At the University of Alabama at Birmingham, the competition is sponsored by the Sparkman Center for Global Health (Sparkman Center for Global Health, 2016). Students register for their teams online, and often the spaces fill within hours after the online registration opens! The teams receive the case on a Tuesday afternoon, and work together to develop an innovative and evidence-based approach to address the case problem. Problems that have been addressed in recent years include obesity in Mexico, child trafficking in Thailand, and open defecation in India. Each team is assigned a faculty mentor who provides up to 1 hour of consultation as the teams work on their problems. The teams present their proposals to a panel of judges on Saturday (4 days after receiving the case), and the winning team receives a monetary award and support to attend the international competition at Emory university. Student evaluations of these competitions have been positive, and their comments have reflected appreciation for the opportunity to learn from students in other disciplines and to think creatively to address current and pressing global health issues.

USING TECHNOLOGY TO FACILITATE SHARING AND COLLABORATION

The availability of the Internet and advances in information technology offer many new opportunities to facilitate collaboration and communication with nurses and students around the globe. There are many global nursing networks that facilitate communication and collaboration. For example, the Pan American Health Organization supports more than 20 nursing networks focused on different areas of nursing specialization, and many of these networks meet via online conferences (Global Nursing Caucus, 2016; ICN, 2016; Pan American Health Organization Human Resources for Health Observatory, 2016).

Ziemba et al. (2016) described an innovative teaching strategy that involves use of the Internet to facilitate sharing between community health nursing students in their school and at a partner nursing school in Haiti. Students at both schools used a similar framework and tool for their community assessment assignment, and they held weekly videoconferences to share their findings and to compare identified health challenges. Despite problems associated with technology and language differences, students evaluated the experience positively and cited numerous strengths, including the opportunity to learn about other cultures and community health problems and solutions in different contexts. Another example of using Internet technology to enhance global learning is encouraging students and faculty to participate in online communities of practice such as the Global Alliance for Nursing and Midwifery (2016) and Global Health Nursing and Midwifery Online (2016).

PROMOTING A GLOBAL HEALTH FOCUS IN RESEARCH INITIATIVES

International nursing research has been defined as "research where investigators and participants are from different countries, rather than research targeting populations by race or ethnicity" (Working Group for the Study of Ethical Issues in International Nursing Research, 2003, p. 2). Chiang-Hanisko, Ross, Ludwick, and Martsolf (2006) described international collaborative research in nursing as "cross-sectional research on nursing phenomena that is conducted in more than one country via a working partnership that share resources, time and talents" (p. 308). George and Meadows-Oliver (2013) suggested that collaborations and partnerships that exist between nurses in low- and high-resource countries require strategic planning and foresight in order for these partnerships to be beneficial for all involved. International research collaborations are challenged by the imbalance of funding focused on low-resource countries. It is estimated that only 10% of global research dollars are spent on countries that carry 90% of the global disease burden, a paradox known as the "10/90 gap" (Stevens, 2004). Schools of nursing can contribute to addressing global research inequities by enhancing global health research opportunities for undergraduate and graduate students. There are many ways to integrate global perspectives in research in both undergraduate- and graduate-level nursing programs.

Undergraduate nursing students can be encouraged to integrate global perspectives in research by means of introductory evidence-based practice courses. In many BSN programs, students first begin to learn how to search for and synthesize critical evidence in existing scientific literature. Although local evidence is important in making clinical decisions for patients, borderless or global evidence that extends beyond nations and disciplines (Hopp & Rittenmeyer, 2012) is equally important in making clinical decisions. Undergraduate students can be assigned to search and synthesize the literature based on a variety of global health-related topics. One example would be the clinical problem of dental caries that disproportionately affects children living in rural areas in low-resource countries. Students would be asked to review the evidence and then develop clinical guidelines to address this issue within the context of limited resources.

Undergraduate students working on scholarly projects might partner with investigators involved in global research partnerships. Students may not be able to travel internationally (due to resource or other constraints), but they could gain a wealth of knowledge about different cultural contexts and global health issues by assisting with various aspects of such a project, including literature review, data analysis, or helping with preparing presentations or publications from the project. Even if the students are highly motivated, they may need considerable assistance from nursing faculty members to identify global health investigators and mentors.

On the master's level, the incorporation of global perspectives in research can help prepare students to translate evidence into practice in a variety of contexts. Students can learn that the strategies to develop, implement, and evaluate patient care delivery may differ significantly from a resource-rich context to a context that is resource-limited. There are certain health indicators for outcomes that all countries share, such as safety and quality. However, emerging technologies and how to manage health systems data can differ greatly from country to country.

On the doctoral level, students can benefit from opportunities to conduct research in diverse international settings, learning about different ethical guidelines and health care delivery systems, as well as global perspectives on health promotion and disease prevention. Additionally, interprofessional collaborations will help doctoral students to develop and implement sustainable global health projects with local and international community partners. Doctoral students also should understand the increasing relevance of global participatory action research. Participatory action research enables action through reflection, attends to power dynamics, ensures that power is shared between researchers and participants, and involves participants in the research (Baum, MacDougall, & Smith, 2006). This method is well-suited for global research collaborations. Doctoral students also should learn about potential sources of support for global research initiatives. For example, the Fogarty International Center at the U.S. National Institutes of Health offers pre- and postdoctoral fellowships in global health (Fogarty International Center, 2016).

Doctoral students engaged in global health research need to be aware of ethical considerations in global health research. The Working Group for the Study of Ethical Issues in International Nursing Research (2003) identified two major factors that cause ethical concern: the level of cultural differences between the countries involved in the research and the capability of exploitation. Guiding principles to overcome these potentially ethical issues include respect for persons, beneficence, justice, respect for community, and contextual caring (Working Group for the Study of Ethical Issues in International Nursing Research, 2003).

SUMMARY

In conclusion, students and nurse educators alike need to be aware of major global health challenges, such as increasing disparities in global burden of disease, climate change, and the future challenges to the sustainable development of global and planetary health. Globalization has a lasting impact on nursing practice. Although travel and migration present opportunities for greater global awareness and understanding, they also usher in challenges, such as the potential for spread of disease that transcends national borders. Nurse educators are in unique positions to prepare students as global citizens who can contribute to global health diplomacy and ensure culturally competent care at local and international levels.

Globalization has had a significant impact on higher education, as evidenced by the increasing interest among students and faculty and the growing recognition of the need to prepare students for work in an increasingly globalized world. Accordingly, schools of nursing must be involved in curriculum changes and pedagogical approaches that support diversity of students and faculty and integrate global perspectives across the curriculum. The definition of global health by the Global Advisory Panel for the Future of Nursing and Global Health can be used to guide the incorporation of global health into nursing education programs. Key concepts of this definition include: planetary health, interprofessional collaboration, individual- as well as population-level health care that addresses health problems, and solutions that transcend national borders. Many groups, such as the National Academy of Medicine (formerly the Institute of Medicine), WHO, and the Interprofessional Education Collaborative, have identified the need to incorporate global health and interprofessional education into health professional educational programs. Nurse educators can use strategies such as competency mapping to ensure that both interprofessional and global health competencies are incorporated into the curriculum at both undergraduate and graduate levels to ensure that graduates are prepared to work in a globalized world and to contribute to planetary health.

REFERENCES

Adams, V. W. (2016). The challenges of USA nursing education to meet local, regional and global need. *Revista Brasileira de Enfermagen, 69*, 417–418. doi:10.1590/0034-7167.2016690301i

Ali, M. K., Grund, J. M., & Koplan, J. P. (2011). Case competitions to engage students in global health. *Lancet, 377*(9776), 1473–1474. doi:10.1016/s0140-6736(10)62186-1

All Party Parliamentary Group on Global Health. (2016). Triple impact: How developing nursing will improve health, promote gender equality and support economic growth. Retrieved from http://www.appg-globalhealth.org.uk

American Academy of Family Physicians. (2012). *Recommended curriculum guidelines for family medicine residents: Global health.* Retrieved from http://www.aafp.org/dam/AAFP/documents/medical_education_residency/program_directors/Reprint287_Global.pdf?cmpid=_van_722

American Association of Colleges of Nursing. (2008). *The essentials of baccalaureate education for professional nursing practice.* Retrieved from http://www.aacn.nche.edu/education-resources/BaccEssentials08.pdf

American Association of Colleges of Nursing. (2011). *The essentials of master's education in nursing.* Retrieved from http://www.aacn.nche.edu/education-resources/MastersEssentials11.pdf

American Association of Colleges of Nursing. (2016). *Policy brief: The changing landscape: Nursing student diversity on the rise.* Retrieved from http://www.aacn.nche.edu/government-affairs/Student-Diversity-FS.pdf

Amerson, R. (2014). Research-based recommendations for implementing international service-learning. *Journal of Professional Nursing, 30*, 175–179. doi:10.1016/j.profnurs.2013.09.006

Anders, B. A., Briggs, D. J., Hai-Jew, S., Caby, Z., & Werick, M. (2011). Creating an online global health course and game. *EDUCAUSE Quarterly, 34*(4). Retrieved from https://www.learntechlib.org/p/110781

Archambault, N. (2010). *Incorporating global health into undergraduate nursing education* (MSN Thesis). Vancouver, BC, Canada: University of British Columbia.

Arthur, M. A., Battat, R., & Brewer, T. F. (2011). Teaching the basics: core competencies in global health. *Infectious Disease Clinics of North America, 25*, 347–358. doi:10.1016/j.idc.2011.02.013

Association of Schools of Public Health. (2011). *Global health competency model final version 1.1.* Retrieved from http://www.aspph.org/educate/models/masters-global-health

Baggett, R. (2009). Feeding children for—and with—peanuts. *Emory University Magazine, Autumn*, p. 18.

Battat, R., Seidman, G., Chadi, N., Chanda, M. Y., Nehme, J., Hulme, J., . . . Brewer, T. F. (2010). Global health competencies and approaches in medical education: A literature review. *BMC Medical Education, 10*, 94. doi:10.1186/1472-6920-10-94

Baum, F., MacDougall, C., & Smith, D. (2006). Participatory action research. *Journal of Epidemiology and Community Health, 60*, 854–857. doi:10.1136/jech.2004.028662

Baumann, S. L. (2013). Global health nursing: Toward a human science-based approach. *Nursing Science Quarterly, 26*(4), 365. doi:10.1177/0894318413500404

Biemiller, L. (2014, February 24). QuickWire: EdX and Facebook team up to offer free education in Rwanda. *Chronicle of Higher Education.* Retrieved from http://www.chronicle.com/blogs/wiredcampus/quickwire-edx-partners-with-facebook-to-offer-courses-in-rwanda/50693

Buy, T., Evert, J., McCarthy, V., Asokan, I., Mehta, A., Miller, K., . . . Wen, S. (2016). *Reflection in global health: An anthology*. San Francisco, CA: Global Health Collaborations Press.

Caldwell, P., & Purtzer, M. A. (2015). Long-term learning in a short-term study abroad program: "Are we really truly helping the community?" *Public Health Nursing, 32*(5), 577–583. doi:10.1111/phn.12168

Cassady, C., Meru, R., Chan, N. M., Engelhardt, J., Fraser, M., & Nixon, S. (2014). Physiotherapy beyond our borders: Investigating ideal competencies for canadian physiotherapists working in resource-poor countries. *Physiotherapy Canada, 66*(1), 15–23. doi:10.3138/ptc.2012-54

Chiang-Hanisko, L., Ross, R., Ludwick, R., & Martsolf, D. (2006). International collaborations in nursing research: Priorities, challenges and rewards. *Journal of Research in Nursing, 11*, 307–322.

Childs, G., Jonew, R., Nugent, K. E., & Cook, P. (2004). Retention of African-American students in baccalaureate nursing programs: Are we doing enough?. *Journal of Professional Nursing, 20*, 129–133.

Clark, M., Raffray, M., Hendricks, K., & Gagnon, A. J. (2016). Global and public health core competencies for nursing education: A systematic review of essential competencies. *Nurse Education Today, 40*, 173–180. doi:10.1016/j.nedt.2016.02.026

Committee on the Robert Wood Johnson Foundation Initiative on the Future of Nursing at the Institute of Medicine. (2011). *The future of nursing: Leading change, advancing health*. Washington, DC: The National Academies Press.

Consortium of Universities for Global Health. (2014). About CUGH. Retrieved from http://www.cugh.org/about

Coursera. (2017). Coursera. Retrieved from http://coursera.org

Crigger, N. J., & Holcomb, L. (2007). Practical strategies for providing culturally sensitive, ethical care in developing nations. *Journal of Transcultural Nursing, 18*(1), 1–70.

Crump, J. A., & Sugarman, J. (2008). Ethical considerations for short-term experiences by trainees in global health. *Journal of the American Medical Association, 300*(12), 12–1456.

Currier, C., Lucas, J., & Saint Arnault, D. (2009). Study abroad and nursing: From cultural to global competence. In R. Lewin (Ed.), *The handbook of practice and research in study abroad*. New York, NY: Routledge/Taylor & Francis.

Dalmida, S. G., Amerson, R., Foster, J., McWhinney-Dehaney, L., Magowe, M., Nicholas, P. K., . . . Leffers, J. (2016). Volunteer service and service learning: Opportunities, partnerships, and United Nations Millennium Development Goals. *Journal of Nursing Scholarship, 48*, 517–526.

Dawson, M., Gakumo, A., Phillips, J., & Wilson, L. (2016). Process for mapping global health competencies in undergraduate and graduate nursing curricula. *Nurse Educator, 41*, 37–40. doi:10.1097/NNE.0000000000000199

Donaldson, M. E., Gadbury-Amyot, C. C., Khajotia, S. S., Nattestad, A., Norton, N. S., Zubiaurre, L. A., & Turner, S. P. (2008). Dental education in a flat world: Advocating for increased global collaboration and standardization. *Journal of Dental Education, 72*, 408–421.

Drain, P. K., Primack, A., Hunt, D. D., Fawzi, W. W., Holmes, K. K., & Gardner, P. (2007). Global health in medical education: A call for more training and opportunities. *Academic Medicine, 82*, 226–230. doi:10.1097/ACM.0b013e3180305cf9

edX. (2017). edX. https://www.edx.org

Emory University Global Health Institute. (2016). Emory global health case competitions. Retrieved from http://www.globalhealth.emory.edu/what/student_programs/case_competitions/index.html

Fisman, D. N., & Laupland, K. B. (2010). The 'One Health' paradigm: Time for infectious diseases clinicians to take note? *Canadian Journal of Infectious Diseases & Medical Microbiology, 21*(3), 3–111.

Fogarty International Center. (2016). Non-NIH funding opportunities for predoctoral and graduate researchers. Retrieved from https://www.fic.nih.gov/Pages/Default.aspx

Frei, J., Alvarez, S. E., & Alexander, M. B. (2010). Ways of seeing: Using the visual arts in nursing education. *Journal of Nursing Education, 49*, 672–676. doi:10.3928/01484834-20100831-04

Freire, P. (1974). *Education for critical consciousness*. New York, NY: Continuum International Publishing Group.

Frenk, J., Chen, L., Bhutta, A. Z., Cohen, J., Crisp, N., Evans, T., . . . Zurayk, H. (2010). Health professionals for a new century: Transforming education to strengthen health systems in an interdependent world. *Lancet, 376*(9756), 1923–1958. doi:10.1016/S0140-6736(10)61854-5

George, E. K., & Meadows-Oliver, M. (2013). Searching for collaboration in international nursing partnerships: A literature review. *International Nursing Review, 60*(1), 31–36. doi:10.1111/j.1466-7657.2012.01034.x

Giannobile, W. V. (2013). Our duty to promote gllobal oral health. *Journal of Dental Research, 92*, 573–574.

Gilchrist, K. L., & Rector, C. (2007). Can you keep them? Strategies to attract and retain nursing students from diverse populations: Best practices in nursing education. *Journal of Transcultural Nursing, 18*(3), 277–285. doi:10.1177/1043659607301305

Global Alliance for Nursing and Midwifery Communities of Practice. (2016). *Working together for health knowledge exchange.* Retrieved from http://knowledge-gateway.org/ganm

Global Health Council. (2016). Photo gallery. Retrieved from http://globalhealth.org/resources/photo -gallery

Global Health Nursing & Midwifery. (2016). GHD online: Global Health Nursing & Midwifery. Retrieved from http://www.ghdonline.org/nursing

Global Network of WHO Collaborating Centers for Nursing and Midwifery Development. (2016). Retrieved from http://www.eerp.usp.br/globalnet

Global Nursing Caucus. (2016). Global Nursing Caucus: *Engaging nurses to advance global health.* Retrieved from http://www.globalnursingcaucus.org

Global One Health Core Competency Working Group. (2013). *One health core competency domains, subdo-mains, and competency examples: Global OHCC Working Group: USAID RESPOND initiative.* Retrieved from https://issuu.com/prakitkitsupee/docs/ohcc_domains_final_respond

Grootjans, J., & Newman, S. (2013). The relevance of globalization to nursing: A concept analysis. *International Nursing Review, 60*(1), 78–85. doi:10.1111/j.1466-7657.2012.01022.x

Hanson, L. (2010). Global citizenship, global health, and the internationalization of curriculum: A study of transformative potential. *Journal of Studies in International Education, 14*(1), 70–88.

Hopp, L., & Rittenmeyer, L. (2012). *Introduction to evidence-based practice: A practical guide for nursing.* Philadelphia, PA: F. A. Davis.

Horton, R., Beaglehole, R., Bonita, R., Raeburn, J., McKee, M., & Wall, S. (2014). From public to planetary health: A manifesto. *Lancet, 383*(9920), 847. doi:10.1016/s0140-6736(14)60409-8

Howard, C. R., Gladding, S. P., Kiguli, S., Andrews, J. S., & John, C. C. (2011). Development of a com-petency-based curriculum in global child health. *Academic Medicine, 86*(4), 521–528. doi:10.1097/ ACM.0b013e31820df4c1

Howard, J. (2012). Service learning reserach: Foundational issues. In S. H. Billig & A. S. Waterman (Eds.), *Studying service learning: Innovations in education research methodology* (pp. 1–12). New York, NY: Routledge Taylor & Francis Group.

Hunter, A., Stanhope, M., Wilson, L., Hatcher, B., Hattar, M., & Messias, D. K. H. P., D. (2013). Global health diplomacy: An integrative review of the literature and implications for nursing. *Nursing Outlook, 61,* 85–92. doi:10.1016/j.outlook.2012.07.013

Institute of Medicine. (1972). *Educating for the health team.* Retrieved from https://nexusipe.org/ informing/resource-center/iom-1972-report-educating-health-team

International Council of Nurses. (2016). *ICN networks.* Retrieved from http://www.icn.ch/networks/ icn-networks/

Interprofessional Education Collaborative. (2016). *Core competencies for interprofessional collaborative practice: 2016 update.* Retrieved from http://www.usi.edu/media/5598895/core-competencies-new-2016.pdf

Interprofessional Education Collaborative Expert Panel. (2011). *Core competencies for interprofessional col-laborative practice: Report of an expert panel.* Retrieved from http://www.aacn.nche.edu/education -resources/IPECReport.pdf

Janes, C. R., & Corbett, K. K. (2009). Anthropology and global health. *Annual Reviews of Anthropology, 38,* 167–183. doi:10.1146/annurev-anthro-091908-164314

Jarvis, P. (1997). The globalization of nurse education within higher education. *Nurse Education Today, 17*(1), 22–30.

Jogerst, K., Callender, B., Adams, V., Evert, J., Fields, E., Hall, T., . . . Wilson, L. (2015). Identifying interprofessional global health competencies for 21st century health professional. *Annals of Global Health, 81*(2), 239–247. doi:10.1016/j.aogh.2015.03.006

Kahn, L. H., Kaplan, B., Monath, T., Woodall, J., & Conti, L. (2014). A manifesto for planetary health— Correspondence. *Lancet, 383,* 1460. doi:10.1016/S0140-6736(14)60709-1

Kirk, M. (2002). The impact of globalization and environmental change on health: Challenges for nurse education. *Nurse Education Today, 22,* 60–71.

Kjellstrom, T., & McMichael, A. J. (2013). Climate change threats to population health and well-being: The imperative of protective solutions that will last. *Global Health Action, 6,* 20816. doi:10.3402/gha .v6i0.20816

Klopper, H. C., & Hill, M. (2015). Global Advisory Panel on the Future of Nursing (GAPFON) and Global Health. *Journal of Nursing Scholarship, 47*(3–4). doi:0.1111/jnu.12118

Koplan J. P., Bond T. C., Merson M. H., Reddy K. S., Rodriguez M. H., Sewankambo N. K., & Wasserheit, J. N. (2009). Towards a common definition of global health. *Lancet, 373*(9679), 1993–1995.

Lencucha, R. (2014). A research-based narrative assignment for global health education. *Advances in Health Sciences Education, 19*(1), 129–142.

Martinez, I. L., Artze-Vega, I., Wells, A. L., Mora, J. C., & Gillis, M. (2015). Twelve tips for teaching social determinants of health in medicine. *Medical Teacher, 37*(7), 647–652. doi:10.3109/01421 59X.2014.975191

Martins de Oliveira, A. K., & Tuohy, D. (2015). Communication and nursing: A study-abroad student's reflections. *British Journal of Nursing, 24*(21), 1080–1084. doi:10.12968/bjon.2015.24.21.1080

Melby, M. K., Loh, L. C., Evert, J., Prater, C., Lin, H., & Khan, O. A. (2016). Beyond medical "missions" to impact-driven short-term experiences in global health (STEGHs): Ethical principles to optimize community benefit and learner experience. *Academic Medicine, 91*(5), 633–638. doi:10.1097/ acm.0000000000001009

Merson, M. H. (2014). University engagement in global health. *New England Journal of Medicine, 370*(18), 1676–1678. doi:10.1056/NEJMp1401124

Michaud, J., & Kates, J. (2013). Global health diplomacy: Advancing foreign policy and global health interests. *Global Health, Science and Practice, 1*(1), 24–28. doi:10.9745/GHSP-D-12-00048

Mill, J., Astle, B. J., Ogilvie, L., & Gastaldo, D. (2010). Linking global citizenship, undergraduate nursing education, and professional nursing: Curricular innovation in the 21st century. *Advances in Nursing Science, 33*(3), E1–E11.

Moore, B., Sorensen, W., Cooper, C., & Daussat, L. (2012). Evaluation of a newly implemented undergraduate global health course in the public university setting. *Journal of General Education, 61*(4), 505–526.

National Black Nurses Association. (2016). National Black Nurses Association NBNA. Retrieved from http://www.nbna.org

NextGenU. (2017). NextGenU. Retrieved from http://nextgenu.org

Nursing Students Without Borders. (2016). *Nursing students without borders.* Retrieved from https:// atuva.student.virginia.edu/organization/nursingstudentswithoutborders/about

Palmer, S., Wing, D., Miles, L., Heaston, S., & de la Cruz, K. (2013). Study abroad programs: Using alumni and graduate students as affiliate faculty. *Nurse Educator, 38*(5), 198–201. doi:10.1097/ NNE.0b013e3182a0e587

Pan American Health Organization. (2016). International nursing networks. Retrieved from http://www .paho.org/hq/index.php?option=com_content&view=article&id=11172&Itemid=41549&lang=en

Pan American Health Organization Human Resources for Health Observatory. (2016). *Redes Internacionales de Enfermeria (International Nursing Networks).* Retrieved from http://www .observatoriorh.org/?q=redes-internacionales-de-enfermeria

Rieger, K. L., & Chernomas, W. M. (2013). Arts-based learning: Analysis of the concept for nursing education. *International Journal of Nursing Education Scholarship, 10*(1), 1–10. doi:10.1515/ijnes-2012-0034

Riner, M. E. (2011). Globally engaged nursing education: An academic program framework. *Nursing Outlook, 59*(6), 308–317. doi:10.1016/j.outlook.2011.04.005

Rodger, S., & Hoffman, J. S. (2010). Where in the world is interprofessional education? A global environmental scan. *Journal of Interprofessional Care, 24*(5), 479–491. doi:10.3109/13561821003721329

Rowson, M., Wilcott, C., Hughes, R., Manini, A., Martin, S., Miranda, J. J., . . . Yudkin, J. S. (2012). Conceptualising global health: Theoretical issues and their relevance for teaching. *Globalization and Health, 8*(36). doi:10.1186/1744-8603-8-36

Saenz, K., & Holcomb, L. (2009). Essential tools for a study abroad nursing course. *Nurse Educator, 34*(4), 172–175. doi:10.1097/NNE.0b013e3181aaba6b

Shishani, K., Allen, C., Shubnikov, E., Salman, K., Laporte, R. E., & Linkov, F. (2012). Nurse educators establishing new venues in global nursing education. *Journal of Professional Nursing, 28*(2), 132–134. doi:10.1016/j.profnurs.2011.11.008

Sparkman Center for Global Health. (2016). UAB Sparkman Center for Global Health. Retrieved from http://www.uab.edu/sparkmancenter

Stevens, P. (2004). *Diseases of poverty and the 10/90 gap.* Retrieved from http://www.who.int/ intellectualproperty/submissions/InternationalPolicyNetwork.pdf

Swider, S. M., Krothe, J., Reyes, D., & Cravetz, M. (2013). The Quad Council practice competencies for public health nursing. *Public Health Nursing, 30*(6), 519–536. doi:10.1111/phn.12090

The Guardian Global Development. (2016). *Global health messages in pictures.* Retrieved from https://www.theguardian.com/global-development/gallery/2011/may/19/global-health-images-in-pictures

Torres, H., Harper, D., & Wilson, L. (2016). *Mixed methods, modified delphi study: Identification of global health competencies for baccalaureate nursing education: Poster presentation.* Paper presented at the Nurses: A Force for Change: Improving Health Systems' Resilience-Global Nursing Caucus, Massachusetts General Hospital, and SEED Global Health, Boston, MA.

Underwood, M., Gleeson, J., Konnert, C., Wong, K., & Valerio, B. (2016). Global host partner perspectives: Utilizing a conceptual model to strengthen collaboration with host partners for international nursing student placements. *Public Health Nursing, 33*(4), 351–359. doi:10.1111/phn.12258

United Nations. (2016). *Sustainable development goals: 17 goals to transform our world.* Retrieved from http://www.un.org/sustainabledevelopment/sustainable-development-goals

University of Alabama at Birmingham Global Health Interest Group. (2016). *UAB Global Health Interest Group—GHIG.* Retrieved from https://www.facebook.com/GHIGatUAB

University of Southern California Institute for Global Health. (2016). *Global health films database.* Retrieved from http://apruglobalhealth.org/ghfilms

Upvall, J. J., Leffers, J. M., & Mitchell, E. M. (2014). Introduction and perspectives of global health. In M. J. Upvall & J. M. Jeffers (Eds.), *Global health nursing: Building and sustaining partnerships* (pp. 1–17). New York, NY: Springer Publishing.

Ventura, C. A. A., Mendes, I. A. C., Wilson, L., deGodoy, S., Tamy-Maury, I., Zarate, R., & Salas, S. (2014). Global health competencies from the perspective of nursing faculty from Brazilian higher education institutions. *Revista Latina-Americana de Enfermagem, 22*(2), 179–186.

Warren, N., Breman, R., Budhathoki, C., Farley, J., & Wilson, L. L. (2015). Perspectives of nursing faculty in Africa on global health nursing competencies. *Nursing Outlook.* doi:10.1016/j.outlook.2015.11.016

Whitmee, S., Haines, A., Beyrer, C., Boltz, F., Capon, A. G., de Souza Dias, B. F., . . . Yach, D. (2015). Safeguarding human health in the Anthropocene epoch: Report of The Rockefeller Foundation-Lancet Commission on planetary health. *Lancet, 386*(10007), 1973–2028. doi:10.1016/S0140-6736(15)60901-1

Wilson, L., Callender, B., Hall, T. L., Jogerst, K., Torres, H., & Velji, A. (2014). Identifying gobal health competencies to prepare 21st century global health professionals: Report from the Global Health Competency Subcommittee of the Consortium of Universities for Global Health. *Journal of Law, Medicine and Ethics, 42,* 26–31. doi:10.1111/jlme.12184

Wilson, L., Harper, D. C., Tami-Maury, I., Zarate, R., Salas, S., Farley, J., . . . Ventura, C. (2012). Global health competencies for nurses in the Americas. *Journal of Professional Nursing, 28*(4), 213–222.

Wilson, L., Mendes, I. A., Klopper, H., Catrambone, C., Al-Maaitah, R., Norton, M. E., & Hill, M. (2016). 'Global health' and 'global nursing': proposed definitions from The Global Advisory Panel on the Future of Nursing. *Journal of Advanced Nursing, 72*(7), 1529–1540. doi:10.1111/jan.12973

Wilson, L., Moran, L., Zarate, R., Warren, N., Ventura, C. A., Tami-Maury, I., & Mendes, I. A. (2016). Qualitative description of global health nursing competencies by nursing faculty in Africa and the Americas. *Revista Latina-Americana de Enfermagem,* 1518–8345 (Electronic). doi:10.1590/1518-8345.0772.2697

Working Group for the Study of Ethical Issues in International Nursing Research. (2003). Ethical considerations in international nursing research: A report from the International Centre for Nursing Ethics. *Nursing Ethics, 10*(2), 122–137.

World Federation of Academic Institutions for Global Health. (2016). World Federation of Academic Institutions for Global Health. Retrieved from wfaigh.org

World Health Organization. (2010a). *Framework for action on interprofessional education & collaborative practice* Retrieved from http://whqlibdoc.who.int/hq/2010/WHO_HRH_HPN_10.3_eng.pdf

World Health Organization. (2010b). *WHA 63.16: Global code of practice on international recruitment of health personnel.* Retrieved from apps.who.int/gb/ebwha/pdf_files/WHA63/A63_R16-en.pdf

World Health Organization. (2011). *Closing the gap: Policy into practice on social determinants of health.* Discussion paper for the World conference on social Determinants of Health. Retrieved from http://www.who.int/sdhconference/Discussion-paper-EN.pdf

World Health Organization. (2013). *World health report 2013: Research for universal health coverage.* Retrieved from http://www.who.int/whr/en

World Health Organization. (2016a). Climate change and human health: Documentary films and videos. Retrieved from http://www.who.int/globalchange/mediacentre/videos/en

World Health Organization. (2016b). Global Health Observatory (GHO) data: Monitoring health for the SDGs. Retrieved from http://www.who.int/gho/en

World Health Organization. (2016c). *Global strategic directions for strengthening nursing and midwifery 2016-2020.* Retrieved from http://www.who.int/hrh/nursing_midwifery/global-strategic -midwifery2016-2020.pdf

Wright, D. J. (2010). Planning a study abroad clinical experience. *Journal of Nursing Education, 49*(5), 280–286. doi:10.3928/01484834-20100115-05

Ziemba, R., Sarkar, N. J., Pickus, B., Dallwig, A., Wan, J. A., & Alcindor, H. (2016). Using international videoconferencing to extend the global reach of community health nursing education. *Public Health Nursing, 33*(4), 360–370. doi:10.1111/phn.12272

Appendix A: Examples of Teaching Materials and Other Documents for a Laboratory Module

APPENDIX A.1 TEACHING ENVIRONMENT SETUP: EQUIPMENT, SUPPLY USE, AND RESET GUIDE

INSERT NAME OF LAB **Setup Instructions**
Equipment and Supplies
Place a copy of the equipment and supply list in each room's teaching box for that lab (see Appendix A.3)
• List all equipment required for the lab (with storage location in room or elsewhere)
• List each supply needed for the lab (with storage location in room or elsewhere)
Equipment and Supply Use and Reset Guide
Outline each step required to set up the lab room using the supplies listed above. Ideally steps should be listed chronologically.

1. Provide instructions to finalize setup prior to lab:
  a. Explain what has to be checked, such as the presence of a fluid reservoir.
  b. Identify final preparation setup steps to complete, such as applying dressings.
  c. List items to lay out for instructor and/or student use, such as syringes and needles.

2. Provide instructions to follow during lab:
  a. Indicate where to find replacement or additional supplies for items used during lab.
  b. Indicate what is reusable and how to harvest for reuse such as refilling and repackaging syringes or emptying and repackaging tubing.
  c. Indicate what is disposable and how to properly dispose of items, including biohazardous waste requirements.

3. Provide instructions to reset at the end of lab for repeated sessions that day:
  a. Identify what the instructor and students need to do to reset the area, such as restocking with new supplies, refilling bags or syringes, or emptying reservoirs.
  b. Identify where to find replacements to restock one-time-use supplies.

(continued)

APPENDIX A.1 TEACHING ENVIRONMENT SETUP: EQUIPMENT, SUPPLY USE, AND RESET GUIDE (*continued*)

4. Provide instructions to close down the room if there is a delay between teaching sessions and at the end of the final teaching session:
 	
   a. List the items that need to be refilled and repackaged or emptied and repackaged.
 	
   b. List activities necessary to prevent degradation of supplies or equipment, such as removing transparent dressings from manikins and emptying reservoirs.
 	
   c. List steps to close the room, such as emptying trash, washing items or manikins, and/or turning off technology.

APPENDIX A.2 LESSON PLAN

INSERT NAME OF LAB Schedule	
TIME	**EVENT or SKILL**
Insert time in minutes or hours	List out each individual event or skill in a separate row in preferred chronological order before the break • Include a breakdown of expected teaching method, such as round table practice, instructor demonstration, or student practice after instructor demonstration
Insert time	**BREAK** (indicate when the break occurs)
Insert time in minutes or hours	List out each individual event or skill in a separate row in preferred chronological order as above
Optional: List specific information the instructor needs to remember to do with equipment or supplies (for example, keep original packaging with feeding tubes and repackage after demonstrating the tubes)	

APPENDIX A.3 TEACHING BOX SUPPLY LIST[a]

ITEM	**LOCATION**
List each item needed to teach the content for that specific lab in a separate row	List storage area for each item
Optional: Give an overview of what the room should look like when the instructor enters the room, such as manikins in bed with supplies from setup document in place (Appendix A.1). Include picture (optional).	

[a]Placed in Teaching Box, see Figure 9.1

APPENDIX A.4 STANDARDIZED LEARNING MODULE OVERVIEW

INSERT NAME OF LAB Key Concepts and Procedures
PREPARATION:
1. List instructions students need to complete prior to attending lab, such as taking an online quiz or completing assigned readings. 2. List supplies and equipment students should bring to lab, such as electronic or printed copy of learning module, supply kits, and student identification cards for attendance. 3. List expectations of students during lab, such as participating in skills practice and using standard precautions and proper body mechanics. 4. List expectations of students at the end of lab, such as cleaning up or repackaging their supplies to take with them. 5. List reminders for students, such as not throwing away reusable supplies. 6. Encourage students to ask staff if they have questions.
Identify if and what supply bag kits students should bring to lab or whether they will receive supplies in lab. If students are supposed to bring a supply kit they have already received, it is helpful to include a picture of the supply kit and/or a list of the required items.

LEARNING OUTCOMES:

At the completion of this module, the student should be able to:

1. [Numerically list all expected student behavioral outcomes using appropriate taxonomy.]

2. [Ideally, list outcomes in the same order that they are presented in the Topic/ Assignment section below.]

REQUIRED READINGS/AUDIOVISUALS:

Books

[List textbook(s) used to develop the teaching content and augment learning, using appropriate reference formatting.]

Journals

[List journal(s) used to develop the teaching content and augment learning, using appropriate reference formatting.]

Websites

[List websites and/or videos used to develop the teaching content and augment learning, using appropriate reference formatting.]

TOPIC	ASSIGNMENTS
List each specific topic in a separate row of the table and include applicable learning outcome(s)	List the specific pages from the textbook or the specific journal or Internet site/video that addresses the topic.

[TOPIC]

Key Concepts

- Present the theoretical concepts that students need to know for each topic discussed in the lab, using either a bulleted or paragraph format (use appropriate reference formatting).

Procedure

In a table format, list the steps for each procedure that applies to the topic area:

Group related steps or sequential actions in the same cell to encourage students to cognitively associate content, either by bulleting or by numbering steps for clarity

Provide a rationale for steps or for grouped concepts

APPENDIX A.5 EXAMPLE PROVIDER'S ORDER

FOR EDUCATIONAL USE ONLY. NOT FOR ACTUAL PATIENT CARE[a]			
Carrington General Hospital			Patient Identification
Provider Order Entry			
Weight:			
Allergies:			
Order#	Order Start Time	Order Stop Time	Order
#0001			List each medication order (standard, one-time and stat) in a separate row. Ensure each medication order has all required elements.
#0002			List each PRN medication order, including reason(s) medication can be given, in a separate row. Ensure each medication order has all required elements. Include the following when required: **High Alert Med: Requires dual signoff**

Signed Electronically: John Q. Public, MD Provider # 12345 Pager # 987-6543

This is not a part of the permanent chart. Working document only. Do not send to Medical Records.

Source: Copyright Education-Innovation-Simulation Learning Environment, School of Nursing, The University of North Carolina at Chapel Hill, 2017. Reprinted by permission, 2017.

[a]In the interest of patient safety and to clearly differentiate simulated documents from actual patient care documents, label these forms and documents "For Educational Use Only. Not for Actual Patient Care."

APPENDIX A.6 EXAMPLE MEDICATION ADMINISTRATION RECORD

FOR EDUCATIONAL USE ONLY. NOT FOR ACTUAL PATIENT CARE[a]

Carrington General Hospital DX: **Weight: 60 kg** **Allergies: No Known Allergies**			Patient Identification	
OMITTED MED CODE N=NPO N/V = NAUSEA/VOMITING R = REFUSED H = HELD O = OFF UNIT C = SEE CHART				
Order Start Time	**Order Stop Time**	**Order**	**Admin Time**	**Initials**
		List each medication order (standard, one-time and stat) in a separate row for each medication administration time. Ensure each medication order has all required elements.		
PRN Medications Reassessment Code: E—med effective A—additional meds needed M—MD notified			Time Given/Initials	Time Reassessed/ Initials/Code
		List each PRN medication order, including reason(s) medication can be given, in a separate row. Ensure each medication order has all required elements. Include the following when required: High Alert Med: Requires dual signoff	_____/___ _____/___ _____/___ _____/___ _____/___	____/___/___ ____/___/___ ____/___/____ ____/___/___ ____/___/___
Injection Site Code: Site #1—Left Deltoid Site #2—Right Deltoid Site #3—Left Vastus Lateralus		Site #4—Right Vastus Lateralus Site #5—Left Upper Quad Site #6—Left Lower Quad Site #7—Right Upper Quad	Site #8—Right Lower Quad Site #9—Left Ventrogluteal Site #10—Right Ventrogluteal	
Initials	**Legal Signature/Title**			

Source: Copyright Education-Innovation-Simulation Learning Environment, School of Nursing, The University of North Carolina at Chapel Hill, 2017. Reprinted by permission, 2017.

[a]In the interest of patient safety and to clearly differentiate simulated documents from actual patient care documents, label these forms and documents "For Educational Use Only. Not for Actual Patient Care."

APPENDIX A.7 EXAMPLE SKILL COMPETENCY EVALUATION CHECKLIST

Evaluation Criteria: miss any 1 bullet in a 1-star item (*), have to redo

miss any 2 bullets out of 2-star items (**), have to redo

miss any 3 bullets out of 3-star items (***), have to redo

NAME OF SKILL	✓/-		
	Eval	Redo 1	Redo 2
List the steps for each section of the skill: • Use bullets (if no specific order is required) or numbers (if a specific order is required) to list all sub-steps that should be accomplished • Use a separate row for different steps • Indicate the level of evaluation criteria after each step or sub-step using the appropriate number of stars (*/**/***)			
	DATE	EVALUATOR NAME	SCORE (circle one)
Evaluation			Skill: Pass (Points) Redo
Redo 1			Skill: Pass (Points) Redo
Redo 2			Skill: Pass (Points) Redo

Source: Copyright Education-Innovation-Simulation Learning Environment, School of Nursing, The University of North Carolina at Chapel Hill (2017). Reprinted by permission (2017).

These documents may be reproduced and modified provided that attribution is clearly stated on any resulting work and it is used for noncommercial, scientific, or educational—including professional development—purposes.

Appendix B: Clinical Teaching Activities and Resources for Students

Minimal supplies are needed for this exercise, and it is an excellent way to engage students during orientation to the clinical setting. Equipment needed includes: a large glass jar or vessel, one bag of large-sized shells, one bag of medium-sized shells, one bag of small shells, and a small bag of sand. Before beginning the exercise, have only the large glass jar in view for students. Ask for four volunteers from the group.

The clinical teacher produces the first bag of large shells and asks a student volunteer to arrange them inside the glass jar. After the student has completed this exercise, the group is asked, "Is the vessel full?" The likely answer will be "no." The faculty member then produces the second bag of medium-sized shells and asks the second student volunteer to arrange these inside the same jar. This student may need to get creative by first removing some of the larger shells, adding the medium size shells into the container, and then replacing/rearranging the large shells again. On completion, the clinical group is again asked, "Is the vessel full?" Usually, by now, the students have become wise to this question and state "no." Sequentially, the faculty member produces the third bag of small shells and has the third volunteer add these to the jar, then the bag of sand is produced and the fourth student volunteer adds the sand. Each time, after the student volunteer has completed his or her task, the student group is asked whether the jar is full. They will likely continue to state that the jar is not full, as they could still add water or other materials.

Students are then asked to brainstorm about what they learned from this exercise, and the relationship that this interactive exercise has to their clinical practice and group functioning. Many valuable analogies can be made using this exercise. The following are only a few key points that students and/or teacher might raise based on the "shell exercise."

- Keep your "big shells," or your nursing priorities, in place. If the small shells were deposited into the jar first, the big shells would not have fit. Similarly, the nurse who gets sidetracked with repeated tasks may lose sight of the "big picture," and nursing priorities are unlikely to be met.

- Students may point out the importance of teamwork, as various student volunteers were required to work together to fill the vessel. They may also point out creative thinking toward patient goals and having to be flexible as a nurse, just as some of the large shells had to be temporarily removed and then replaced in the jar in order to make room for some of the smaller items.

- Students may articulate that the well-rounded nurse (in other words, the full jar) is made up of many different qualities, such as knowledge, technical skill, caring, the ability to educate the patient and family, patient advocacy, communication skills, and so forth. An observation may be made that the jar was not full when it contained only large, or only large- and medium-sized shells, but that a *variety* of shells were needed for it to be full. Similarly, the nurse needs knowledge and a variety of competencies to make a difference to patients and their care.

- Students might raise the issue of reflection on one's professional practice and the importance of consciously reflecting on one's professional growth at regular intervals, just as the clinical group reflected on whether the jar was full during regular points within the shell exercise.

- Students may comment on the aesthetically pleasing end result of a jar filled with an array of shells and sand, and faculty members may draw an analogy to the beauty of developing the art and science of nursing.

APPENDIX B.2: SAMPLE CLINICAL SETTING ORIENTATION TREASURE HUNT

Fire stations

Crash carts

Alarms/codes

Biohazardous waste management system

Staff bathroom

Report room

Pneumatic tube system

Patient refreshments

Ice machine, cups, plastic utensils, straws

Bladder scanner

Skin care supplies

Mechanical lifts

Sliding board for patient transfer

Medications and supplies associated with medication administration

Isolation supplies

Laundry hampers

Where to dispose:

Soiled transfer sheets

Used equipment for cleaning

Used patient meal trays

Portable BP machines, manual BP cuff

Pulse oximeter

Linens: sheets, towels, patient gowns, nonslip footwear

Sequential compression devices

Lift equipment and transfer sheets

Glucometers

Medication system

Glucometer docking port

Quick references:

Nursing policies

Accepted abbreviations

Mission statement of agency

Other site-specific information

Medical records: provider orders, history, progress notes, diagnostics and lab reports, consultations, and so on

Electronic medical record system, other forms of documentation

Pharmacology references

Patient education references

In an empty patient room, find:

Gloves

Computer for charting

Call bell

Familiarize yourself with bed operations

Sink, toilet, shower

Sharps containers

Thermometers

Suction and oxygen equipment

Saline flushes

Saline/water for irrigation

Nasogastric and other tubes

Primary and secondary intravenous tubing

Suction catheters

Catheter sets

Personal care items (shampoo, toothpaste, etc.)

Oxygen tubing/nasal cannula and so on

Tape

Dressing change supplies

Urinals

Specimen containers

BP, blood pressure.

APPENDIX B.3: ORGANIZATIONAL TOOL FOR NURSING STUDENTS: CLINICAL TIMELINE EXAMPLE 1

Time	Clinical Activity
0800–0830	Meet in patient resource room. Preconference with your fellow students and clinical teacher.
0830–0845	Introduce yourself to the staff nurse as well as the nursing assistant. Communicate what you will and will not be involved in during the clinical experience with respect to patient care. Be specific in what time you will be leaving the unit and obtain a patient update from the staff nurse.
0845–0930	Introduce yourself to the patient, establish priorities, revisit your time sequence plan for the day; check the chart for any new orders, and check the medication records for any new medications or changes to previously ordered medications. Obtain baseline patient assessments and document accordingly. Brief morning care, nutrition, intake, and output.
0930–1300	Medications, skills, nursing rounds, therapies, and treatments (e.g., deep breathing and coughing, ambulation, turning and positioning, toileting, pain management, patient education, glucometer readings, hygiene). Linen changes, attend to room environment. Keep documentation in e-chart current. Review medical records to learn more about patient, plan of care, and modifications of treatment plan. Attend team/family conferences. Enter patient documentation as you go—remember this is the only way other members of the health care team can have access to the information you have gathered. Report to your student buddy and the staff nurse prior to your morning break and lunch. Have your e-charting cosigned by the clinical teacher prior to [time].
1300–1400	Nursing rounds and/or postconference, shift wrap up, report off (handoff) to the staff. Do not start new procedures during this time.

APPENDIX B.4: ORGANIZATIONAL TOOL FOR NURSING STUDENTS: CLINICAL TIMELINE EXAMPLE 2

Time	Nursing Activity	Meds	Comments/Notes
0700	Report and preconference		
0800	Obtain patient's VS and document Safety equipment check E-chart: (a) brief assessment, (b) activities and interventions, (c) intake (oral/IV), (d) output if applicable, (e) vascular access device if applicable, (f) pain assessment, (g) neurological assessment if applicable		After getting report: Chart for new orders Review MAR Check overnight VS and physical assessment
0900	Patient physical assessment and documentation E-chart: (a) intake and output, (b) vascular access device, (c) activities and interventions, (d) pain		
1000	Patient rounds E-chart: (a) intake and output, (b) vascular access device, (c) activities and interventions, (d) pain		
1100	Patient rounds E-chart: (a) intake and output, (b) vascular access device, (c) activities and interventions, (d) pain		
1200	Patient rounds Obtain patient's VS and document Neurological check if applicable E-chart: (a) intake and output, (b) vascular access device, (c) activities and interventions, (d) pain, (e) VS		Prior to leaving unit: Make sure all documentation is current Chart, MAR check! Safety check! Report to your buddy and registered nurses (handoff)

MAR, medication administration record; VS, vital signs.

Appendix C: Caputi's Alternative Approach to Clinical Evaluation

Teaching and evaluating student learning and performance in the clinical setting is one of the most challenging aspects of nursing education. However, no matter the setting or unique challenges the setting presents, there is one important principle that oversees clinical evaluation—is the student performing at a passing level related to the student learning outcomes? Therefore, when developing and implementing a clinical evaluation tool (CET), it is important to consider all learning outcomes, not just those that relate to physical contact with the patient (Caputi, 2010a).

It can be difficult to ensure students are engaging in student learning outcomes that are not readily observable. Because teachers need to ensure safe patient care is delivered by all students, many learning outcomes may not be evaluated completely. Evaluation of such learning outcomes may result from assessing care plans, typically written by students and graded by faculty away from the clinical setting following the actual experience. A major purpose of the clinical experience is to provide learning in actual patient contexts. Removing the evaluation of student performance to outside that context is less than desirable. Students are no longer able to return to the setting to collect further information to answer questions teachers may pose, and teachers are no longer in the setting to verify information.

To remedy these and other weaknesses in clinical education, Caputi's perspective requires evaluating students in the clinical setting with a CET that is both valid and reliable (Caputi, 2010b). Clinical teachers provide guidance to assist students to think like a nurse as they demonstrate achievement of all student learning outcomes reflected on the CET. However, to provide one-to-one guidance on all learning outcomes for all students in the clinical setting is difficult.

A new perspective is one that examines student learning outcomes performed in the clinical setting with student activities tied directly to the behaviors on the CET. These behaviors reflect the course student learning outcomes and competencies. If a course has both a theory component and a clinical component, the same student learning outcomes and competencies are applied to both learning environments. Once those student learning outcomes and competencies are written, they become the CET. Using them as the CET ensures consistency between theory and clinical.

For example, many courses require students to demonstrate knowledge about and performance of learning outcomes related to major areas such as safety, evidence-based practice, caring, informatics, teamwork/collaboration, clinical judgment, and others. If the theory component of a course expects a particular level of behavior about these major concepts as expressed through student learning outcomes and competencies, then the student's ability to apply these same behaviors during clinical is desirable. Unfortunately, what tends to happen is clinical teachers guide learning and assessment of psychomotor and technological skills, then rely on other means of documentation for the other concepts—such as a written care plan or reflection journal. This can be remedied with a CET that has activities tied to the CET behaviors. This provides a valid tool because the activities evaluated are related directly to the competencies on the CET. To ensure inter-rater reliability of the activity, grading rubrics are used.

For example, a course has a student learning outcome of: Engage in clinical judgment to make patient-centered care decisions with expected behaviors (competencies) of:

a. Use clinical judgment to make management decisions to ensure accurate and safe care in all nursing actions, including addressing anticipated changes in the patient's condition.
b. Use clinical judgment when implementing all steps of the nursing process while integrating best-available evidence in the care of adult patients with complex health issues.
c. Anticipate risks, and predict and manage potential complications when caring for adult patients with complex health issues.
d. Prioritize patient care.

How will the faculty determine if each student has satisfactorily completed all four competencies for this student learning outcome? Caputi's approach is to include activities students are required to complete during the clinical experience. The faculty members teaching the course now have an established focus of expectations for each of these competencies—the same focus and expectations for all students. This helps to ensure reliability. Because the activities are specifically aligned with the competencies, the tool becomes valid in that it is evaluating what the course is teaching. The following example demonstrates this approach: the learning activities align with each of these four competencies.

Course Student Learning Outcome: Engage in clinical judgment to make patient-centered care decisions

Competencies demonstrating the Course Student Learning Outcome has been achieved:

a. Use clinical judgment to make management decisions to ensure accurate and safe care in all nursing actions, including addressing anticipated changes in the patient's condition.
b. Use clinical judgment when implementing all steps of the nursing process while integrating best available evidence in the care of adult patients with complex health issues.

Tool: Apply and analyze Clinical Judgment (Uses Tanner's [2006] steps of the Clinical Judgment Model)

Choose two events that occurred during the experience in the clinical setting that required you to engage in clinical judgment.

For each event, complete the following tool to guide your thinking.

| Overview of the Problem: |
| Background: |
| Noticing: |
| Interpreting: |
| Responding: |
| Reflection-in-Action |
| Reflection-on-Action |

Explain the following:

1. How did you use the Clinical Judgment Model?
2. How did the model assist in you in arriving at decisions?
3. What available evidence did you use when completing the "responding" section of the tool?
4. Do you use another approach for thinking? Explain.

GRADING RUBRIC FOR APPLYING CRITICAL THINKING

Performance Criteria	S	NI	U
Clear and accurate answers to all questions on tool.	Clearly and accurately answers all questions on tool.	Clearly and accurately answers some but not all questions on tool.	Unable to clearly and accurately answer all questions on tool.

NI, needs improvement; S, satisfactory; U, unsatisfactory.

c. Anticipate risks, and predict and manage potential complications when caring for adult patients with complex health issues.

Tool: Predict and Manage Potential Complications
For each patient answer these questions:

1. What are you on alert for today with this patient?
2. What are the important assessments to make?
3. What complications may occur? What could go wrong?
4. What interventions will prevent complications?
5. How will you prioritize implementation of nursing interventions? Explain.
6. What actions will you take for each complication should it occur?

GRADING RUBRIC TO PREDICT AND MANAGE POTENTIAL COMPLICATIONS

Performance Criteria	S	NI	U
Able to identify the potential complications.	Clearly identifies potential complications.	Description of potential complications for this patient is scant.	Unable to identify potential complications.

(continued)

(continued)

Performance Criteria	S	NI	U
Able to identify the important assessment data to monitor for this patient.	Clearly identifies the important assessment data to monitor for this patient.	Description of the important assessment data to monitor for this patient is scant.	Unable to identify the important assessment data to monitor for this patient.
Able to identify all factors influencing the most important data to monitor.	Clearly identifies all factors influencing the most important data to monitor.	Description of all factors influencing the most important data to monitor is scant.	Unable to identify the most important data to monitor.
Able to prioritize planned interventions.	Clearly identifies ways to prioritize planned interventions.	Superficially discusses ways to prioritize planned interventions.	Unable to prioritize planned interventions.
Able to plan actions to take if complications occur.	Clearly identifies actions to take if complications occur.	Superficially discusses actions to take if complications occur.	Unable to discuss actions to take if complications occur.

NI, needs improvement; S, satisfactory; U, unsatisfactory.

d. Prioritize patient care.

Tool: Prioritizing Patient Needs

Refer to your concept map for patient care. Categorize the identified patient needs using the following criteria (National Council State Boards of Nursing [NCSBN], n.d.). Explain your rationale.

1. First-order priority need—immediate threat to health, safety, or survival.
2. Second-order priority need—actual problem for which immediate help has been requested by the patient or family.
3. Third-order priority need—actual or potential issue of which the patient or family is not aware.
4. Fourth-order priority need—actual or potential issue that is anticipated in the future and for which help will be needed.

First-Priority Needs With Rationale

_____

_____

Second-Priority Needs With Rationale

_____

_____

Third-Priority Needs With Rationale

_____

_____

Fourth-Priority Needs With Rationale

_____

_____

GRADING RUBRIC FOR PRIORITIZING PATIENT NEEDS

Performance Criteria	S	NI	U
Prioritizes patient needs	Prioritization of needs is correct.	Prioritization is correct in some but not all identified patient needs.	Unable to accurately prioritize patient needs.
Provides rationales	Rationales are clear and accurate.	Rationales are superficial and are not clearly explained.	Unable to provide any correct rationales.

NI, needs improvement; S, satisfactory; U, unsatisfactory.

SUMMARY

In summary, the purpose of this approach for evaluation of students' behaviors or competencies in the clinical setting is to provide a more objective evaluation tool. With this approach students are required to complete specific activities that demonstrate their ability to meet the expected outcomes of the clinical course. By using these tools and grading rubrics, faculty are less reliant on subjective evaluations based totally on observation. Faculty may not be able to make all the necessary observations of each student because of the demands to oversee student care to ensure patient safety. The burden of proof of meeting the expected behaviors is now on the student rather than on the faculty's opportunity, or lack thereof, to observe every student performing every expected behavior on the CET.

REFERENCES

Caputi, L. (2010a). Evaluating student in the clinical setting. In L. Caputi (Ed.), _Teaching nursing: The art and science_ (pp. 152–174). Glen Ellyn, IL: College of DuPage Press.

Caputi, L. (2010b). Transforming clinical education: The Caputi clinical activities portfolio®. In L. Caputi (Ed.), _Teaching nursing: The art and science_ (pp. 216–255). Glen Ellyn, IL: College of DuPage Press.

National Council State Boards of Nursing. (n.d.). _Transition to practice: Outline of NCSBN's transition to practice._ Chicago, IL: Author. Retrieved from https://www.ncsbn.org/1603.htm

Tanner, C. (2006). Thinking like a nurse: A research-based model of clinical judgment in nursing. _Journal of Nursing Education, 45_(6), 204–211.

Appendix D: Resources for Nurse Educators

APPENDIX D.1: CERTIFICATION FOR NURSE EDUCATORS

Mission of Certification Program

The National League for Nursing's Academic Nurse Educator Certification Program "promotes excellence in the advanced specialty role of the academic nurse educator."

Goals of Certification:

- "Distinguish academic nursing education as a specialty area of practice and an advanced practice role within professional nursing.
- Recognize the academic nurse educator's specialized knowledge, skills, and abilities and excellence in practice.
- Strengthen the core competencies of nurse educator practice.
- Contribute to nurse educators' professional development."

From National League for Nursing. (2017). *Certification for nurse educators (CNE)*. Retrieved from www.nln.org/professional-development-programs/Certification-for-Nurse-Educators

APPENDIX D.2: CERTIFIED NURSE EDUCATORᶜᴹ EXAMINATION CONTENT AREAS AND PERCENT OF TEST ITEMS

Facilitate Learning, 22%
Facilitate Learner Development and Socialization, 14%
Use Assessment and Evaluation Strategies, 17%
Participate in Curriculum Design and Evaluation of Program Outcomes, 17%
Pursue Continuous Quality Improvement in the Academic Nurse Educator Role, 9%
Engage in Scholarship, Service, and Leadership, 21%

From National League for Nursing. (2016). *Certified nurse educator (CNE) 2016 candidate handbook*. Retrieved from www.nln.org/professional-development-programs/Certification-for-Nurse-Educators/handbook

APPENDIX D.3: CORE COMPETENCIES OF NURSE EDUCATORS AND SAMPLE ACTIVITIES FOR EACH COMPETENCY

Competency	Sample Activities
Facilitate learning	Develop innovative teaching-learning activities
	Base teaching strategies on Educational Theory and evidence
	Use information technologies in teaching
Facilitate learner development and socialization	Assist students to develop as nurses and integrate expected values and behaviors
	Identify individual learning styles and needs for culturally diverse, at-risk, or physically challenged learners
	Assist learners to engage in thoughtful constructive self- or peer evaluation
Use assessment and evaluation strategies	Create appropriate assessment instruments to evaluate learner outcomes
	Design tools for assessing clinical practice
	Provide input for the development of program policies related to admission, progression, or graduation
Participate in curriculum design and evaluation of program outcomes	Design curricula that reflect trends while preparing graduates to function in the health care environment
	Develop or revise courses reflecting theoretical framework of curriculum
	Support educational goals through community partnerships
Pursue continuous quality improvement in the nurse educator role	Develop and maintain competence in the nurse educator role (e.g., by attending conferences, seminars, workshops)
	Mentor and support faculty colleagues in the role of academic nurse educator
	Use feedback from peers, learners, and others for improvement
Function as a change agent and leader	Provide leadership in the nursing program or other organization
	Work on a special panel or in a think tank for an educational issue
	Represent nursing education on an interdisciplinary work group
Engage in scholarship	Develop an area of expertise within the academic educator role
	Implement scholarly activities
	Share expertise with colleagues (e.g., through publications and presentations)

Competency	Sample Activities
Function within the educational environment	Collaborate with other disciplines to enhance the academic environment
	Participate in committee work on the departmental or institutional level
	Develop collaborations and partnerships within the academic institution and with clinical agencies

Source: Adapted from Wittmann-Price, R. A., Godshall, M., & Wilson, L. (2013). *Certified nursing educator (CNE) manual* (2nd ed., pp. 15–16). New York, NY: Springer Publishing. Reprinted by permission, 2013.

APPENDIX D.4: SELECTED NURSING AND HIGHER EDUCATION ORGANIZATIONS

American Academy of Nursing	Serves the public and nursing profession by advancing health policy and practice. Academy's members, known as Fellows, are nursing's most accomplished leaders in education, practice, administration, and research.	http://www.aannet.org/home
American Association of Colleges of Nursing	Represents baccalaureate and higher-degree nursing programs. Promotes quality nursing education. Offers faculty development programs and webinars. Collects data about nursing education programs, faculty, and students, and analyzes trends in nursing education. Publishes position papers.	www.aacn.nche.edu
American Association of Community Colleges	Provides advocacy for community colleges at the national level. Works closely with states on policy.	www.aacc.nche.edu
American Association of University Professors	Focuses on advancing academic freedom and shared governance. Defines fundamental professional values and standards for higher education and faculty.	www.aaup.org

(continued)

American Association of University Women	Promotes equity and education for women and girls. Advocates for fundamental educational, social, economic, and political issues.	www.aauw.org
American Council on Education	Represents presidents of accredited, degree-granting institutions (2- and 4-year colleges, private and public universities, and nonprofit schools) in the United States. Focuses on higher education challenges, with the goal to improve access and better prepare students.	www.acenet.edu/Pages/default.aspx
Association of American Colleges and Universities	Focuses on promoting high-quality undergraduate liberal education. Website contains links to resources on liberal education, general education, curriculum, faculty work, assessment, diversity, and others.	www.aacu.org/about/index.cfm
Association of Black Nursing Faculty, Inc.	Provides a group for Black professional nurses with similar interests and concerns to promote health-related issues and nursing education. Assists members in professional development and provides continuing education.	www.abnf.net
Association of Community Health Nursing Educators	Focuses on promoting excellence in community and public health nursing education, research, and practice.	www.achne.org/i4a/pages/index.cfm?pageid=1
EDUCAUSE	Advances higher education through use of information technology. Focuses on issues and emerging trends and technologies affecting higher education.	www.educause.edu

Interprofessional Education Collaborative (IPEC)	Collaborative of schools of health professions to promote efforts that advance interprofessional learning experiences to prepare future health professionals for team-based care and improved population health outcomes. These organizations that represent higher education in allopathic and osteopathic medicine, dentistry, nursing, pharmacy, and public health created core competencies for interprofessional collaborative practice to guide curricula development across health professions schools.	https://www.ipecollaborative.org/about-ipec.html
Multimedia Educational Resource for Learning and Online Teaching (MERLOT)	Includes repository of resources and information for faculty development and to download for use in teaching. Publishes *Journal of Online Learning and Teaching*.	www.merlot.org
National League for Nursing	Promotes excellence in nursing education at all levels. Offers faculty development programs, webinars, and annual educational conference. Sponsors certification program for nurse educators (CNE). Publishes position papers on nursing education and has a grant program for nursing education research. The NLN Commission for Nursing Education Accreditation (CNEA) accredits nursing programs.	www.nln.org

(continued)

National Organization of Nurse Practitioner Faculties	Focuses on promoting quality nurse practitioner (NP) education at national and international levels. Leading organization for NP faculty in US and globally.	www.nonpf.com
National Student Nurses Association	Serves as organization for nursing students with goal of enhancing their professional development and promoting transition into the profession.	www.nsna.org
Organization for Associate Degree Nursing (OADN)	Is dedicated to enhancing the quality of associate degree (AD) nursing. Advocates for AD nursing and promotes academic progression of AD nursing graduates in furthering their education.	www.oadn.org
POD Network	Focuses on faculty, instructional, and organizational development in higher education.	www.podnetwork.org
Quality and Safety Education for Nurses (QSEN)	Collaborative of nurses and other health care professionals focused on education, practice, and scholarship to improve quality and safety of health care. Identified knowledge, skills, and attitudes (KSAs) necessary to continuously improve quality and safety of health care. Website is a central repository of information on core QSEN competencies, KSAs, teaching strategies, and faculty development resources.	http://qsen.org/about-qsen

Sigma Theta Tau International Honor Society of Nursing	Supports learning and professional development of nurses worldwide. Membership is by invitation to baccalaureate and graduate nursing students with excellence in scholarship and to nurse leaders with exceptional achievements in nursing. Offers conferences for sharing research and publishes *Journal of Nursing Scholarship*, among other resources.	www.nursingsociety.org

Index